Binging with Babish fans, rejoice!

If you have ever watched *Seinfeld* and wondered what made the Soup Nazi's wild mushroom soup so good, or been curious about what *The Godfather*'s cannoli tastes like, then this is the book for you. In every episode, creator and host Andrew Rea painstakingly recreates some of film and television's most iconic dishes with startling accuracy, such as using squab, wild boar, and rabbit to craft the pigeon pie from *Game of Thrones*. He replicates classic dishes like Kevin's homemade chili from *The Office* (spilt straight onto a carpet), shrimp gumbo from *Forrest Gump*, and crème brûlée from *Amélie*. He also tackles those dishes you can't help but wonder about, such as the krabby patty from *Spongebob* and Buddy's pasta, smothered in sweets, from *Elf*. Rea's art is in taking the previously enigmatic dishes from TV and movies and breathing life—and flavor—into them, dissecting how they would be made from screen cues and creating an accessible recipe. The recipes are woven together with never-told-before stories about how *Binging with Babish* began, making this book a must-have for fans.

BINGING
— WITH —
BABISH

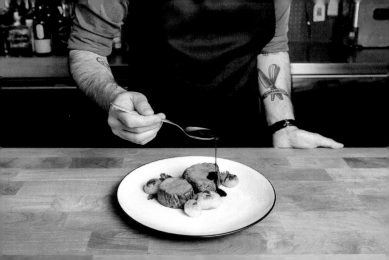

BINGING
— WITH —
BABISH

100 Recipes Recreated from
Your Favorite Movies and TV Shows

ANDREW REA

FOREWORD BY JON FAVREAU
PHOTOGRAPHY BY EVAN SUNG

HOUGHTON MIFFLIN HARCOURT
BOSTON   NEW YORK

hmhbooks.com

Library of Congress Cataloging-in-Publication Data
Names: Rea, Andrew, author. | Sung, Evan, photographer.
Title: Binging with Babish : 100 recipes recreated from your favorite movies
and TV shows / Andrew Rea ; photography by Evan Sung.
Description: New York, New York : Houghton Mifflin Harcourt Publishing
Company, [2019] | Includes index.
Identifiers: LCCN 2019013137 (print) | LCCN 2019014076 (ebook) |
ISBN 9781328592385 (ebook) | ISBN 9781328589897 (paper over board)
Subjects: LCSH: Cooking. | Television programs—Plots, themes, etc. | Motion
pictures—Plots, themes, etc. | Food in motion pictures. | LCGFT: Literary cookbooks.
Classification: LCC TX714 (ebook) | LCC TX714 .R385 2019 (print) | DDC 641.5—dc23
LC record available at https://lccn.loc.gov/2019013137

Book design by Allison Chi
Printed in the United States of America
9 2021
4500817338

To my mother: Everything I've ever made is steeped in your love and memory

-TABLE OF- CONTENTS

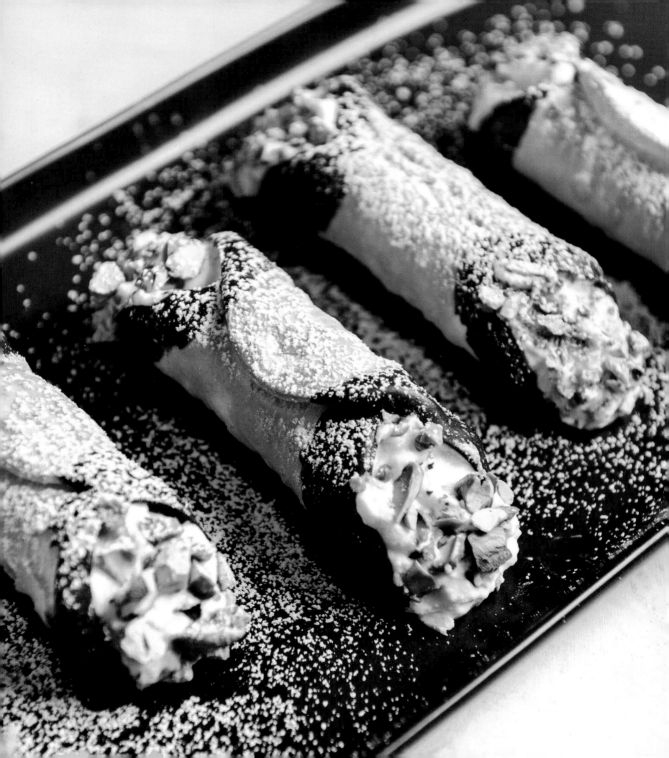

I've often touted myself as something of a one-man-band. To some extent, it's true: I still cook, shoot, edit, color, animate, and perform the voice-over for every episode of *Binging*. But like any burgeoning enterprise, an ever-growing team of creatives, collaborators, obsessives, and partners begin turning the screws in the increasingly complex machinations of what started out as an after-work hobby. This book, the show(s), and my career would not exist without them, and while they deserve an entire chapter dedicated to their tireless contributions, I remembered that this is a cookbook, and maybe I should just relax a little. So here goes.

First up is my family—whenever I need encouragement, love, or a swift kick in the ass, they've been there with unrelenting support and honesty. My mother died when I was eleven, and I responded to the pain and confusion by becoming a total prick. Despite my predictably bad behavior, a rapidly changing world, and his own grief and heartache, my father, Douglas Rea, was unflappable in his efforts to instill a sense of kindness, morality, and work ethic in his wayward son. I wouldn't be the man nor the storyteller I am today without him. My brother David, in addition to raising a beautiful family (and being nothing short of a genius), has always been there for me with words of wisdom and a glass of brown liquor when I've needed it most. Barb, Kelly, Christopher, Everett, Donna, Kathy, Bob, Lauren, Josh, and the rest are a small but passionate and connected family that I can't imagine my life without, and I can't wait to see what comes next for each of us.

Next are my friends and colleagues—the line between which is growing blurrier as we speak. Sawyer Jacobs, my best friend and business partner, has grown from being an invaluable member of my team into practically my common law husband. Despite knowing him for almost two decades at the time of this writing, he relentlessly surprises me with acts of wild creativity and intelligence, and there is no one else I'd even want to imagine taking this journey with. *Binging* would have stayed a pastime forever were it not for the patience and moral support of my former roommate and forever my dearest friend, Rashid Duroseau. I'm lucky enough to have remained thick as thieves with my roommates from college, Eddie Liu and Steven Farrell, the latter of whom has helped me shoot four episodes in his home (any of the ones to do with BBQ, fittingly). Though they've moved halfway across the world, Jon Magel and

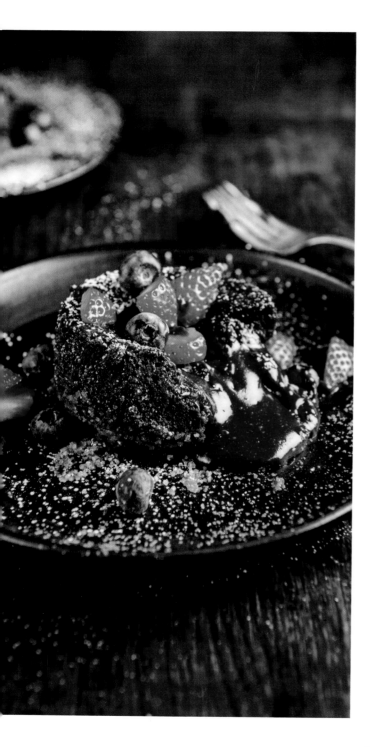

Diana Dayrit continue to be the confidants, role models, and dear friends they've been for nine years now—I would not be the man I am today without them. Kevin Grosch, Keith Johnson, Brad Cash, and all the folks at Made In Network have been instrumental to the channel's success, not to mention Ben Davis, Miles Gidaly, Eve Attermann, and the rest of the team at WME. The show has certainly been helped by those who have been kind enough to appear on it: Sean Evans, Maisie Williams, Masaharu Morimoto, Brad Leone, Alvin Cailan, Roy Choi, and many others. Jon Favreau will be a recipient of my endless thanks not only for appearing on the show, but for writing the absolutely stunning foreword for this book. No book is possible without its publisher, but this one's beauty, thoughtfulness, and singularity wouldn't be possible without Justin Schwartz, Evan Sung, Erin Merhar, Maya Rossi, Susan Choung, and Allison Chi.

The biggest thanks, however, is owed to you. Yes, you, the one who bought the book, who watched a video, who told a friend, who supported me on Patreon, and who commented, liked, and subscribed. We live in an incredible time of democratized self-expression, where almost anyone with something to say has been given a voice. Audiences now choose, support, and decide the fate of the very content they watch, and I am in a constant state of disbelief that you've chosen to lift me up so dizzyingly high. I've lived the vast majority of my life in fear—fear of being rejected, mocked, and disliked—but you've made me unafraid to be my truest self. My entire world as I know it would not be possible without you, and I will spend the rest of my life working to try and earn everything you've given me.

My kids asked me one day if I had heard of *Binging with Babish*. I hadn't. My children share my appreciation of cooking-related content and are always pointing out cool videos to watch online. They sat me down and I immediately began to binge *Binging with Babish*.

I felt a connection to Andrew as I watched his playlist of cooking vignettes. There was something very unique about what he was doing. He was a content creator, but he was also a film fan. He didn't show his face, but his videos weren't just a sped-up close-up of disembodied hands. The pace was swift and succinct, but he actually went into great depth about technique. Above all, it was obsessive.

The one unifying characteristic I found as I trained under chefs is that they're all obsessive. They are fixated on details and will relentlessly dissect and organize. Directors, especially those involved with visual effects, tend to share this proclivity. It was no surprise when I learned that Andrew's background also included a career in visual effects and film before *Babish* was born.

I was taken in by how meticulously he re-created recipes from movies and how he, like I, appreciated the impact food could have in the right story.

I was also taken in by the care with which he re-created the recipes from my film *Chef*.

I was flattered by the deluge of views they received and the amount of people who actually replicated the steps shown in the film and meticulously documented by Andrew in his tutorials.

Much like with cooking, we go into the field of storytelling because we want to connect with others on an emotional level. The stylized rituals of both of these disciplines are complex, but their goal is simple. We seek to communicate on a very pure level. Emotion, memory, and sensation are all intertwined on that rare occasion that you hit it right. Andrew not only points his audience to the moments in film where all of those things come together, he also shows them how to create these experiences in real life. He encourages his fans not just to continue watching his channel for his next video but also to turn off the screen and embark on a journey of learning and connecting with real people in real life. This might be the best lesson *Binging with Babish* has taught.

—JON FAVREAU

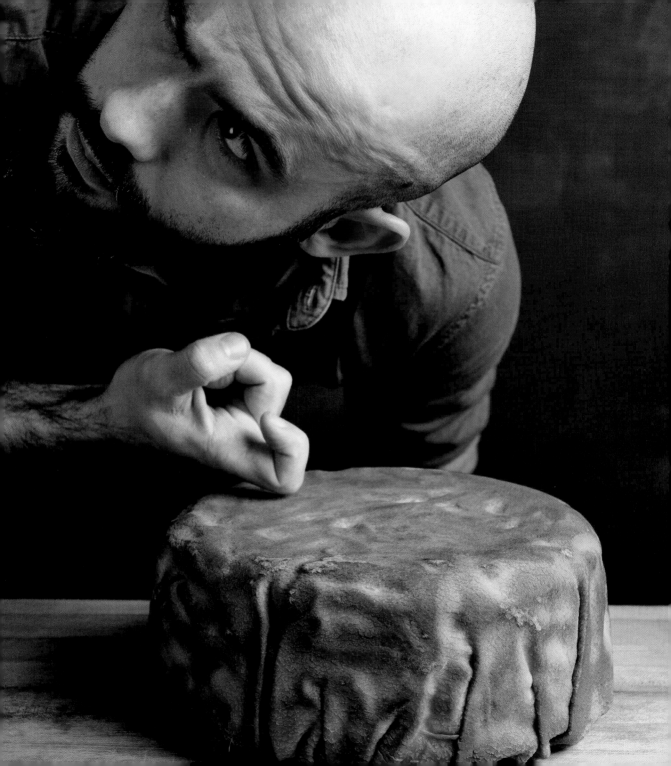

I never meant to become a YouTuber. The proof is in the name: *Binging with Babish*? The most common question I've gotten since starting the show has consistently been, "Who the hell is Babish?" The answer, dear reader, is an ancillary character from eight total episodes of the seminal NBC classic *The West Wing*, portrayed by Oliver Platt. I named my Reddit handle after his character, Oliver Babish, as a joke. I named my cooking show after my Reddit handle, as a joke. Now that joke is my entire brand and professional identity. Life is funny sometimes.

As far back as I can remember, my focus and energy were always torn between food and film. My mother taught me to cook before I started to properly form memories, and I was making what can only charitably be called "short films" the same day my dad brought home our first MiniDV camera. I thought I was hot shit, both at making shaky, camera-edited class projects and whipping up undercooked chicken breasts stuffed with artichoke hearts and cream cheese. When the day finally came to choose one over the other (AKA deciding where to go to college), I chose film—you know, the way-more-secure career path. Even as I stayed up late writing crappy scripts about hit men and drug deals gone bad, I tried to hone my ability as a cook. I was lucky enough to have a roommate equally deluded about his culinary skills, and we sullied our dorm's communal kitchen with experiments ranging from acidic, undercooked tomato sauces to rubbery, salty homemade jerky. It was even worse when I cooked for family or significant others, showcasing the shortcoming of many kitchen newcomers—attempting to cook well above my pay grade. Burnt-on-the-outside, raw-on-the-inside homemade English muffins with scrambled hollandaise sauce. Roasts that were somehow both falling apart and thirst provokingly dry. I probably used the word *reduction* more often in casual conversation than I used contractions. It wasn't until after a fateful breakfast in 2009 that I started taking things seriously. I had four of my best friends in town, the first time we had been under the same roof since high school, and I was determined to make them the hangover brunch of their dreams after a night of debauchery. My friends stumbled bleary-eyed out of bed to the sound of me clattering away in the kitchen, hopeful that they might get the greasy-spoon experience their bodies needed. Instead, they were met with a plate of sous vide quail eggs, asparagus, and truffle oil crostini, a few of which they managed to choke down before sheepishly asking if there was a diner nearby. Over chilaquiles and beers, red-faced with embarrassment, I realized that I had always tried to be inventive with a craft I didn't yet fully understand. I was secretly hoping that I harbored some kind of Mozart-like prodigious knowledge, but in reality, I was waving a stick around and wondering why the orchestra sounded so bad. I resolved to get ahold of the basics so I could make food that impresses with its flavor rather than its concept. You know, the kind of cooking people actually like.

For some reason it took nearly fifteen years for me to put food and film together, and it happened quite by accident. I had given up my Hollywood megastar dreams, gotten a day job in post-production, and focused on something I knew I was good at—storytelling. I took every documentary gig I could get my hands on, toiling until twilight after work, often with something bubbling away in the background on the stovetop. One of the documentaries I edited got in to the TriBeCa Film Festival, but overall, my contributions to the field went unnoticed. Moreover, I was slipping into a deep depression, resigning myself to the belief that I didn't have anything unique to share with the world. I stopped applying myself at work, seeking out new projects, being an attentive and present partner, and most alarming, I stopped cooking. This eventually culminated in spending two weeks in bed feigning food poisoning, because I couldn't bear to get up and face the looming reality that, despite my tireless efforts, my voice would never be heard. This was the rock

> ## "THE SHOW IS MORE THAN JUST A COOKING SHOW. IT'S BEEN THE MEANS TO EXPRESS MYSELF CREATIVELY."

bottom I had so often heard about, the tipping point at which no one can help you but yourself. So began the process I like to think of as the ever-widening of my then-perilously-small comfort zone. The first step was to see a therapist, something I urge anyone currently battling depression to seek out immediately. Next was to find a more fulfilling creative outlet and as I picked up the whisk once more, I decided that might end up being food photography. So the following step was investing in myself in the form of a five-thousand-dollar loan to amp up my abilities as a freelancer: a Sony a7S II camera, a smattering of cheap lenses, a light, and a microphone. I decided to test out my new toys in my oddly-perfectly-lit kitchen, whipping up a smoothie out of vegetables in the fridge.

I hit *stop* on the camera, ripped out the memory card, and was editing it within a minute. It wasn't until after I had cut together a rough facsimile of a cooking show, sassily scored to "Cream on Chrome" by Ratatat (this would end up being the precursor to *BwB*), that I realized I was having fun. I hadn't had fun, in any capacity, in years.

The most difficult part was yet to come: I had to burn everything to the ground. Which is just a metaphor, I'm not an arsonist, relax. With the expanding of my comfort zone came maybe the most challenging step yet, which was a step inward. I realized that I was perpetually unhappy, and as is often the case with those in denial, I hadn't the foggiest idea why. I was making progress in therapy, but I needed to undergo catastrophic change. What I did next, you should know, is not advisable—please do not try this at home. I had read about psychedelics being used in clinical trials to treat PTSD and severe depression, and it got me curious about the twisted, desiccated little fungi I had trepidatiously purchased and kept in my desk at work. Then, one night before therapy, I decided to choke down two of the unpalatable little buggers, just to see what would happen. I arrived early, shot the shit with my therapist to show him that I was cognizant and aware, and said, "So listen, Doc, you should know I'm tripping face on mushrooms right now. You know

what to do." He laughed, asked if I needed water, and proceeded to ask me questions that rocked my very foundation. In a forty-five-minute chitchat, I came to the unshakable conclusion that I was in a broken marriage, something I was unable to accomplish in the thirteen years it had spanned prior to that evening. I spent the next few days on the couch, unable to eat, crushed under the weight of my discovery. I told my wife how I felt that week, and a month later we had moved out of Queens and gone our separate ways.

Now, you might be asking yourself, "I was certain I bought a cookbook, so why am I being subjected to your life story?" Well, to me, the show is more than just a cooking show. It's been the means to express myself creatively and personally for nearly three years at the time of this writing. It's how I pulled myself out of the depths of depression and how I've connected with new friends and reconnected with old. It's been my anchor as I continue the Sisyphean endeavor of expanding my comfort zone. It's reminded me that I've got a story to tell, and sharing that story with all of you has been the defining experience of my life. I hope that the show, this book, or the recipes within encourage you to try telling a story of your own, be it to the din of the world or in the quiet of dinner with someone you love. You never know how it might affect them, or maybe more important, yourself.

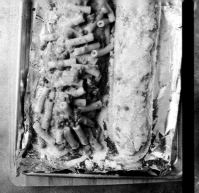
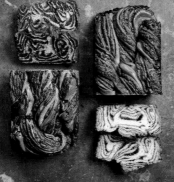
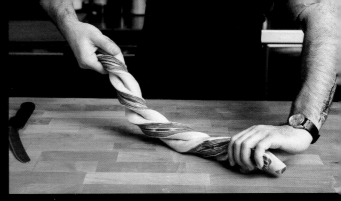
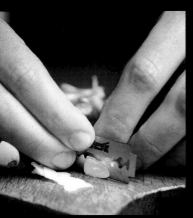
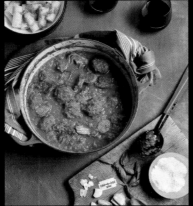
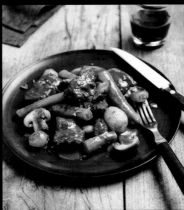
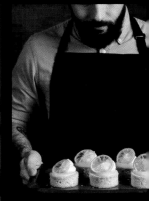
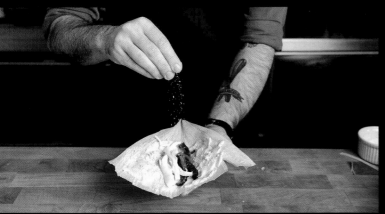
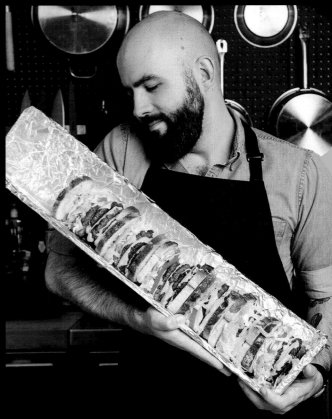
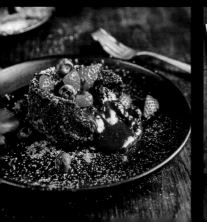
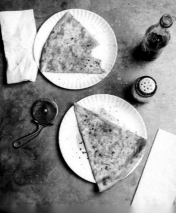

— THE —
RECIPES

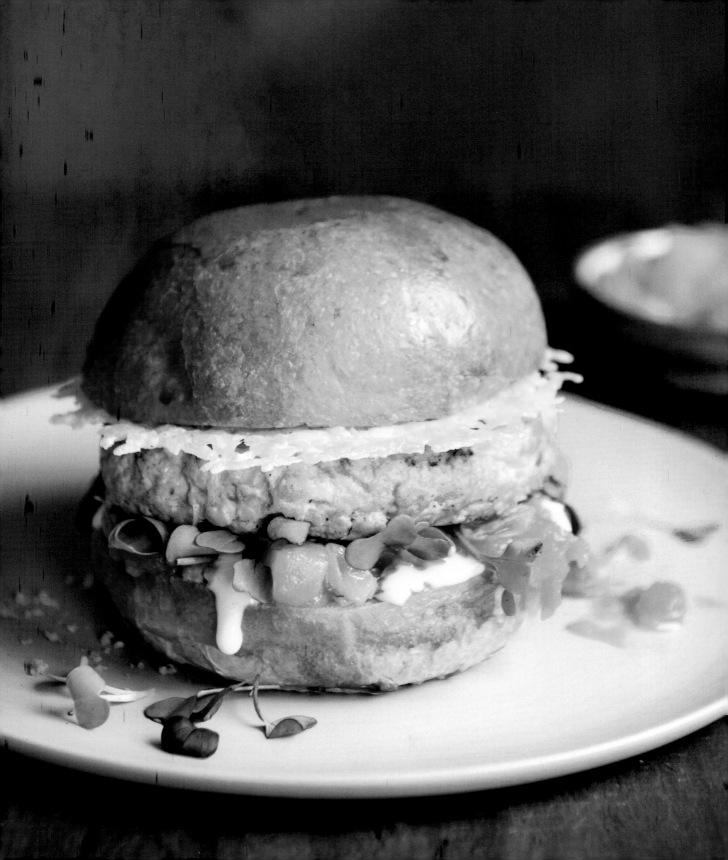

TRAEGER TURKEY BURGER

SERVES 4

Well, folks, this is it: the accidental genesis. The camera test that evolved into my hobby, then into my passion project, then into my career and life as I know it. Into the book you're now reading. As you may have read in the introduction, I had purchased a camera and a small LED light and was futzing around with them in the kitchen. By virtue of my tiny Queens apartment, my kitchen was also my living room—and as had become habit, I would play Netflix in the background as one plays music. The soundtrack that night: *Parks and Recreation*. As I clumsily (and perhaps dangerously) attempted to tape parchment paper over the light in an effort to diffuse it, I overheard Rob Lowe's character rattling off the trendy ingredients draped atop his organic turkey burger, and the proverbial light bulb stuttered to life over my head. Not the "I'm going to make a career out of pop culture cooking" light bulb you might be imagining—more like a "hey, would that taste good? Maybe I should try to make that for my next dinner party" kind of bulb. Eventually, I realized it might be fun to document the burger's creation, and I endeavored to source

the ingredients the following evening after work. Even in New York City, this was no mean feat; exactly where does one source microgreens at eight p.m. on a weeknight? Was papaya in season (does papaya have a season)? Not just brioche buns, but gluten-free brioche buns? After spotting daikon radish sprouts at Fairway and convincing Bareburger to sell me some of their gluten-free brioche buns, I made it home by ten p.m. and was cooking by eleven. I had spent the day at work researching recipes when my bosses weren't looking, so I was ready to hit the ground running. I didn't know it yet, but my life was about to change dramatically thanks to this fussy little burger.

VERDICT: Chris's burger is, without a doubt, the best turkey burger I've ever had. The flavors actually (surprisingly) work quite well together, and I can't honestly say it would be better off without any particular element. One taste of a plain Ron Swanson burger, however, and it all becomes clear: you can dress up turkey as resplendently as you like, but it will never be beef.

(recipe continues)

1 small eggplant

Extra-virgin olive oil, for drizzling

1 teaspoon anchovy paste

1 tablespoon soy sauce

1 teaspoon Marmite (available at Whole Foods and specialty markets)

1½ pounds ground turkey breast

Kosher salt and freshly ground black pepper

1 tablespoon vegetable oil

4 brioche buns (gluten-free, if you want to stay true to Chris Traeger's recipe)

Papaya Chutney (recipe follows)

Microgreens

Cheese Crisps (recipe follows)

Black Truffle Aioli (recipe follows)

PREHEAT THE oven to 400°F.

CUT THE top off the eggplant, halve lengthwise, and score crosshatches into the flesh. Transfer to a rimmed baking sheet, drizzle with olive oil, and place the eggplant cut-side down. Bake for 30 to 40 minutes, until golden brown and soft. Set aside until cool enough to handle, then scoop the eggplant flesh into a large bowl.

ADD THE anchovy paste, soy sauce, and Marmite and whisk until well combined. Add the turkey and gently fold together using a rubber spatula until well incorporated. Form the turkey mixture into four patties, pressing a divot into the center of each to prevent the burgers from puffing up during cooking. Season the patties generously with salt and pepper.

IN A large nonstick skillet, heat the vegetable oil over medium-high heat. Add the patties to the skillet and sear on both sides until the internal temperature registers 165°F, 5 to 7 minutes total.

TOAST THE brioche buns. Dress the bottom buns with the chutney and top with the microgreens. Place the turkey patties on the microgreens and top with the cheese crisps. Dress the top buns with the aioli, then close the burgers and serve.

PAPAYA CHUTNEY

MAKES ABOUT 1 CUP

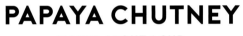

1 medium papaya, peeled, halved, and seeded

⅓ cup apple cider vinegar

⅓ cup golden raisins

Pinch of saffron threads

Kosher salt and freshly ground black pepper

CUT THE papaya into ½-inch pieces. Transfer the papaya to a small saucepan and add the vinegar, raisins, and saffron. Bring to a simmer and cook for about 20 minutes, until thickened. Season with salt and pepper. Remove from the heat and let cool.

BLACK TRUFFLE AIOLI

MAKES ABOUT 1½ CUPS

4 large egg yolks
Juice of ½ lemon
1 cup canola oil
¼ cup black truffle oil

COMBINE THE egg yolks and lemon juice in an immersion blender cup. (Alternatively, use a food processor or standing blender.) Combine the canola oil and truffle oil in a liquid measuring cup and, with the blender running on high, slowly stream the oil mixture down the side of the blender cup. Blend until the mixture is emulsified and has thickened to the consistency of a loose mayonnaise. Transfer to a bowl, cover, and refrigerate until ready to use or overnight.

CHEESE CRISPS

MAKES 4 CRISPS

6 ounces Fontina cheese, shredded
6 ounces Parmesan cheese, grated

PREHEAT THE oven to 400°F. Line a baking sheet with a silicone baking mat or other non-stick pan liner.

COMBINE THE two cheeses in a small bowl. Arrange the cheese mixture in four even piles on the prepared baking sheet. Bake until golden brown and set. Remove the cheese crisps from the pan with a thin spatula and let cool on a wire rack.

FUN FACT

I accidentally burnt the shit out of the gluten-free brioche bun during toasting, but by that point it was nearly two a.m., and I was in no mood to haggle with the manager at Bareburger all over again the next day. So I carefully scraped off the blackened crust and angled it toward the camera so you couldn't see the gouges on both sides of the bun.

TIMPANO

SERVES 8 TO 10

I had never intended to make more than one episode of *Binging with Babish*. The proof is in the name—it's a stupid name, picked arbitrarily based on my Reddit handle and a food-/TV-relevant alliteration. But the *Parks and Rec* burger cook-off received a few thousand views and some resoundingly positive feedback, which was more than enough to rally me into making another, and this time I had my sights set on one of the most magnificent dishes ever featured on film. Re-creating the towering *timpano* from *Big Night* was certainly the most difficult episode to produce, in part due to the complexity of the recipe, but more by virtue of having to work ten hours during the day. But, folks, this is how my mind operates—once I've settled on doing something (which, at the time, was rare), I am going to do it, no matter how inefficient or ill-advised that something is. It was that dog-with-a-bone mentality that kept me up making pasta until five a.m., saw me off to work at eight, and sent me back into the fray of assembling the pasta-filled monstrosity the moment I got back home. While it might've been one of the most labor-intensive episodes to date, it's also one of my fondest memories ever: my friends and coworkers came over for an impromptu dinner party, and waited in drunken revelry while the great Calabrian beast stewed in the oven. When it finally emerged from its cast-iron cage, they clapped. When the first steaming slice was cut, they cheered. If the couple of thousand views and dozen positive comments on the *Parks and Rec* burger were gasoline, this was rocket fuel. I had never felt so validated as a home cook, and even after the sleepless night spent making pasta and the party winding down in my house, I couldn't help but begin editing the episode that same night. I was hooked. And I think I can safely say that if that *timpano*, after all the work of both creating and filming it, had exploded/leaked/sagged/burned in front of all my friends, you wouldn't be reading this sentence. I'd have taken up skateboarding or knitting or something.

VERDICT: If you're a passionate home cook, you owe it to yourself to try making *timpano* at least (if not only) once in your life. It might be a mélange of familiar ingredients presented in a different form, but like any great dish, it's greater than the sum of its parts. The sense of accomplishment that comes from cracking it open like a great wheel of Parmesan, the excitement on your guests' faces, the knowing that you built it entirely from scratch—it's an unparalleled kitchen experience.

(recipe continues)

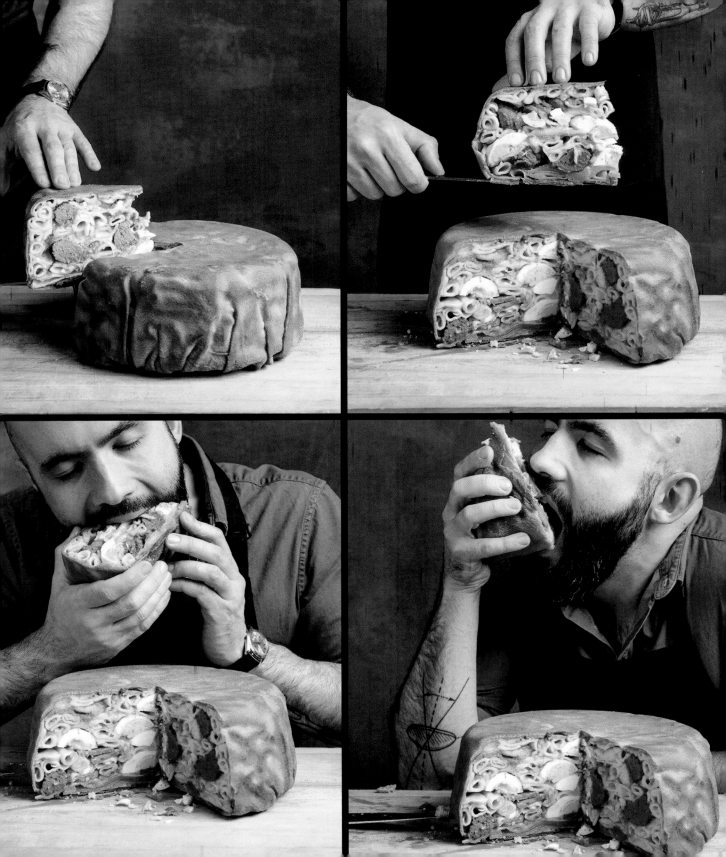

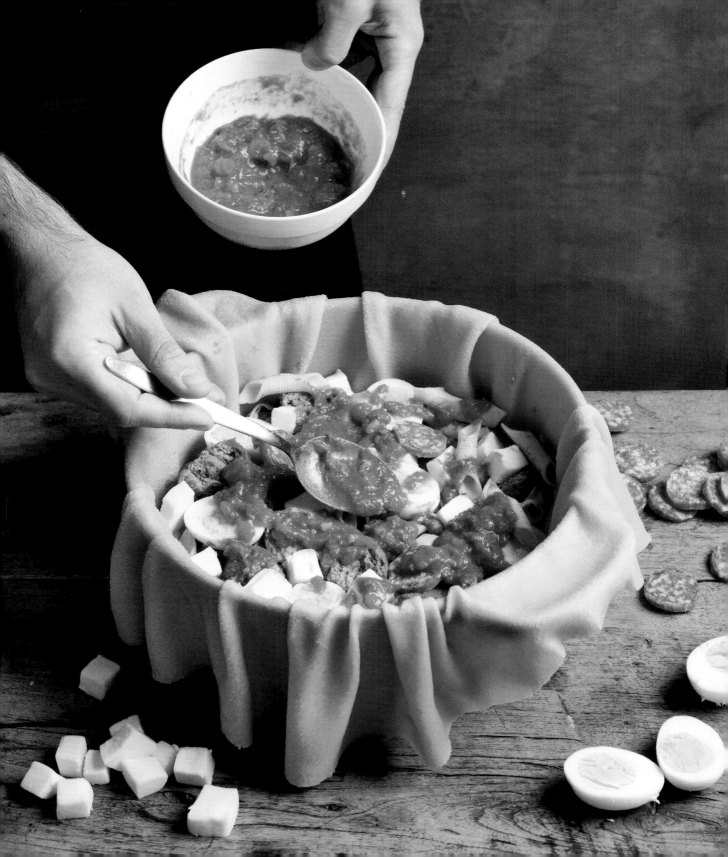

Meatballs (recipe follows)

Prison Gravy (see page 47)

24 ounces fresh garganelli pasta, homemade (recipe follows) or store-bought

2 tablespoons extra-virgin olive oil

Fresh Pasta (recipe follows)

All-purpose flour, for dusting

12 hard-boiled large eggs, halved lengthwise

½ pound aged provolone cheese, grated

1 pound low-moisture mozzarella cheese, cut into 1-inch cubes

1 pound Genoa salami, sliced into ¼-inch rounds

Whole nutmeg, for serving

TRANSFER THE meatballs to the pot of sauce for the final hour of cooking. Remove the meatballs and set them aside until ready to assemble the timpano. Remove the sausage and beef shank and reserve them for another use. Keep the sauce warm.

PREHEAT THE oven to 375°F.

BRING A large pot of salted water to a boil over high heat. Cook the garganelli for about 3 minutes, or until al dente. Drain, then toss with a few tablespoons of the sauce and set aside.

COAT THE interior of a 5-quart enameled Dutch oven with the olive oil. Unwrap the pasta dough and dust it with flour. On a well-floured work surface, begin rolling it out into a large disc, flouring it as necessary to keep it from sticking, then roll it out to ⅛ inch thick. Roll the round of dough around a rolling pin, then unroll into the Dutch oven, pressing it down into the corners and making sure there are at least 8 inches of overhang around the Dutch oven.

FILL THE pasta dough with one-quarter of the cooked garganelli and ¼ cup of the sauce, then layer with one-quarter of each of the fillings: hard-boiled eggs, meatballs, cheeses, and salami. Repeat, reserving some of the provolone for the end, until the Dutch oven is filled to the brim. Sprinkle the reserved provolone over the top to help prevent the timpano from leaking after it's inverted. Fold the overhanging dough over the top and press down to seal. For a softer crust, cover the Dutch oven; for a crispier crust, leave uncovered. Bake for about 2 hours, until the internal temperature registers at least 125°F and the exterior is golden brown. Remove from the oven and let the timpano rest for 1 hour.

PLACE A large cutting board or plate over the top of the Dutch oven and invert the timpano onto it. Slice the timpano into wedges. For each serving, ladle some of the sauce onto a plate, top with a wedge of the timpano, and grate nutmeg over the top.

(recipe continues)

MEATBALLS

MAKES 18 TO 24 MEATBALLS

3 ounces torn Italian bread

½ cup buttermilk, plus more as needed

1 medium onion, minced

4 ounces fatty pancetta, finely minced

4 ounces Parmesan cheese, grated

4 large egg yolks

½ cup homemade veal demi-glace, or ½ cup chicken stock mixed with 4 (¼-ounce) packets unflavored powdered gelatin

½ cup loosely packed fresh parsley leaves, minced

4 garlic cloves, finely minced

1 tablespoon minced fresh oregano

1½ teaspoons kosher salt

¾ teaspoon freshly ground black pepper

1 pound ground beef chuck

½ pound ground short ribs

1 pound ground pork

1 pound ground veal

3 tablespoons leaf lard or vegetable oil

Prison Gravy (see page 47)

IN THE bowl of a stand mixer, combine the bread with the buttermilk, tossing to coat. Let stand, tossing occasionally, until the bread is completely moist, about 10 minutes. Squeeze the bread between your fingers or mash with a spoon to make sure there are no dry spots; if there are dry spots that refuse to moisten, add more buttermilk 1 tablespoon at a time until the bread is moist throughout. Add the onion, pancetta, Parmesan, egg yolks, demi-glace, parsley, garlic, oregano, salt, and pepper.

USING THE paddle attachment, beat on low speed, gradually increasing to medium-high, until thoroughly blended, stopping to scrape down the sides as necessary. Add one-third each of the chuck, short rib, pork, and veal and beat on medium-high speed until thoroughly blended.

REMOVE THE bowl from the stand mixer and add the remaining meat. Gently mix the meatball mixture by hand, breaking up the ground meat with your fingers, just until the ingredients are thoroughly distributed throughout; avoid mixing any more than is necessary for even distribution. Form into golf ball–size meatballs.

IN A large cast-iron skillet, melt the leaf lard over medium-high heat. Add the meatballs and sear on all sides. Set aside until ready to add to the timpano.

FRESH PASTA

MAKES ABOUT 1 POUND

15 ounces tipo 00 flour or all-purpose flour

2 large eggs plus 6 large egg yolks

2 tablespoons extra-virgin olive oil

2 teaspoons kosher salt

MOUND THE flour onto a wooden work surface or baking mat. Make a large well in the center of the flour. Pour the eggs, egg yolks, olive oil, and salt into the well. Beat with a fork until a thick slurry forms. Begin working in the flour with your hands to form a shaggy dough. Knead for 5 minutes, or until smooth and not tacky. Wrap the dough in plastic wrap and let rest for 30 minutes.

HOMEMADE GARGANELLI

MAKES ABOUT 2 POUNDS

20 ounces tipo 00 flour (or all-purpose), plus more for dusting

4 large eggs plus 8 large egg yolks

2 teaspoons kosher salt

MOUND THE flour onto a wooden work surface or baking mat. Make a large well in the center of the flour. Pour the eggs, egg yolks, and salt into the well and beat with a fork until a thick slurry forms. Begin working in the flour with your hands to form a shaggy dough. Knead for 5 minutes, or until smooth and tacky but not sticky. Wrap the dough in plastic wrap and let rest for 30 minutes.

LINE A baking sheet with a clean kitchen towel and dust it liberally with flour.

DIVIDE THE dough into 6 equal pieces using a bench scraper. Working with one piece at a time (keep the rest covered with plastic wrap until ready to use), roll the dough into a rectangular shape on a well-floured surface until it's thin enough that you can see the outline of your hand through the dough. Using a pizza or pasta cutter, trim the edges off the pasta sheet to form it into a rectangle. Cut the rectangle into 2-inch squares. Wrap each square diagonally around a small wooden dowel, then press against a gnocchi stripper to form garganelli. Remove the garganelli from the dowel and transfer it to the towel. Repeat with the remaining pieces of dough, spacing the garganelli apart on the towel as you go. If desired, let the garganelli dry out overnight. (You won't cook the pasta until you're ready to assemble the timpano.)

FUN FACT

This was my first time introducing nutmeg into a savory Italian situation, and I haven't looked back since. Freshly grated nutmeg has the ability to awaken dormant qualities of cheeses, sauces, and meats—try it in your next lasagna!

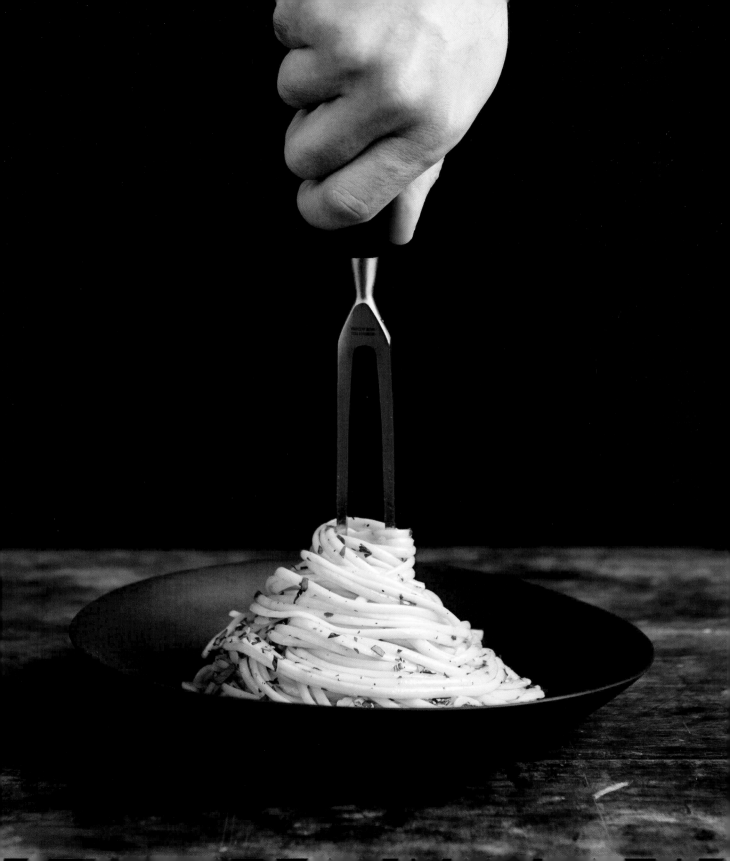

PASTA AGLIO E OLIO

SERVES 2

There's a reason the image of a twirl of pasta around a carving fork has been permanently emblazoned on my left forearm: this has been, far and away, the most important episode of the show. The idea came to me around 7:30 p.m. as I was gearing up to leave work, and it dawned on me that while I already had all the necessary ingredients at home, I would need to buy a carving fork. *Binging with Babish* does, after all, prioritize accuracy above most anything else. I managed to find the one kitchen supply shop still open, a place in Chelsea called Whisk, and managed to find their only carving fork available: a Messermeister knife and fork set, ringing in at $65. Being deeply in debt at the time, I had a big decision to make: *Do I just plate up the pasta as I normally would, hoping that viewers will give me a pass? Or do I buy this carving fork, that I'll likely only use once, with money I don't have, all for the sake of doing it the way the guy in the movie did?* The shop was closing its doors, the manager was getting frustrated with me standing and staring at the carving fork set just a few feet from the checkout counter, and the scales finally tipped. With that decision, my priorities were set, and would become a crucial part of my show's format.

As important as that experience was for me personally (eventually culminating in actually meeting Jon Favreau), the importance of this episode extends far beyond my seemingly meaningless credit card–funded purchase. It became, and continues to be, an influential dish for burgeoning home cooks around the world. Every single day, I get tagged in photos across social networks, first-time chefs exclaiming that they tried making something for the first time and loved it. It has encouraged those who might not have otherwise tried their hand with a pot and pan to step outside their comfort zone, take a risk, reap the rewards. It's one of the aspects of my career for which I am most grateful, and that I am most humbled and most enlivened by.

VERDICT: Pasta aglio e olio is something very special: eight simple ingredients (nine, if you count boiling water) coming together to make something greater than the sum of their parts. While it takes a bit of practice to get it just right—a creamy, emulsified sauce with sweet, blond garlic—it is very forgiving and will almost always produce a delicious result.

(recipe continues)

Kosher salt

½ pound linguine

½ cup good-quality extra-virgin olive oil

6 large garlic cloves, thinly sliced

1 teaspoon red pepper flakes

½ lemon, seeded

½ cup fresh flat-leaf parsley, finely chopped

Freshly ground black pepper

HEAVILY SALT a large pot of water and bring to a boil. Add the pasta and cook about 1 minute less than the suggested cooking time on the package, or until very al dente.

IN A large sauté pan, heat the olive oil over medium-low heat until barely shimmering. Add the garlic and cook, stirring continuously, until softened and turning golden on the edges, about 2 minutes. Add the red pepper flakes and reduce the heat to medium-low.

DRAIN THE pasta, reserving about ¼ cup of the pasta cooking water. Add the pasta and reserved cooking water to the sauté pan. Squeeze the juice from the lemon over the top, add the parsley, and toss well to combine. If the sauce is too watery, cook until the pasta has absorbed more of the liquid, 1 to 3 minutes.

TASTE AND season with salt and pepper. Twirl the spaghetti into two nests with a carving fork, transfer to shallow bowls, and serve.

FUN FACT

This episode was one of two that received scathing reviews from a group of real Italian chefs on YouTube. While I'd be quick to remind them that this is a show with an emphasis on accurate re-creation of the foods from fiction, I also welcome their criticism and encourage you to check it out as well. *Binging with Babish* is, after all, a learning experience— for both you and me!

NEW YORK–STYLE PIZZA

MAKES TWO 14-INCH PIZZAS

This was the first instance of *Binging with Babish* veering into "kind of a stretch" (pun intended) territory: there was no recipe, no culinary specificity to the media. Just a montage of New Yorkers enjoying slice after slice of hot, cheesy, stretchy, thin-crust pizza—one that I distinctly remember making me extremely hungry when I repeatedly watched it as a child. So in this episode, technique had to come to the forefront. I read every nerdy dissertation on the internet about the difficulty of making pizza at home, consulted my homemade-pizza-obsessed friend (we all have one of those . . . right?), and eventually settled on what remains my favorite method to this day: measured ingredients for accuracy and repeatability, using a food processor for rapid kneading and gluten formation, an overnight ferment for flavor and texture, and a two-stone oven setup for concentrated heat. You can definitely go to greater lengths to achieve that impossibly thin, crispy, chewy, restaurant-style crust at home, but provided you have a day in advance to make the dough, this one comes together with pretty minimal effort. The most important takeaway here is the overnight ferment: not only does this develop the dough's flavor, it allows for natural gluten development to occur while keeping the dough relaxed, so it's super-easy to roll and stretch out into a pie.

VERDICT: This is an incredibly reliable and relatively easy way to create New York–style pizza at home. My end product in the episode, as commenters have pointed out, turned out pretty crust-heavy. To prevent this, stretch your dough out as wide as possible while leaving a very narrow border of slightly thicker dough on its circumference.

New York–Style Pizza Dough (recipe follows)
¼ cup semolina flour
All-purpose flour, for dusting

Pizza Sauce (recipe follows)
8 ounces low-moisture whole-milk mozzarella, shredded

(recipe continues)

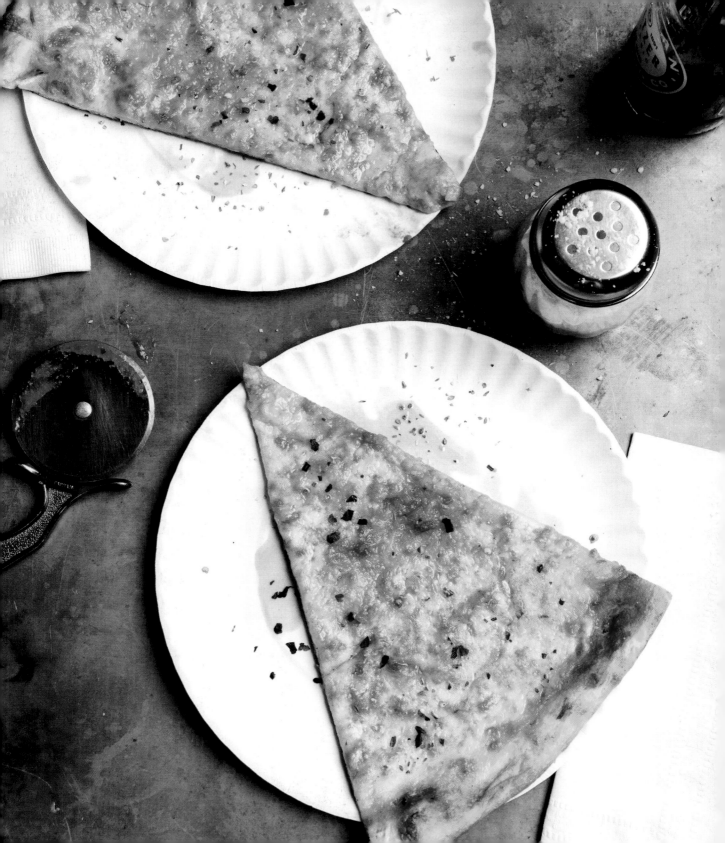

DIVIDE THE chilled dough into two equal pieces. Wrap individually in plastic wrap and let rest at room temperature for 1 hour.

PLACE A pizza stone on the top rack of the oven and preheat the oven to 550°F (or the highest setting) for 1 hour.

DUST A pizza peel with half the semolina flour. Generously dust a work surface with all-purpose flour and place one piece of the dough on top. Pressing gently with your fingertips, push the dough out to form an 8-inch round, leaving the edge slightly thicker. Pick up the round of dough and drape it over your knuckles, letting gravity stretch it. Pass the dough hand over hand until you have about a 14-inch round. Transfer the dough to the prepared pizza peel and reshape it into a circle, if necessary, leaving the edge slightly thicker.

LADLE ABOUT ½ cup of the pizza sauce onto the dough and spread until evenly coated, making sure to leave a ½-inch border exposed. Scatter half the mozzarella over the sauce. Slide the pizza onto the preheated pizza stone and bake until the crust is well browned and the cheese is bubbling and browned in spots, about 12 minutes. Using the pizza peel, transfer the pie to a large cutting board or pizza pan. Slice into 6 wedges and serve. Repeat with the remaining dough, sauce, and cheese to make a second pizza.

FUN FACT
This was the first episode I made as a newly minted single man—you may notice that a ring on my left hand is no longer visible for the first time. Is that a fun fact? I dunno.

NEW YORK–STYLE PIZZA DOUGH
MAKES TWO 14-INCH PIZZAS

- 16 ounces bread flour (about 3¾ cups), plus more for dusting
- 1 tablespoon sugar
- 2 teaspoons kosher salt
- ½ teaspoon active dry yeast
- 1¼ cups ice water
- 1 tablespoon vegetable oil, plus more for greasing

IN A food processor, pulse together the bread flour, sugar, salt, and the yeast until well combined. In a liquid measuring cup, combine the ice water and 1 tablespoon of vegetable oil and, with the machine running, slowly drizzle the mixture in through the feed tube until a ball of sticky dough forms. Transfer to an oiled work surface and knead until smooth, about 2 minutes. Transfer to an oiled bowl, cover with plastic wrap, and refrigerate overnight before using.

(recipe continues)

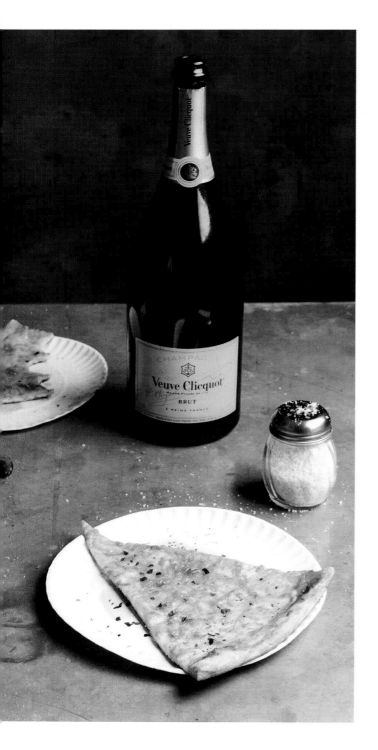

PIZZA SAUCE

MAKES 3½ CUPS

1 (28-ounce) can whole peeled tomatoes, with their juices

2 medium garlic cloves, minced

1 teaspoon kosher salt

1 teaspoon dried oregano

½ teaspoon red pepper flakes

½ teaspoon dried basil

½ teaspoon sugar

IN A food processor, combine the tomatoes and their juices, garlic, salt, oregano, red pepper flakes, basil, and sugar. Process until smooth. Set aside until ready to use.

PHILLY CHEESESTEAK SANDWICHES

MAKES 2

This was the very first episode to come out of my new apartment in Harlem, after an almost four-month gap encompassing a major upheaval in my personal life: getting divorced. I had to move apartments, build out a whole new kitchen, build up a whole new life. I was almost certain that I would give up on the show. I agonized over camera angles, backdrops, and work surfaces—painting and repainting my walls, filming in front of every available surface in the apartment, rearranging my lighting in countless different iterations. My previous apartment, with its white walls, backsplash, and work surface, had been a dream to shoot in. This new apartment, with its black cabinetry and lime-green walls, was proving to be a challenge I wasn't sure I could surmount. Eventually, finally, I settled on the angle that might now be most familiar to you: butcher block work surface, flanked by a stove and a bar. The obstacles didn't end with the production design, however: try as I might, I couldn't settle on a cheesesteak recipe I was happy with. I'd get the look right—thin, crumbly beef, melty cheese, pebble-bottomed roll—but the taste wouldn't be right. I'd get the flavor right, but it would start looking like some steak melt from Quiznos. It took some time and reflection to realize, but the fears surrounding the show were running parallel to the fears surrounding my frightening new reality. I was on my own for the first time in thirteen years, and was as terrified to put myself out there as I had been back in high school. The show continued to entangle itself in my personal life as I realized that even if the end result wasn't perfect, I couldn't allow myself to be paralyzed by fear. Bet you didn't know that there was life-altering turmoil and self-realization behind this sandwich.

VERDICT: While not a truly authentic Philly cheesesteak, this is an outstanding home substitute. Opt for high-quality, fatty meat and a soft, dense, squishy roll—the rest is up to you—but you can expect me to scoff if you put ketchup and mayo on it, as they do in the movie.

(recipe continues)

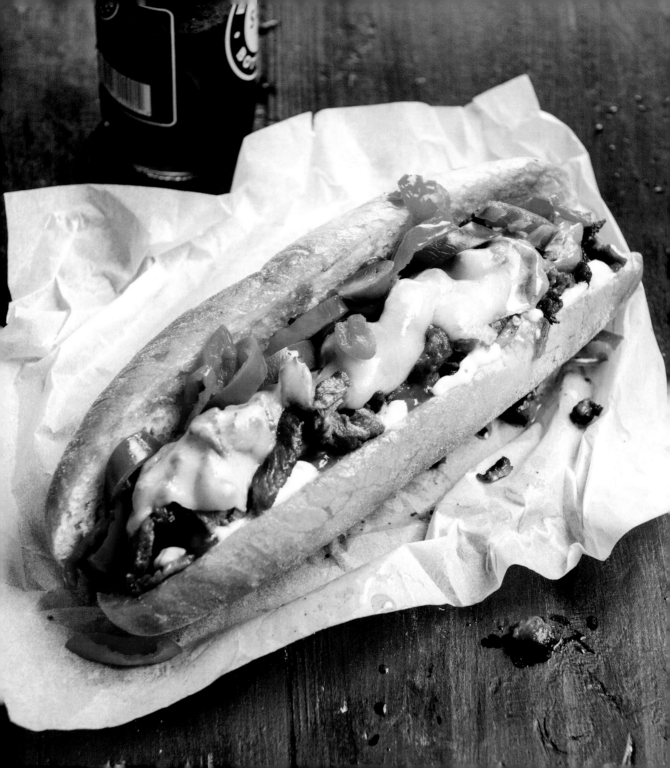

1 teaspoon kosher salt

1 (24-ounce) boneless rib eye steak

2 tablespoons vegetable oil

4 slices provolone cheese

2 dense, squishy hoagie rolls, split open

2 tablespoons ketchup

2 tablespoons mayonnaise

2 ounces sweet and hot peppers, sliced

SPRINKLE THE salt all over the rib eye and transfer to a wire rack set on a baking sheet. Freeze for 30 minutes, or until the steak is firm to the touch. With a very sharp knife, slice the rib eye as thinly as possible, leaving any fat intact.

IN A large cast-iron skillet, heat the vegetable oil over medium-high heat until shimmering. Add half the beef in an even layer—don't crowd the pan. Cook, undisturbed, for 2 to 3 minutes, until browned and crispy. Flip and cook until evenly browned and crisp. Arrange the beef in a long pile in the center of the pan and top with 2 slices of the cheese. Reduce the heat to medium-low and cook until the cheese has melted.

DRESS ONE roll with half the ketchup and mayo, and top with the cooked beef and half the peppers. Cut the cheesesteak in half and serve. Repeat with remaining ingredients for the second sandwich.

FUN FACT

This is one of the two episodes featuring the key light coming from camera right—after the following apple pie episode, you can see the light shift to the other side of the frame. This might seem trivial, but it was a decision months in the making that I literally lost sleep over.

APPLE PIE

MAKES ONE 9-INCH PIE

Pie is the central focus of a surprising number of pop culture mainstays. When it's not being used as a sex toy by hormonally crazed teen-agers, it's being flung into faces for comedic effect, draped with American cheese by socio-paths, or made into a creative and emotional outlet for a repressed heroine. Here we have the first example of an episode inspired by multiple appearances in film and television—not to mention my first time ever baking a pie. I was understandably nervous diving into this recipe as well, but after the warm recep-tion given to the Philly cheesesteak episode, I resolved to continue stepping outside my comfort zone. I opted for the food proces-sor piecrust recipe, which seemed to stream-line the normally intuition-reliant process by which the finicky pastry is made. While my latticework left a great deal to be desired, I was surprised to be rewarded with a rich, flaky crust made with relative ease. The dreaded soggy bottom (which normally plagues lattice-top pies) was also delightfully absent, thanks to the preheated baking sheet (or pizza stone) upon which the pie is baked.

VERDICT: Like the *Teenage Mutant Ninja Turtle* pizza (see page 31), this is a relatively foolproof recipe for dipping one's toes into the beguiling world of baking. The crust is somewhat forgiving, opening up the opportu-nity for experimenting with spices and differ-ent kinds of washes (egg, egg white, milk).

2½ pounds baking apples, such as Granny Smith or Honeycrisp, peeled, cored, and sliced into ½-inch wedges

2 tablespoons sugar, plus more for sprinkling

2 tablespoons all-purpose flour, plus more for dusting

¼ teaspoon ground cinnamon

¼ teaspoon ground allspice

¼ teaspoon freshly grated nutmeg

¼ teaspoon ground ginger

Pie Dough (recipe follows)

1 large egg white, beaten

(recipe continues)

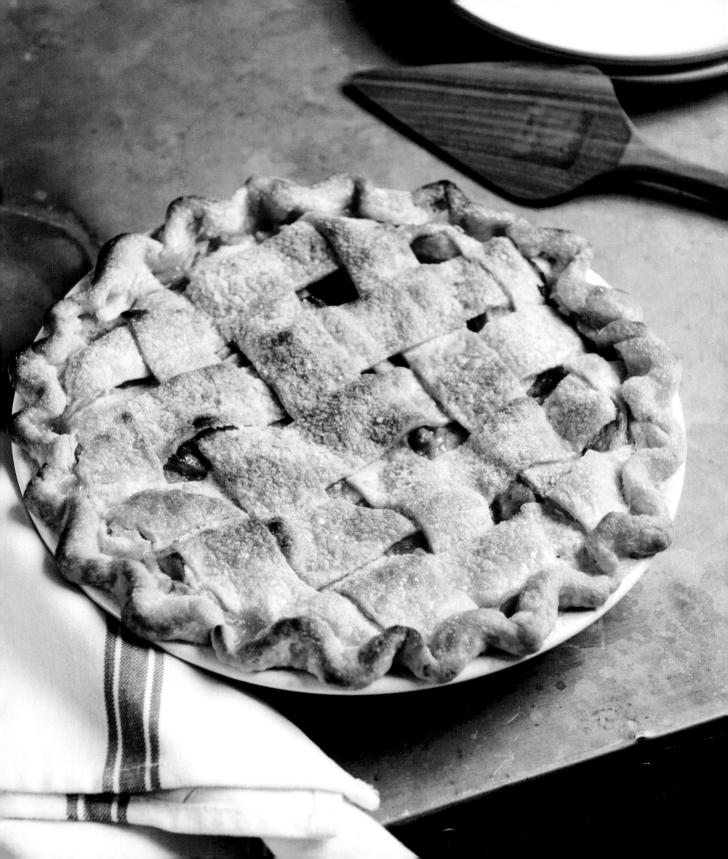

IN A large bowl, toss the apples with the sugar, flour, and spices. Set aside.

TRANSFER THE dough to a floured work surface. Dust the dough with flour and pound it lightly with a rolling pin. Divide it into two equal pieces and gently roll one out to a 13-inch round. Roll the dough round onto your rolling pin and unroll it over a 9-inch pie plate. Without stretching the dough, ease it into the pie plate, leaving a 1-inch overhang all around. Wrap the pie plate with plastic wrap and refrigerate for 10 to 15 minutes. Roll the second piece of dough out to a 10-inch round and cut it into ten 1-inch-wide strips for the lattice top.

PLACE AN aluminum baking sheet in the oven and preheat the oven to 500°F. Transfer the apples to the pie plate and press down gently. Place 5 of the lattice strips across the top of your pie, spacing them evenly, lifting 2 strips at a time and interweaving the strips in the opposite direction. Trim off the excess dough and tuck it underneath the edge. Crimp the edge every inch or so using your fingers. Brush the edge and lattice with the beaten egg white and sprinkle sugar over the top. Transfer the pie plate to the preheated baking sheet, reduce the oven temperature to 400°F, and bake until the crust is deep brown and crisp, 30 to 45 minutes. Remove the pie from the oven and let cool on a wire rack for at least 4 hours.

SLICE INTO wedges and serve.

PIE DOUGH

MAKES ONE 9-INCH PIE CRUST PLUS LATTICE TOP

12½ ounces all-purpose flour (about a scant 3 cups), plus more for dusting

¾ cup sugar

1 teaspoon kosher salt

1 cup (2 sticks) unsalted butter, cubed and chilled

¾ to 1 cup ice water

IN A food processor, combine the flour, sugar, and salt. Pulse to combine. Add the butter and pulse until the mixture resembles wet sand. Transfer to a large bowl. Sprinkle in ¾ cup of the ice water and gently fold in using a rubber spatula. Add more ice water if necessary until a shaggy dough forms.

TURN THE dough out onto a work surface and pat it into a disk. Liberally dust the dough with flour, wrap it in plastic wrap, and refrigerate for at least 2 hours or up to 2 days.

FUN FACT

This is the only voice-over I ever did stoned. Being an occasional cannabis user, it was inevitable that I'd eventually try to deliver a pithy narration while under the influence of the sticky icky, and it taught me one thing: I am not capable of doing a voice-over stoned.

THE MOISTMAKER SANDWICH

MAKES 1 SANDWICH, PLUS ENOUGH FILLINGS TO SERVE 10

Monica Geller had a simple but genius idea: nestle a slice of gravy-soaked bread in the middle of a Thanksgiving leftovers sandwich. The result not only drove Ross to near madness, it became the first real windfall for *Binging with Babish*. Reddit, in many ways, acts as a tastemaker for the rest of the internet—so when this episode began climbing the ranks of /r/videos, it wasn't long before it was being posted elsewhere, as well as written up by the *Huffington Post* and *Entertainment Weekly*. It was the first time I thought, *Okay, maybe I've got something worth pursuing here.* I was still working a full-time job (and would continue to for another year), but I resolved to put out an episode every Tuesday at nine a.m. And if the Moistmaker was any indication, this was another full-time job; its construction required the making of an entire Thanksgiving meal from scratch. Freshly tattooed and cooking in my pajamas, day one consisted of spatchcocking and dry-brining the turkey, a

technique popularized by my personal food idol, J. Kenji López-Alt. Not only does dry-brining deeply flavor the meat and desiccate the skin (making it extra crisp), spatchcocking the bird allows it to cook in nearly half the time it would take whole. Yes, you heard me right, folks—half. Imagine cutting an extra two or so hours out of the whirlwind clusterfuck that is Thanksgiving prep, while being able to make turkey stock from scratch in the process. All you need is a strong pair of kitchen shears.

VERDICT: This recipe yields, well, a full Thanksgiving dinner. Each technique is thoughtful and reliable, and if you're crazy enough to make the whole thing explicitly for a sandwich, you'll end up with a superlative one. The so-called "Moistmaker" does just that: introduces gravy to the sandwich without making it sloppy, keeping everything moist and flavorful.

---

3 slices hearty white sandwich bread

Turkey Gravy (recipe follows)

Sliced Roast Turkey and Sage-Sausage Stuffing (recipe follows)

Cranberry Sauce (recipe follows)

LIGHTLY TOAST the bread. Soak one piece of the toast in the gravy. Assemble a triple-decker sandwich with the roast turkey and some of the gravy, some stuffing, and some cranberry sauce, placing the gravy-soaked bread in the middle of the layers. Transfer to a plate and serve.

(recipe continues)

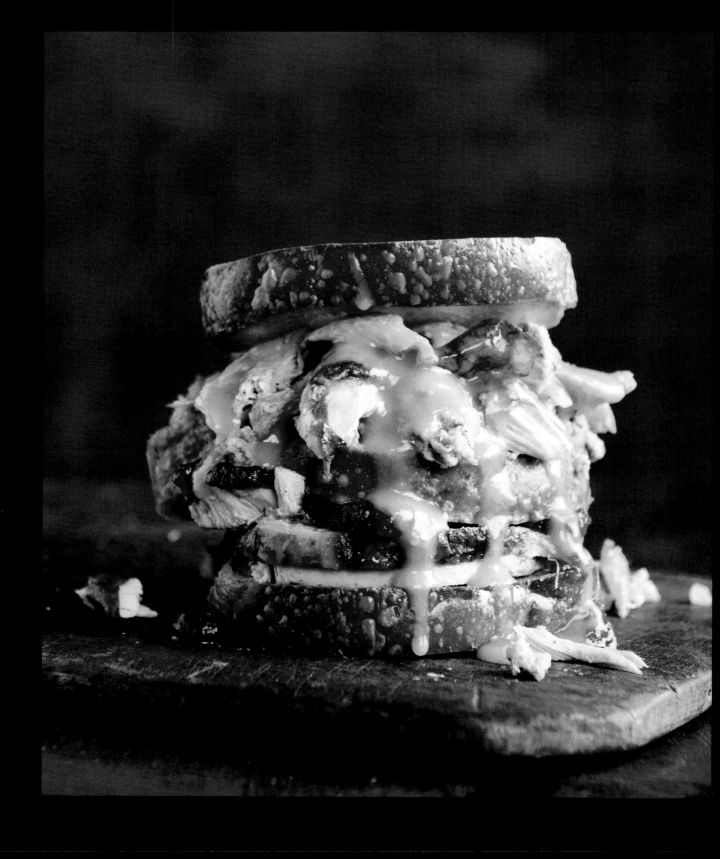

ROAST TURKEY

MAKES 1 TURKEY

---

1 fresh turkey, any size, trimmed of extra fat and giblets removed

2 cups kosher salt, plus more for seasoning

1 tablespoon baking powder

TURKEY STOCK

1 tablespoon vegetable oil

1 turkey backbone and wishbone, reserved from Roast Turkey, cut into 2-inch lengths

2 large carrots, cut into 3-inch lengths

1 onion, quartered

2 celery stalks, cut into 3-inch lengths

5 to 10 sprigs fresh thyme

1 parsnip, peeled and halved

1 turnip, peeled and quartered

1 tablespoon whole black peppercorns

Handful of fresh parsley

1 head garlic, halved crosswise

1 bay leaf

SAGE-SAUSAGE STUFFING

2 loaves white country bread, cut into ½ to 1-inch cubes

1 pound plain pork sausage, casings removed

2 tablespoons bacon fat (optional)

1 large yellow onion, chopped

6 celery stalks, chopped

¼ cup minced fresh sage

2 tablespoons minced fresh thyme leaves

Chopped fresh parsley

3 large eggs, beaten

Kosher salt and freshly ground black pepper

Unsalted butter, for greasing

1 cup chopped carrots

2 cups chopped onions

1 cup chopped celery

LINE A rimmed baking sheet with aluminum foil.

PLACE THE turkey on the baking sheet. Using a sturdy pair of poultry shears, cut along each side of the turkey backbone. Remove the backbone and reserve it for the Turkey Stock. Using a very sharp paring knife, cut around the wishbone, remove it from the bird, and reserve it for the Turkey Stock. Using the poultry shears again, cut deep into the center of the breastbone from the back, so it's easier to crack. Flip the bird over and press down between the breasts to flatten the turkey. Whisk together the salt and baking powder in a medium bowl until well combined. Liberally sprinkle the salt mixture all over the bird until it looks like it's been covered in a light snowfall. Refrigerate, uncovered, overnight.

(recipe continues)

TURKEY STOCK

IN A large saucepan, heat the vegetable oil over high heat until nearly smoking. Add the turkey backbone pieces and sear until well browned on both sides, about 7 minutes. Add the carrots, onion, celery, thyme, parsnip, turnip, peppercorns, parsley, garlic, and bay leaf. Add cold water to cover and bring to a gentle boil. Reduce the heat to keep the stock at a bare simmer and cook, skimming the surface of the stock as necessary for the first 30 minutes, until the stock is brown and deeply flavorful, 4 to 12 hours. You want to end up with 6 cups of stock, so add water as necessary if it reduces too far. Strain the stock through a colander or sieve lined with cheesecloth and discard the solids. Return the stock to the saucepan and keep warm over low heat.

SAGE–SAUSAGE STUFFING

PREHEAT THE oven to 200°F.

PLACE THE bread cubes on two rimmed baking sheets and bake for 1 to 2 hours, until crisp. Transfer the croutons to a large bowl and set aside.

HEAT A large, high-sided sauté pan over medium-high heat. Add the sausage and cook, stirring and breaking up the meat, until browned and plenty of fond (the layer of cooked-on browned bits) has formed on the bottom of the pan, about 5 minutes. Using a slotted spoon, transfer the sausage to the bowl with the croutons, reserving the sausage fat in the pan. Add bacon fat (if using) to the pan and let it melt, then add the onion. Cook the onion over medium heat, stirring, for 2 to 3 minutes, then add the celery, sage, and thyme. Cook, stirring, until the celery has softened, 3 minutes more. Transfer to the bowl with the croutons.

ADD THE parsley and eggs to the bowl and stir to combine. Add 2 to 4 cups of the warm stock, enough that the croutons are soaked but still retain their shape. Season with salt and pepper. (Reserve the remaining stock for making Turkey Gravy, opposite page. It will keep in an airtight container in the refrigerator for up to 3 days.)

GENEROUSLY BUTTER a 9 x 13-inch baking dish.

TRANSFER THE stuffing to the baking dish, cover with aluminum foil, and refrigerate until ready to bake, up to overnight. This can be done as far in advance as the night before baking, but in any case bring to room temperature before putting it in the oven.

WHEN READY to bake the turkey, preheat the oven to 400°F. Line a baking sheet with foil.

BRUSH THE salt mixture off the turkey entirely and transfer the bird to a wire rack. Scatter the chopped vegetables on the prepared baking sheet and place the turkey on the rack on top. Roast until the internal temperature registers 155°F for the breast and 175°F for the thighs, 1½ to 2 hours, depending on the size of the turkey. During the last 30 minutes, transfer the stuffing to the oven with the turkey and bake, covered, for 20 minutes. Remove the foil and bake for 10 minutes more. Remove the stuffing from the oven. Remove the turkey from the oven and let rest for 30 minutes before carving.

TURKEY GRAVY

MAKES 2 CUPS

---

3 tablespoons unsalted butter

3 tablespoons all-purpose flour

2 cups Turkey Stock (opposite page), warmed

1 tablespoon soy sauce

Kosher salt and freshly ground black pepper

IN A medium saucepan, melt the butter over medium heat until foaming. Add the flour and cook, whisking, for about 1 minute, until the raw flour smell dissipates. While whisking continuously, slowly stream in the stock and whisk until completely combined. Reduce the heat to maintain a bare simmer and cook until the gravy reaches your desired thickness. Remove from the heat, stir in the soy sauce, and season with salt and pepper. Stir well and keep warm.

CRANBERRY SAUCE

MAKES ABOUT 4 CUPS

---

1 pound fresh cranberries

1 cup sugar

¼ cup red wine

1 cinnamon stick

½ teaspoon freshly grated nutmeg

Juice of ½ orange

1 (3-inch) strip orange zest (peeled with a vegetable peeler)

IN A medium saucepan, combine all the ingredients and 1½ cups water. Bring to a simmer and cook until the sauce reaches a thick, syrupy consistency, about 30 minutes.

REMOVE THE cinnamon stick and strip of orange zest and discard. Transfer the sauce to a bowl. Cover and refrigerate until ready to serve.

FUN FACT

The Moistmaker you see onscreen is actually the third I assembled from the Thanksgiving dinner. The first one was never captured, as there was no memory card in the camera, and the second was out of focus.

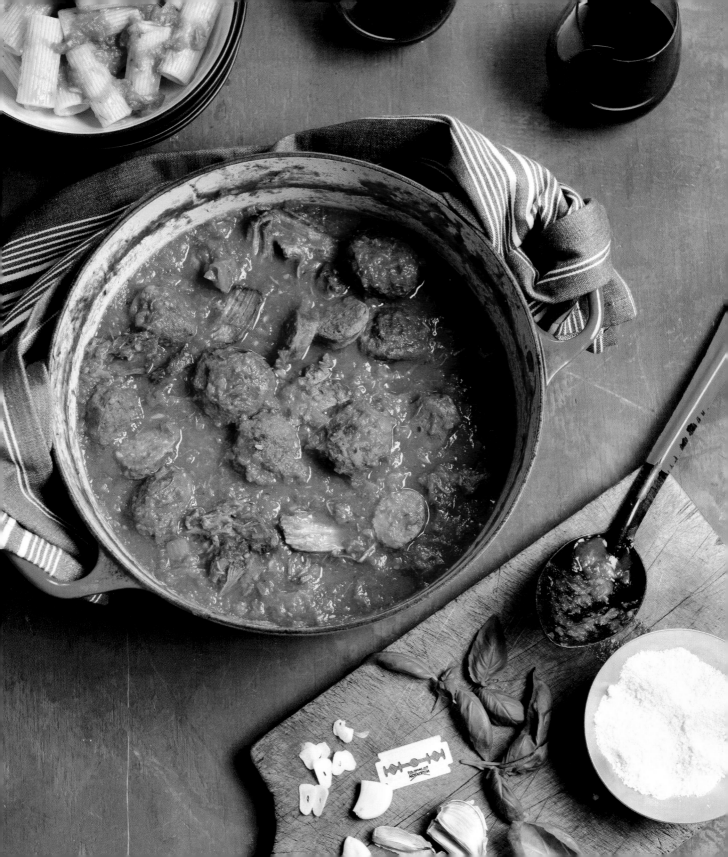

PRISON GRAVY

SERVES 12

Mobsters may be plagued with tacky style, rampant drug use, and short lifespans, but they certainly know how to eat. Even in prison, they can crank out a competent Sunday gravy without breaking a sweat. The only curiosity here, and the main motivation behind the episode, is Paulie's method of slicing garlic wafer-thin with a safety razor. Supposedly, this makes the garlic "liquefy in the pan with just a little oil." Folks, garlic doesn't liquefy, no matter how thin you slice it. In fact, most of the time, it just burns immediately. Now obviously I'm not going to do something as stupid as to contradict Paulie, so the recipe stands, but I recommend that you mince your garlic as usual. I mean, why do you want the garlic to dissolve? Garlic is awesome. Anyway, I'm getting off track here—the more important

takeaway from this recipe is togetherness. Sunday gravy can really only be made as a gigantic meal, and even though it freezes excellently, it's best enjoyed with friends and family. The day after shooting this episode, I brought the leftovers into work and made little meatball sandwiches for everyone. It's an Italian mind-set we could all benefit from: use quality ingredients, treat food with love and patience, and share it with those you care about.

VERDICT: This is about as traditional and familiar as Italian red sauce gets—rich, fatty meat lovingly braised in slowly sweetening San Marzano tomatoes, imbued with garlic and onion. Accept no substitutes.

---

1 tablespoon vegetable oil

1 pound sweet Italian sausage

1 pound hot Italian sausage

1 pound bone-in beef shank

1 pound veal neck bones with some meat attached

1 tablespoon extra-virgin olive oil, plus more if needed

3 garlic cloves, sliced paper-thin with a single-edged razor blade

3 small onions (key word: small), finely chopped

1 tablespoon tomato paste

½ cup red wine

3 (28-ounce) cans whole peeled DOP San Marzano tomatoes, with their juices, crushed with a wooden spoon or run through a food mill

2 large sprigs fresh basil

1 large carrot, cut into thirds

(ingredients continue)

1 pound Meatballs (see page 26), cooked

Kosher salt and freshly ground black pepper

3 pounds durum semolina pasta (preferably with ridges, such as rigatoni rigate), cooked al dente, for serving

Butter, for serving (optional)

Freshly grated Parmesan cheese, for serving (optional)

IN A large nonreactive (such as stainless steel or enameled cast-iron) pot, heat the vegetable oil over medium-high heat until shimmering. Sear the sausage, beef, and veal in batches until well browned and fond (the layer of cooked-on browned bits) has formed on the bottom of the pot, about 5 minutes. Transfer the meat to a plate and set aside.

IN THE same pot, heat the olive oil until shimmering. Add the garlic and cook for 30 seconds, until softened. Add the onions and tomato paste and cook, stirring, until the onions are translucent, about 2 minutes. Add the wine, stirring and scraping up all the browned bits from the bottom of the pot. Pour in the tomatoes and their juices and return the browned meats to the pot. Add the basil and carrot and bring the sauce to a bare simmer.

REDUCE THE heat and let the sauce simmer for about 4 hours total, stirring and scraping the bottom occasionally (don't let anything

stick—it will scorch and ruin your sauce). Add the meatballs for the final hour of cooking.

DISCARD THE carrot and bones, and season the sauce with salt and pepper. For each serving, coat some freshly cooked pasta with a spoonful of sauce; stir in butter or olive oil for a richer sauce. Top with some of the meat and more "gravy," sprinkle with Parmesan, and serve.

THE SAUCE can be frozen for up to 2 months and reheats exceptionally well.

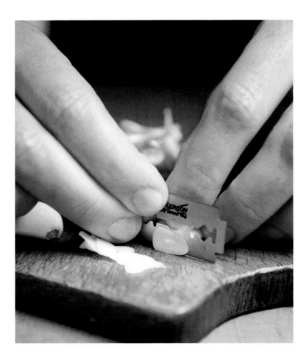

LATE-NIGHT SANDWICH

MAKES 1 SANDWICH

This seemingly simple sandwich has some serious culinary chops behind it: in the film's DVD extras, there's a charming video of Thomas Keller himself teaching Adam Sandler the subtle ways a chef would amp up a BLT. For this episode of *Binging with Babish*, however, I knew folks wouldn't just want to watch me eat a runny-cheesy-bacony egg sandwich— it seemed like the perfect opportunity to show how to bake bread. I settled on a method somewhere between traditional and no-knead bread, an ultra-high-hydration loaf that relies on machine kneading and an extra-long rise to become manageable.

VERDICT: Baking your own bread for the first time is an accomplishment in itself, and making a sandwich out of said bread makes it taste all the more satisfying. Even if you can't bake your own bread, this is a damned fine sandwich, elevated by thoughtful construction and a few simple touches.

2 slices Country Loaf (recipe follows)

2 slices Monterey Jack cheese

2 tablespoons mayonnaise

1 large tomato, sliced

Kosher salt

4 slices bacon, cooked

1 large egg, fried sunny-side up

3 butter lettuce leaves, rinsed and dried

Beer, for serving

PREHEAT THE oven to 400°F. Line a baking sheet with aluminum foil.

PLACE THE bread on the prepared baking sheet. Top one slice with the cheese. Bake for 3 to 5 minutes, until the bread is lightly browned and the cheese has melted. Remove from the oven and transfer the bread to a cutting board. Spread the mayo on the untoasted side of the cheeseless slice of bread, top with 4 slices of tomato, and season them lightly with salt. Add the bacon, egg, and lettuce, then close the sandwich with the second slice of bread, cheese-side down. Cut in half, stare at the cross-section in wonderment, and enjoy with a tall, cold beer.

(recipe continues)

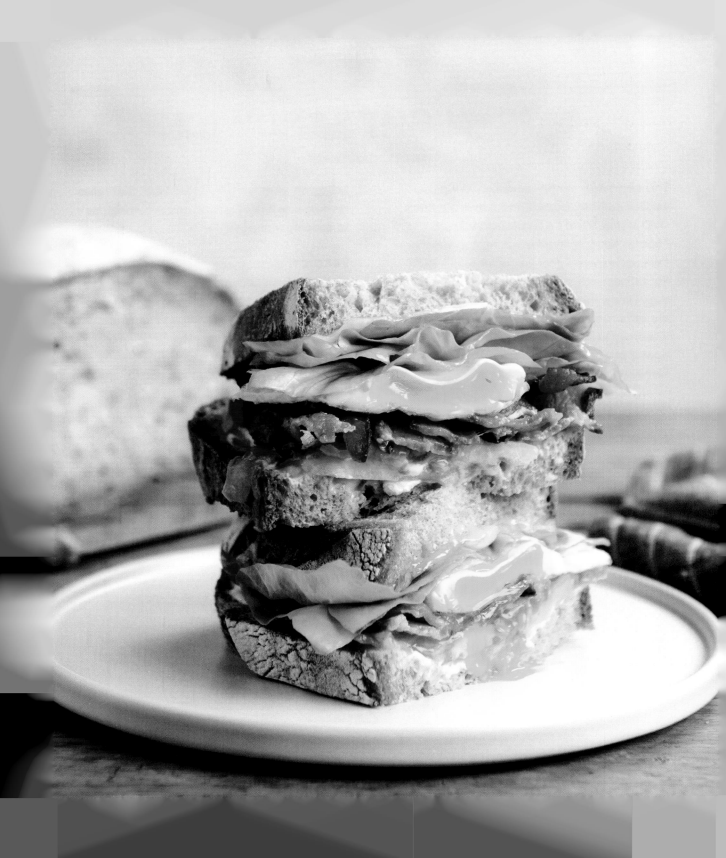

COUNTRY LOAF

MAKES 1 LOAF

½ teaspoon active dry yeast

2⅓ cups room-temperature water

24½ ounces bread flour (about 6¼ cups)

4½ ounces whole wheat flour (about 1¼ cups),
  plus more for dusting

2½ ounces rye flour (about ⅔ cup)

2 tablespoons honey

Neutral vegetable oil, for greasing

WAKE UP super early because that's the first
rule of bread baking. In the bowl of a stand
mixer, dissolve the yeast in 1 cup of the room
temperature water. Add 5 ounces of the bread
flour and the whole wheat flour. Stir with a
rubber spatula until a wet, sticky dough forms.
Cover the bowl tightly with plastic wrap and let
ferment at room temperature for 5 to 16 hours.
(A longer ferment will yield more flavorful
bread.) Go back to sleep.

ADD THE remaining 19½ ounces bread flour,
1⅓ cups water, the rye flour, and the honey to
the dough. Mix lightly with a rubber spatula,
then transfer to the bowl of a stand mixer fitted with the dough hook. Knead the dough for
15 minutes on medium-low speed, or until the
dough is sticky and very loose.

TRANSFER THE dough to a lightly oiled bowl.
Cover the bowl with plastic wrap and let the
dough rise at room temperature for 2 hours,
or until nearly tripled in size. Heavily flour a
work surface. Turn out the dough, pulling the
edges into the center to create a smooth top

for your bread. Line a colander with cheesecloth and dust the cloth heavily with flour.
Transfer the dough, smooth-side down, to the
cheesecloth-lined colander; wrap with plastic
wrap and let the dough rise for 45 minutes, or
until nearly doubled in size.

PREHEAT THE oven to 450°F with a pizza
stone on the upper-middle rack. Line a pizza
peel with parchment paper and lightly dust the
parchment with flour.

TURN THE dough out onto the floured parchment. Score a cross into the top of the dough
about ¼-inch deep vertically then horizontally
with a razor blade or very sharp bread knife.
(This allows the dough to rise in the oven without splitting the crust.) Spritz the dough generously with water from a spray bottle. Using the
pizza peel, slide the dough-topped parchment
onto the pizza stone in the oven. Bake for 35 to
45 minutes, until the bread is deeply browned
and sounds hollow when tapped on the bottom.
Remove the loaf from the oven, transfer to a
wire rack, and let cool for at least 3 hours before
slicing. Store any leftover bread in a bread box
or wrapped in a towel or paper bag at room
temperature.

FUN FACT
The loaf you see on the show
is actually my fourth attempt.
Bread is a bastard.

EGGS WOODHOUSE

SERVES 1

At this point, the show was growing in popularity, and I was starting to become inundated with requests. Chief among them was Eggs Woodhouse, a purposefully over-the-top creation for the titular spoiled-brat secret agent in *Archer*. With the holidays approaching, however, consuming such a decadent and expensive meal somehow felt . . . wrong. I didn't want to end up like the entitled spy for whom the dish was intended, so the episode became "Eggs Woodhouse (For Good)," prompting viewers to give charitably to Hour Children, an NGO I had done some video work for in the past. Feeling vindicated, I went off to Dean & DeLuca to gawk at the cost of Ibérico ham ($80/pound), osetra caviar ($120/ounce), and black winter truffles ($100/ounce). All told, this messy gloop of extravagance set me back around $350, and was hardly even eaten. I can tell you, however, that I made one hell of an omelet the next day.

VERDICT: This mountain of excess has a number of competing flavors and textures, virtually none of them playing nicely together. It is also absent any kind of crunch, solidity, or acidity, so its richness becomes overwhelming. Try incorporating one or two of these luxuriant elements into your usual eggs Benedict instead.

---

2 whole artichokes, steamed and trimmed down to the hearts

½ cup Creamed Spinach (recipe follows)

2 large eggs, poached

¼ pound thinly sliced Ibérico ham, cut into thin strips

Hollandaise Sauce (recipe follows)

1 small black truffle

Pinch of paprika

Pinch of Kashmiri saffron

Generous spoonful of beluga or osetra caviar

ARRANGE THE artichoke hearts on a warm plate and top each with ¼ cup of the spinach and a poached egg. Mound the ham on top, drizzle with the hollandaise, and shave the entire black truffle over the top. Sprinkle with the paprika and saffron, top each egg with caviar, and serve.

(recipe continues)

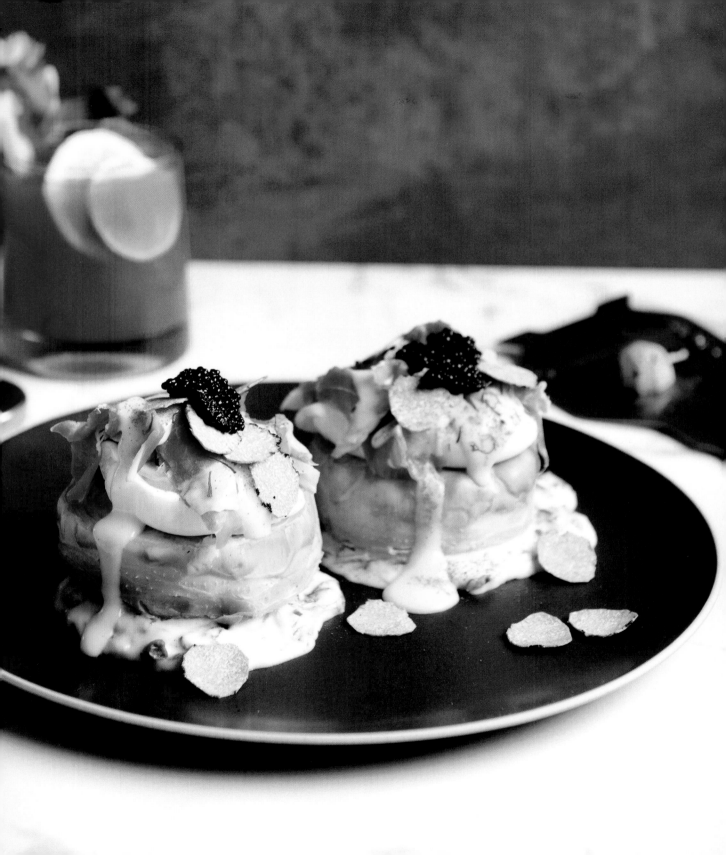

CREAMED SPINACH

MAKES ABOUT 1 CUP

1 tablespoon extra-virgin olive oil
1 cup spinach, rinsed and dried
3 tablespoons unsalted butter
3 tablespoons all-purpose flour
½ cup whole milk
Kosher salt and freshly ground black pepper

IN A large sauté pan, heat the olive oil over medium-high heat until shimmering. Add the spinach and cook, stirring, until bright green and wilted, about 2 minutes. Remove the pan from the heat.

IN A small saucepan, melt the butter over medium-high heat. Once the butter begins to bubble, add the flour and whisk to combine. Cook, stirring, until the raw flour smell dissipates, 30 to 60 seconds. While whisking continuously, add the milk in a steady stream and whisk until completely incorporated. Cook over medium-low heat until the béchamel is thickened, about 3 minutes.

ADD THE béchamel to the spinach and simmer for about 1 minute, until the flavors are incorporated. Season with salt and pepper.

HOLLANDAISE SAUCE

MAKES ABOUT 1 CUP

½ cup (1 stick) unsalted butter
4 large egg yolks
Juice of ½ lemon
Kosher salt

IN A small saucepan, melt the butter over medium heat and heat until it comes to a boil. Remove from the heat but keep hot.

PLACE THE egg yolks and lemon juice in a blender or the cup of an immersion blender. Pulse a few times to combine. With the blender running, slowly stream in the melted butter and blend until a thick sauce forms, about 15 seconds. Transfer the hollandaise to a saucepan, season with salt, cover, and keep warm until ready to serve.

FUN FACT
The first truffle I bought turned out to be fake. I found a truffle dealer in Queens, and being inexperienced with the fancy fungus at the time, overpaid for a virtually flavorless Chinese truffle. Buyer, beware.

BUDDY'S PASTA

SERVES 2

The Jon Favreau saga continues: despite knowing there's no way it could possibly taste good, I had throngs of commenters requesting candy-laden pasta from the veteran filmmaker's Christmas comedy. It presented an excellent opportunity, however, to demonstrate the way to properly sauce pasta. Far too often in life, we just dump sauce on finished pasta and call it a day. We can elevate even simple spaghetti and red sauce, however, by finishing it in the pan—the starch from the cooking water helps the sauce adhere to the pasta, butter and olive oil add richness, and tossing allows the sauce to aerate and emulsify. While I can't in good conscience recommend that you try the recipe below, I do hope that you'll try saucing up your pasta differently and reap the rewards!

VERDICT: Ew.

BUDDY'S VERSION

Kosher salt

½ pound spaghetti

½ cup jarred tomato sauce

Handful of chocolate chips

Handful of M&M's

1 chocolate fudge Pop-Tart, crumbled

Handful of mini marshmallows

Maple syrup, for serving

Caramel sauce, for serving

Chocolate sauce, for serving

BABISH'S VERSION

Kosher salt

½ pound spaghetti

½ cup jarred tomato sauce

Kosher salt and freshly ground black pepper

1 tablespoon unsalted butter

Extra-virgin olive oil, for drizzling

BUDDY'S VERSION

IN A large pot of salted boiling water, cook the spaghetti according to the package directions. Drain.

IN A large sauté pan, heat the tomato sauce over medium-high heat until bubbling, about 1 minute. Toss the pasta with the tomato sauce,

(recipe continues)

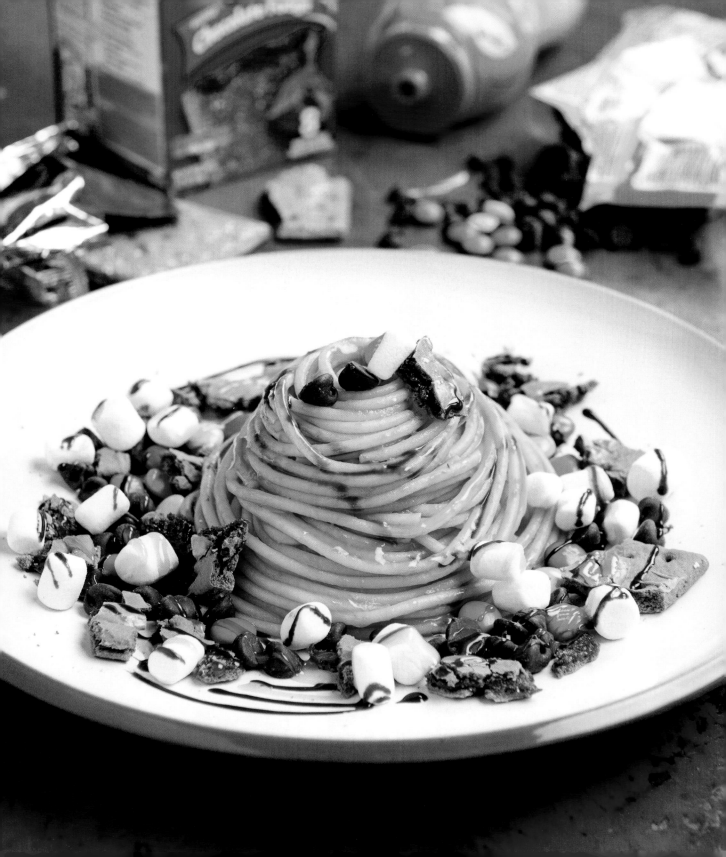

then transfer to a shallow bowl. Top the pasta with the chocolate chips, M&M's, Pop-Tart pieces, and mini marshmallows. Drizzle with maple syrup, caramel sauce, and chocolate sauce, and serve.

BABISH'S VERSION

IN A large pot of salted boiling water, cook the spaghetti for about 1 minute less than the suggested cooking time on the package, or until very al dente.

MEANWHILE, IN a large sauté pan, heat the tomato sauce over medium-high heat until bubbling, about 1 minute.

DRAIN THE pasta, reserving ½ cup of the pasta cooking water, then add both to the sauce. Toss the pasta in the sauce and cook, stirring frequently, for about 1 minute. Season with salt and pepper. Add the butter and a drizzle of olive oil, and toss the pasta high in the pan to aerate and emulsify the sauce. Twirl the spaghetti into a nest with a carving fork, transfer to a shallow bowl, and serve.

FUN FACT

I ended up having to eat this pasta four times: twice for the episode (no memory card in the camera), once for NowThis News, and once for BuzzFeed. Never again.

BIG KAHUNA BURGER

MAKES 1 DOUBLE BURGER

Finally, *Binging with Babish* got its chance to enter the Tarantino Comic Universe. The Big Kahuna Burger, most prominently featured in *Pulp Fiction*, also required the most creative license; the burger in question is clearly a simple fast-food cheeseburger. Happily, this allowed me to show off the smash method, a technique employed by restaurants and diners since the burger's inception. Pressing—nearly smearing—the meat down onto a ripping-hot griddle creates a thin, crispy patty that cooks so quickly, it remains impossibly juicy. But a simple fast-food burger wasn't going to cut it; Big Kahuna Burger being a "Hawaiian burger joint," there wasn't any way I was making this without some pineapple in

it. I am, like many, averse to pineapple used in concert with cheese. I don't judge others for their preferences, but do have my own. I wasn't overjoyed with the end product, but it certainly didn't disgust me as much as I had hypothesized. Then again, you probably could've put a birthday candle in that smashburger, and I still would've eaten it.

VERDICT: The smashburger is an effective, foolproof way to make restaurant-quality burgers at home, all while appeasing friends who might be afraid of "undercooked" meat. Whether to load it up with cheese, teriyaki sauce, and pineapple rings is your choice, and I applaud you for making it.

2 tablespoons unsalted butter

1 red onion, sliced into rings

3 thin pineapple slices

4 ounces ground beef

Kosher salt and freshly ground black pepper

1 tablespoon vegetable oil

2 slices Monterey Jack cheese

1 King's Hawaiian hamburger bun, split sides toasted in butter

1½ teaspoons ketchup

1½ teaspoons teriyaki sauce

IN A sauté pan, melt 1 tablespoon of the butter over medium heat until foaming. Add the onion and cook slowly over low heat, tossing continuously, until soft and caramelized, about 30 minutes. Remove from the heat and transfer the onion to a small bowl. Set aside.

WIPE OUT the pan and melt the remaining 1 tablespoon butter over medium heat until sizzling. Add the pineapple and cook until lightly charred on both sides, about 1 minute per side. Remove from the heat and set aside.

DIVIDE THE ground beef into two equal portions and roll them into balls. Season with salt and pepper. In a large cast-iron skillet, heat the vegetable oil over high heat until smoking. Place the beef balls several inches apart in the skillet and smash each down using a large spatula. Press down firmly on the spatula with a rolling pin or the handle of another spatula until the patties are thin and craggy. Cook until the bottoms are charred and crispy, about 1 minute. Flip and immediately top each patty with a slice of cheese. Remove from the heat but leave the patties in the pan while you assemble the burgers so the cheese can melt completely.

DRESS THE bun with the ketchup and teriyaki sauce, stack the patties on the bottom bun, then add the caramelized onion and pineapple. Close the burger and serve.

FUN FACT

The smoke produced from making these burgers frustrated me to the point of removing my smoke detectors, which I realized months later I had never replaced. Do not do this. Use your exhaust fan judiciously and open a window.

VENICE BEACH FISH TACOS

SERVES 4 TO 6

This recipe was a fun one to track down—though the name of the restaurant at which Peter and Sydney are dining is never mentioned, a little research reveals that it is James' Beach in Venice, California. At the time, I had never even been to LA, much less to James' Beach, so it was a simple matter of reading their menu. I may have also placed a few calls to the restaurant, each time pretending to be someone with a very specific food allergy, so as to find out what was/wasn't in the various accouterments. It's probably the hardest journalism I've ever done. The tacos turned out delicious, and I was delighted to hear Sydney specify that the restaurant makes their tortillas in-house, as I had recently discovered the joys of making one's own tortillas. Cleaner-tasting, tenderer, and all-around better than their store-bought counterparts, homemade tortillas are a revelation on taco night.

VERDICT: This one's a keeper—mahimahi is a relatively simple fish, elevated by complex flavors in the guacamole and salsa verde. Even if you're not in the mood for fish tacos, homemade tortillas are an experience worth having over and over again.

---

2 pounds skin-on mahimahi fillets

Juice of 1 lime

2 teaspoons kosher salt

2 teaspoons freshly ground black pepper

1 tablespoon extra-virgin olive oil, plus more for drizzling

1 teaspoon freshly ground toasted cumin seeds

Homemade Tortillas (recipe follows), warmed

Refried Black Beans (recipe follows)

Pico de Gallo (recipe follows)

Tomatillo Salsa (recipe follows)

Guacamole (recipe follows)

IN A resealable plastic bag, combine the fish fillets, lime juice, salt, pepper, a drizzle of olive oil, and the cumin. Seal the bag and marinate in the refrigerator for 15 minutes to 4 hours. (This is a good time to make the toppings.)

REMOVE THE tortillas that are warming in the oven, wrap them in a clean towel to keep warm, and increase the oven temperature to 350°F.

IN A large ovenproof skillet, heat the olive oil over high heat until shimmering. Sear the marinated fish until lightly browned, about 2 minutes per side. Transfer the pan to the oven and bake for about 30 minutes, or until the internal temperature of the fish registers 135°F. Remove the fish from the oven and transfer to a plate. Remove the skins from the fillets and discard or reserve for another use.

ASSEMBLE TACOS with the tortillas, fish, black beans, pico, salsa, and guacamole, and enjoy.

REFRIED BLACK BEANS

MAKES ABOUT 3 CUPS

16 ounces dried black beans
1 tablespoon vegetable oil
1 medium onion, chopped
1 garlic clove, minced
Kosher salt and freshly ground black pepper

IN A large saucepan, bring 3 cups water to a boil. Remove from the heat, add the beans, and cover. Let soak for about 1½ hours. (This is a good time to make the remaining toppings.)

IN THE same saucepan, bring the beans and soaking liquid to a boil over medium heat.

Reduce the heat to maintain a low simmer and cook for 1 hour, or until the beans are softened. Drain the beans and set aside.

IN A large skillet, heat the vegetable oil over medium-high heat. Add the onion and cook for about 2 minutes. Add the garlic and cook until fragrant. Add the beans and stir to combine. Mash the beans using a large nonslotted spatula. Season with salt and pepper. Remove from the heat and set aside until ready to serve.

PICO DE GALLO

MAKES 2 CUPS

4 tomatoes, cored and diced
½ onion, diced
¼ cup minced fresh cilantro
½ jalapeño, seeded (or keep the seeds in for more heat) and diced
Juice of 1 lime
Kosher salt and freshly ground black pepper

IN A medium bowl, combine the tomatoes, onion, cilantro, jalapeño, and lime juice. Season with salt and pepper. Stir to combine and set aside until ready to serve.

(recipe continues)

TOMATILLO SALSA (SALSA VERDE)

MAKES 2 CUPS

1½ pounds tomatillos (about 10 small), husked, rinsed well, and halved

Extra-virgin olive oil, for drizzling

½ medium onion, diced

¼ cup fresh cilantro leaves, minced

½ jalapeño, seeded if desired, minced

Juice of 1 lime

Kosher salt and freshly ground black pepper

PREHEAT THE broiler. Place a rimmed baking sheet on the top rack of the oven to preheat for about 5 minutes.

IN A large bowl, toss the tomatillos with the olive oil, then carefully arrange them on the preheated baking sheet, cut-sides down. Broil for 5 to 10 minutes, until the skins are blistered and brown. Transfer to a blender and add the onion, cilantro, jalapeño, and lime juice. Blend until still slightly chunky. Season with salt and pepper. Transfer to a bowl and set aside until ready to serve.

GUACAMOLE

MAKES ABOUT 4 CUPS

4 medium avocados

½ jalapeño, seeded (or keep the seeds in for more heat) and minced

¼ Spanish onion, chopped

2 garlic cloves, minced

Juice of ½ lime

2 tablespoons fresh cilantro, chopped

Kosher salt and freshly ground black pepper

Cumin seeds, toasted and ground

HALVE THE avocados and remove the pits. Score the avocado flesh with a butter knife and scoop into a large bowl. Add the jalapeño, onion, garlic, lime juice, and cilantro. Season with salt, pepper, and cumin. Mash with a fork until creamy and scoopable but still chunky.

HOMEMADE TORTILLAS

MAKES TEN 8-INCH TORTILLAS

8½ ounces all-purpose flour (about 1¾ cups), plus more for dusting

1 teaspoon kosher salt

2 tablespoons baking powder

3 tablespoons lard

¾ cup warm water (110°F)

PLACE THE flour, salt, and baking powder in a food processor. Pulse to combine. Add the lard and process until the mixture resembles wet sand. With the machine running, drizzle in the warm water and process until a ball of dough forms. Remove the dough, wrap in plastic wrap, and let rest at room temperature for 30 minutes.

PREHEAT THE oven to 250°F.

HEAT A small skillet over high heat until ripping hot.

GENEROUSLY FLOUR a work surface. Take a golf-ball-size piece of the dough and roll it out to about an 8-inch round. Cook in the hot skillet for about 30 seconds on the first side, until large bubbles form, then flip and cook for 1 minute, until browned. Transfer to a plate and repeat with the remaining dough. Wrap the finished tortillas in aluminum foil and keep warm in the oven.

FUN FACT

I did eventually visit James' Beach, and I'm proud to say that my sight-unseen tacos were a close approximation. Personally, I'm more about Baja fish tacos—while indigenous to Mexico, if you're still in Venice, you can get great ones at Sunny Spot.

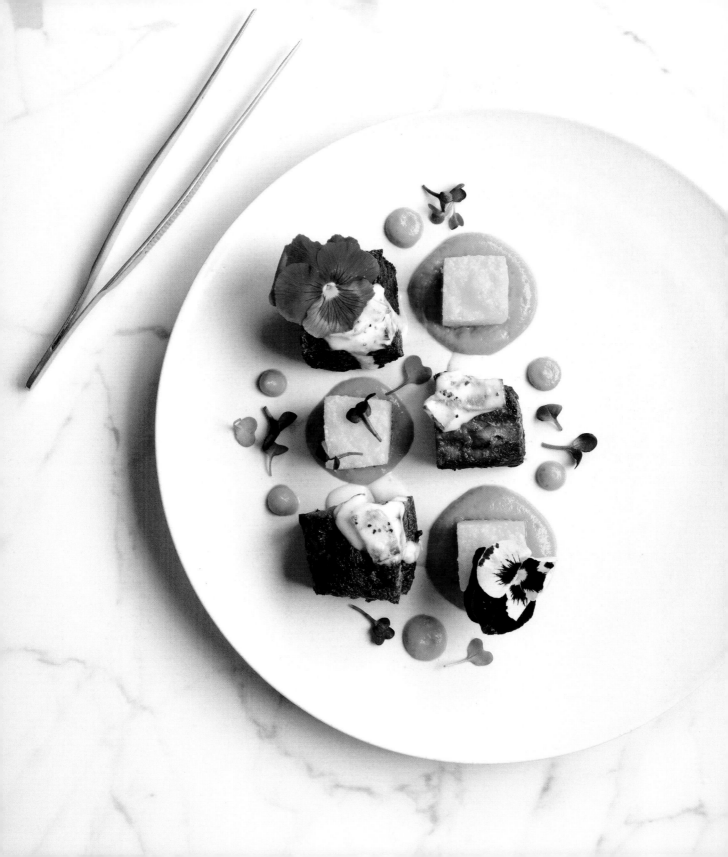

MILK STEAK

SERVES 4

This episode presented what may be, to this day, the biggest culinary challenge faced by the show: how exactly do you make an appetizing dish out of steak cooked in milk? The answer lay in an old Italian technique for braising pork in milk, allowing the milk fats to solidify and separate, resulting in an unappetizing-looking but delicious sauce. This method is rarely used with beef, so when I threw caution to the wind and gave it a try, I was met with mixed results. I decided to puree the decidedly disagreeable cooking liquid into a sauce, which had an equally off-putting yellow color from the oven-browned milk fats. Even though the beef on its own tasted fantastic, I nearly binned the concept altogether, until I dreamt up a new way to incorporate even more milk into the dish: gravy. The salty bacon gravy cut through the rich, herbaceous beef, the rosemary–pea shoot "gel" provided a bright, fresh contrast, and the fried Parmesan polenta cubes were the proverbial cherry on top. It's definitely the biggest leap taken in the show's history, and probably one of the dishes I'm proudest of—even if the plating needs some work.

VERDICT: This dish is a means to an end—a desperate ploy to get beef and milk to play nice together. It's philosophically difficult to recommend actually attempting it at home, in that it's an overcomplicated stunt, albeit a tasty one.

½ pound bacon, chopped

2 boneless short ribs, cut into 2-inch pieces

2¾ cups whole milk

1 small bunch fresh sage leaves

1 sprig fresh rosemary

1 carrot, chopped into 4 pieces

2 garlic cloves

1 tablespoon all-purpose flour

Kosher salt and freshly ground black pepper

Parmesan Polenta Cubes (recipe follows)

Extra-virgin olive oil, for drizzling

1 tablespoon freshly grated Parmesan cheese

Rosemary–Pea Shoot "Gel" (recipe follows)

Mustard microgreens, for garnish

Edible flowers, for garnish (optional)

(recipe continues)

PREHEAT THE oven to 350°F.

IN A large ovenproof skillet, combine the bacon and ¼ cup water and bring to a simmer over medium heat. Simmer the bacon until the water has evaporated and all the fat has rendered from the bacon, about 7 minutes. Drain the bacon on paper towels and pour off all but 2 tablespoons of the fat from the skillet into a heatproof container. Set the bacon and excess fat aside for the gravy.

HEAT THE skillet over medium-high heat until smoking. Add the short ribs and sear until browned all over, about 3 minutes per side. Reduce the heat and add 2 cups of the milk, stirring and scraping up all the browned bits from the bottom of the pan. Add the sage, rosemary, carrot, and garlic, nestling them between the short ribs. Partially cover the pot and transfer to the oven. Braise for about 2 hours, until the short ribs are butter-knife tender.

MEANWHILE, IN a small saucepan, heat 2 tablespoons of the reserved bacon fat over medium heat until shimmering. Add the flour and cook, whisking continuously, until the raw flour smell has dissipated. While whisking continuously, slowly stream in the remaining ¾ cup milk and whisk until completely incorporated. Add the bacon and cook for 5 to 10 minutes, until the gravy has thickened. Taste and season with salt and pepper, if necessary. Remove from the heat and keep the gravy warm until ready to serve.

REMOVE THE short ribs from the oven, transfer to a plate, and let cool slightly.

MEANWHILE, INCREASE the oven temperature to 400°F. Line a baking sheet with aluminum foil.

ARRANGE THE polenta cubes on the lined baking sheet and drizzle on all sides with olive oil. Top with the Parmesan and bake for 15 to 20 minutes, flipping as necessary, until crisp.

USING A very sharp knife, trim the beef into perfect 1½-inch cubes. For each serving, decorate the plate as desired with rosemary–pea shoot "gel." Arrange the short ribs and polenta cubes on top. Dollop each beef cube with gravy, garnish with microgreens and edible flowers, if desired, and serve.

PARMESAN POLENTA CUBES
MAKES ABOUT TWELVE 1-INCH CUBES

Neutral vegetable oil, for greasing
1 tablespoon kosher salt, plus more as needed
½ cup coarse polenta
½ cup freshly grated Parmesan cheese

GREASE A 9-inch square baking dish with vegetable oil.

IN A medium saucepan, combine 2 cups water and the salt and bring to a rolling boil over high heat. While whisking, slowly stream in the polenta and whisk continuously until thickened, about 2 minutes. Reduce the heat to low, cover, and cook for about 30 minutes, until the polenta is creamy and tender. Stir in the Parmesan. Taste and season with salt, if necessary. Pour the polenta into the prepared baking dish. Cover and refrigerate for at least 2 hours, or until completely firm.

UNMOLD FROM the baking dish, cut into 1-inch cubes, and set aside until ready to use.

ROSEMARY– PEA SHOOT "GEL"

MAKES ½ CUP

4 ounces fresh peas

1 ounce fresh pea shoots

Leaves from 1 sprig fresh rosemary, finely chopped

COMBINE THE peas, pea shoots, and rosemary in a high-powered blender and blend on high speed until completely smooth, adding water if necessary. Transfer to a squeeze bottle, if desired, and refrigerate until ready to serve. Return to room temperature before serving.

FUN FACT
Nearly five hours were spent trying to source edible flowers for the Babish-version milk steak. I scoured every gourmet grocery I could find, only to end up spotting them at a relatively ratty supermarket here in the city.

JAKE'S PERFECT SANDWICH

MAKES 1 SANDWICH, LARGE ENOUGH TO SERVE 4

Jake the Dog channels the realm of creation above him to build the sandwich of his dreams, a towering mishmash of meat and condiments that would make Rodney Dangerfield proud. This sandwich had been hotly requested by commenters for some time, and with a large new audience, that voice was being heard louder than ever. But how to tackle such cartoonish concepts as "lobster soul" and "bird from the window"? Lobster soul felt, to me, like an "essence" of the pricey crustacean, so I opted for an aioli imbued with lobster flavor. Bird from the window was just that: a songbird snatched from its perch, transformed instantaneously into an amorphous blob of

meat. The closest equivalent I could conjure up was a whole boneless Cornish game hen, a mild enough piece of poultry that I could at least mimic in form. The rest was pretty well spelled out for me—leave it to *Adventure Time* to incorporate sous vide into a gag.

VERDICT: The so-called "perfect sandwich" is pretty far from that—for starters, unless you're a shape-shifting cartoon dog, it's not physically possible to take a bite of. The flavors are a bit confused, but not offensive. Lose the "bird" and the cucumbers, slice up the steak into manageable/chewable pieces, and you might have yourself a pretty perfect sandwich.

---

1 boneless rib eye steak, roughly the size of your bread (about 1½ pounds)

2 sprigs fresh thyme

2 sprigs fresh rosemary

1½ teaspoons kosher salt

1 teaspoon freshly ground black pepper

1 lobster tail

1 cup vegetable oil

Juice of 1 lemon

3 large egg yolks

1 Cornish game hen, deboned, or 2 boneless chicken thighs

6 slices bacon, cooked and fat reserved

1 large, long sourdough loaf, halved lengthwise

3 tablespoons cream cheese

3 tablespoons fresh dill leaves

1 dill pickle, thinly sliced

1 hard-boiled large egg, sliced

10 thin slices cucumber

1 Vidalia onion, 3 thin rounds sliced off and the rest reserved for inducing tears

8 thin slices plum tomato

2 teaspoons human tears

(recipe continues)

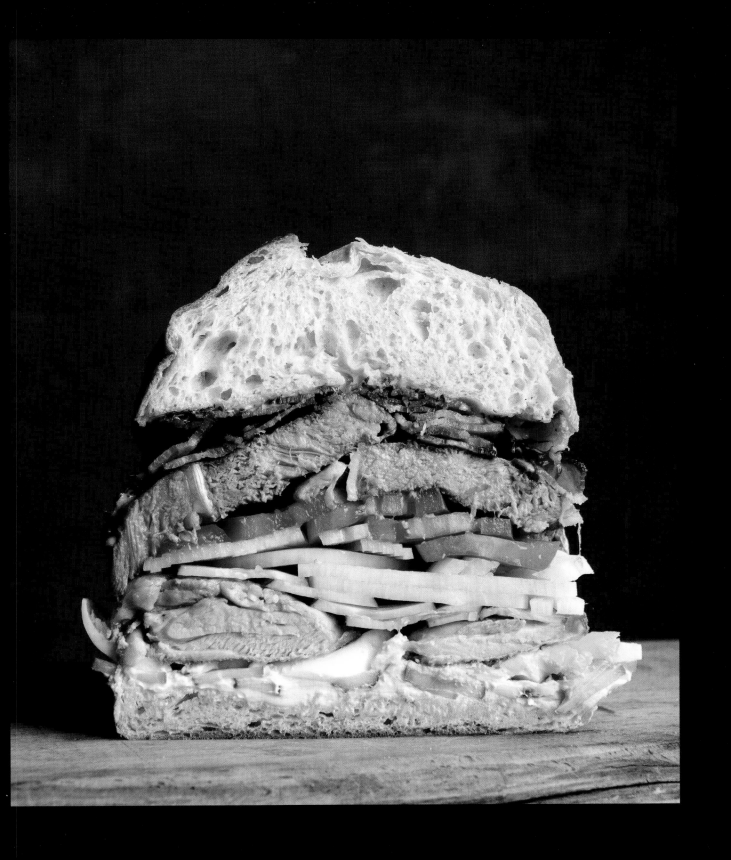

IN A sous vide bag, combine the rib eye, thyme, rosemary, 1 teaspoon of the salt, and the pepper. Vacuum seal and submerge in a sous vide bath set at 135°F for 2 hours. Remove from the bath and set aside.

PREHEAT THE oven to 350°F.

IN A large pot fitted with a steamer insert, bring about 1 inch of water to a simmer over medium-high heat. Place the lobster tail in the steamer. Cover, reduce the heat, and steam for about 8 minutes, or until completely cooked. Remove from the heat. When the lobster is cool enough to handle, remove the meat from the tail and reserve for another use (or add it to this sandwich, if desired). Break the shell into pieces and transfer to a high-powered blender. Add the vegetable oil and blend until the shell is finely ground, 30 to 60 seconds. Pour the lobster oil into a small saucepan and bring to a simmer. Simmer until the oil is reddish and fragrant, about 15 minutes, then strain through a fine-mesh sieve; discard the solids. Set the lobster oil aside to cool completely.

IN THE cup of an immersion blender (or in a food processor or standing blender), combine the lemon juice and egg yolks. Blend briefly to combine. With the blender running, slowly pour the lobster oil down the side of the cup and blend until the mixture is thick and emulsified. Refrigerate the lobster aioli until ready to use.

HEAT A cast-iron skillet over medium-high heat until shimmering. Brush the Cornish game hen with some reserved bacon fat, season with the remaining ½ teaspoon salt, and place skin-side down in the skillet. Cook until golden, about 3 minutes. Flip, then transfer the skillet to the oven and bake until the internal temperature registers 165°F, about 10 minutes. Remove from the oven.

TO ASSEMBLE the sandwich, torch the cut sides of the bread with a culinary torch (only for accuracy—I recommend toasting the bread in the oven or under the broiler instead). Spread the cream cheese on both cut sides of the bread. Sprinkle the dill on the top half of the bread, then slather with some of the lobster aioli. On the bottom half, shingle the slices of pickle and egg. Top with the Cornish game hen, cucumber, onion, tomato, and steak. Use the remaining onion to make yourself cry, then drizzle the tears over the steak. Top with the bacon.

CLOSE THE sandwich, cut in half, and serve.

FUN FACT

This was the first episode to change up the show's intro from the (copyrighted) *Frasier* theme song to the floating-clip-camera-move now featured in every episode. It was also the first episode to be monetized, so it set in motion the wheels that allowed me to eventually make *Binging with Babish* my full-time job.

CUBANO SANDWICHES

MAKES 4 SANDWICHES, WITH ENOUGH LEFTOVER PORK TO SERVE AN ADDITIONAL 4 TO 6

Few food stories are quite so mouth-watering as Jon Favreau's love-letter scene to the Cubano sandwich in *Chef*. Life lessons are handed out alongside the slow-roasted pork as Chef Carl Casper teaches his son a few things about respect, food, and the love that binds them both together. From John Leguizamo's marination dance, to the camera staring longingly at the first Cubano being pressed to melty completion to Carl's rant about the passion for food he wants to share with his son, it's nothing short of a few minutes of perfect culinary cinema. There's a reason you want to cook after watching *Chef* (beyond its ability to make you hungry): it enlivens you to use food as a means by which to grow closer to those around you. Food is one of the few universal languages, a shared experience by which we can all become closer, and it deserves to be done right. I guess that's two sandwiches in this book with turmoil and personal growth lying in wait just under their cheesy surfaces (see: *Philly Cheesesteak Sandwiches, page 35*).

VERDICT: As far as sandwiches go, this one is pretty much as good as it gets. The flavor of the pork is astounding, only complemented by the cured flavor of the ham, the tang of the pickles and mustard, and the richness of the cheese. Cuban-style bread is essential for a genuine experience, but if you can't find it, just use the lightest, softest, squishiest submarine roll you can find.

1 loaf Cubano bread

4 tablespoons (½ stick) unsalted butter, at room temperature

2 tablespoons vegetable oil

12 slices Roast Pork (recipe follows)

8 thick slices deli ham

12 slices Swiss cheese

Dill pickles, thinly sliced

¼ cup Dijon mustard

(recipe continues)

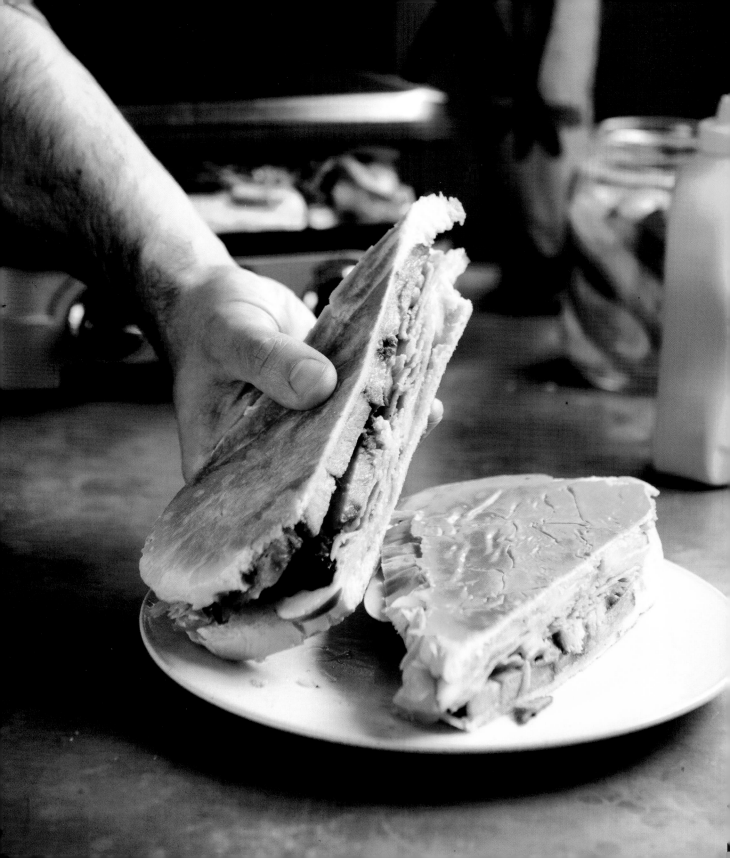

HEAT A plancha or a panini press with flat plates. Split the bread lengthwise, then quarter it crosswise to create the bread for 4 sandwiches. Butter the split sides with 2 tablespoons of the butter and toast butter-side down on the hot plancha (or in the panini press with flat plates). Set aside; leave the plancha on.

IN A large nonstick skillet, heat 1 tablespoon of the vegetable oil over medium-high heat. Working in batches to avoid overlapping, sear half the pork and half the ham on both sides. Transfer to a plate. Repeat with the remaining oil, pork, and ham.

FOR EACH sandwich, on the bottom halves of the bread pile on 3 slices of the pork, 2 slices of the ham, 3 slices of the cheese, and a few pickle slices. Spread the top halves with mustard, then smear the remaining butter on the outside of the bread. Close the sandwiches and press each one on the plancha (or in the panini press) for 2 to 3 minutes, until the bread is deeply browned and the cheese has melted. Cut the Cubanos in half on an angle and serve.

ROAST PORK

MAKES ABOUT 4 POUNDS

1 large bone-in pork shoulder (about 5 pounds)

4 cups orange juice

½ cup rice vinegar

½ cup spiced rum

½ cup kosher salt

¼ cup packed dark brown sugar

4 garlic cloves, minced

2 sprigs fresh oregano, coarsely chopped

2 sprigs fresh rosemary, coarsely chopped

2 sprigs fresh thyme, coarsely chopped

2 sprigs fresh sage, coarsely chopped

3 bay leaves

MOJO MARINADE

½ cup extra-virgin olive oil

Zest and juice of 3 oranges

Zest and juice of 6 limes, juiced rinds reserved

½ cup chopped fresh cilantro

¼ cup chopped fresh mint leaves

2 sprigs fresh oregano, coarsely chopped

4 garlic cloves, minced

2 tablespoons freshly ground toasted cumin seeds

1 tablespoon kosher salt

1 tablespoon freshly ground black pepper

USING A very sharp knife, remove any excess fat from the pork shoulder and score the fat cap on top at 1-inch intervals. In a large stainless-steel bowl, whisk together the orange juice,

(recipe continues)

2 cups water, the vinegar, rum, salt, brown sugar, garlic, oregano, rosemary, thyme, sage, and bay leaves. Transfer the pork shoulder to the bowl and submerge in the brine. Cover and refrigerate for 12 to 24 hours.

DRAIN THE pork shoulder and return it to the bowl.

WHISK TOGETHER all the ingredients for the marinade in a medium bowl. Pour the marinade over the pork shoulder and massage it into the meat for 1 minute. Cover the bowl and refrigerate for 2 hours.

PREHEAT THE oven to 350°F. Set a wire rack on a rimmed baking sheet.

SET THE pork on the rack and reserve the marinade in the bowl. Pick off and discard any large pieces of herbs from the pork. Brush the pork with the marinade and roast for 2½ hours, until the internal temperature registers 165°F at the thickest part of the pork shoulder. Remove from the oven and tent the roast with aluminum foil. Let rest for 30 minutes or refrigerate until ready to assemble the sandwiches. Slice some of the roast pork about ¼ inch thick and reserve the rest for another use. (It can be refrigerated for up to 3 days.)

FUN FACT
Jon Favreau tweeted the video with the single caption "Empingao," a phrase used by his and Leguizamo's characters to describe the sandwich. It's Cuban slang for "next level," "amazing," or "awesome."

RAMEN

**MAKES ENOUGH NOODLES TO SERVE 4,
PLUS ENOUGH BROTH, PORK, AND TARE TO SERVE 12 OR MORE**

They call it a "ramen western" for a reason: *Tampopo* has all the melodrama and stilted action of a spaghetti western, yet is not only set in Japan, its plot revolves around the very noodle itself. Ramen is a complex dish with a storied past, endless variations, and utter proliferation in its originating country. Happily, during the scene in question, we are treated to some insight into a very specific type of ramen, and are taught by a "ramen master" to appreciate it for all its subtleties. In what is presumably a shoyu-style (soy sauce–based chicken broth) ramen, we see the "jewels

of fat glittering on the surface . . . seaweed slowly sinking . . . spring onions floating . . ." and perhaps gain a new level of respect for the time and expertise that goes into every bowl of this storied soup.

VERDICT: Real ramen is a labor-intensive endeavor, and getting it truly "right" may take a lifetime. But like most challenging dishes, it's exciting to see your efforts come to fruition in a complex and satisfying way. If you've got the time and energy, this is more than worth trying at least once.

Ramen Broth (recipe follows)

Tare (recipe follows)

Ramen Noodles (recipe follows), or 1 pound store-bought fresh ramen noodles (available in the refrigerated section at Asian markets)

Chashu Pork (recipe follows), thinly sliced

Kamaboko (Japanese fish cake, sliced; available at Asian markets), for serving

Chopped scallions, for serving

Menma (braised bamboo shoots; available at Asian markets), for serving

1 sheet nori (dried seaweed), cut into 2 x 4-inch rectangles

Sesame oil, for serving

TRANSFER THE chilled broth to a large pot and bring to a rolling boil over high heat. Meanwhile, bring a large pot of water to a boil over high heat for the noodles.

FOR EACH serving, pour 1 to 2 tablespoons of the tare into a bowl suitable for ramen.

(recipe continues)

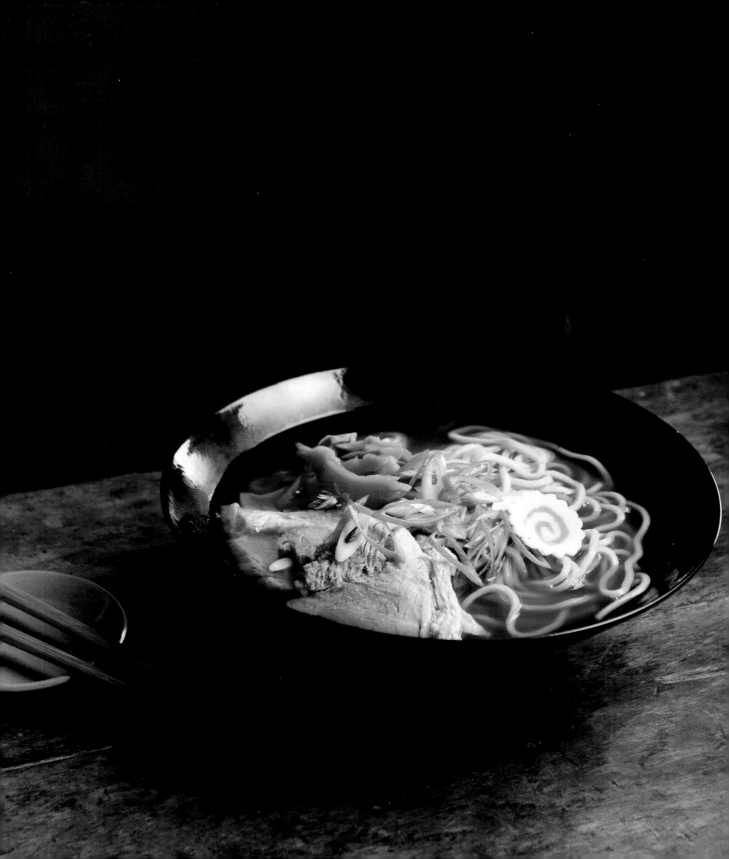

FOR EACH serving, cook 8 ounces of the noodles in the boiling water for no more than 30 seconds. Drain well and transfer to the serving bowl. Arrange a few slices of the pork on the side of the noodles. Add a few slices of kamaboko, some scallions, menma, and 1 rectangle of nori. Ladle in enough boiling broth to barely cover the noodles, drizzle with sesame oil, and serve, being sure to slurp.

RAMEN BROTH

MAKES ABOUT 3 QUARTS

NOTE: *Requires 24 hours soaking time plus overnight chilling.*

4 (5 x 8-inch) pieces kombu (dried kelp; available at Asian markets)

2 pounds chicken wings

1 pound chicken feet, nails cut off

¼ pound pork spareribs

1 whole head garlic, halved crosswise

1 large scallion, cut into 6-inch pieces

1 whole onion, halved

1 cup bonito flakes (smoked dried tuna; available at Asian markets)

1 cup dried anchovies (available at Asian markets)

IN A large stockpot, soak the kombu in 4 quarts water for 24 hours. Remove and discard the kombu.

ADD THE chicken wings, chicken feet, ribs, garlic, scallion, and onion. Bring to a bare simmer over low heat and cook for 4 hours, keeping the broth below 200°F. Skim off any foam that rises to the surface as necessary. Add the bonito and dried anchovies and simmer for 1 hour more. Strain the broth, discarding the solids, and let cool. Cover and refrigerate overnight before using.

RAMEN NOODLES

MAKES ABOUT 1 POUND

½ cup baking soda

8½ ounces bread flour (about 2 cups)

1 ounce vital wheat gluten (about ¼ cup; available at health food stores and online)

½ cup warm water

Cornstarch, for dusting

PREHEAT THE oven to 225°F. Line a rimmed baking sheet with aluminum foil.

SPREAD THE baking soda over the foil. Bake for about 1 hour. Remove from the oven and let cool, taking care to avoid contact with skin until the baking soda is mixed into the dough, as it may cause irritation.

IN A large bowl, combine the bread flour and vital wheat gluten. Dissolve 1 tablespoon of the baked baking soda in the warm water, then pour the mixture into the bowl. Stir to combine until a dough forms. (Let the remaining baked baking soda cool and store in an airtight container for another use.) Turn the dough out onto a work surface and knead for about 5 minutes. Wrap the dough in plastic wrap and let rest for 1 hour.

(recipe continues)

LINE A baking sheet with parchment paper. Roll the dough out, then run it through successively narrower settings on a pasta machine until it can fit into the pasta cutter. Run the dough through the spaghetti cutting attachment and then toss the noodles with some cornstarch. Transfer the noodles to the lined baking sheet, cover with plastic wrap, and refrigerate overnight before using.

CHASHU PORK AND TARE

MAKES ABOUT 3 POUNDS OF CHASHU AND 2½ CUPS OF TARE

PORK

3 pounds pork belly and/or boneless pork shoulder

1 tablespoon vegetable oil (optional)

1 cup mirin

1 cup sake

½ cup soy sauce

1 whole shallot, halved

1 (2-inch) knob fresh ginger, peeled and chopped

6 garlic cloves, crushed

TARE

1 tablespoon vegetable oil (optional)

½ cup dried anchovies

2 cups soy sauce

1 (5 x 8-inch) piece kombu (dried kelp; available at Asian markets)

½ cup bonito flakes (smoked dried tuna; available at Asian markets)

¼ cup sake

¼ cup mirin

1 tablespoon brown sugar

PORK

PREHEAT THE oven to 275°F.

PLACE THE pork belly in a large baking dish.

IF USING pork shoulder, in a large skillet, heat the vegetable oil over high heat until shimmering. Add the pork shoulder and sear until well browned on all sides, about 2 minutes per side.

TRANSFER THE pork shoulder to the baking dish with the pork belly. Set the skillet aside to use for the tare; do not rinse it.

IN A medium bowl, whisk together the mirin, sake, soy sauce, shallot, ginger, and garlic. Pour into the baking dish and cover partially with a lid or aluminum foil. Braise in the oven for about 3 hours, or until the pork is tender.

TARE

MEANWHILE, HEAT the skillet you used to sear the pork shoulder over medium heat until the remaining fat and browned bits in the pan sizzle. (If you didn't use pork shoulder, heat the vegetable oil over medium heat until shimmering.) Add the dried anchovies and cook, stirring, until very fragrant, about 2 minutes. Add the soy sauce and stir, scraping up all the browned bits from the bottom of the skillet. Break the kombu into pieces and add them to the skillet. Reduce the heat and simmer for about 10 minutes.

ADD THE bonito and remove the skillet from the heat. Cover and let steep for 5 minutes. Strain the liquid into a heatproof measuring cup and set aside.

WIPE OUT the skillet and place it over medium heat. Add the sake, mirin, and brown sugar and stir to combine. Bring to a boil to cook off the alcohol. Return the soy sauce mixture to the pan and stir to combine. Remove the tare from the heat and set aside until ready to use.

REMOVE THE pork from the oven and let cool, then refrigerate for at least 3 hours to firm up the pork before using.

FUN FACT

I burnt the shit out of my hands on the baked baking soda. Don't touch it after it comes out of the oven!

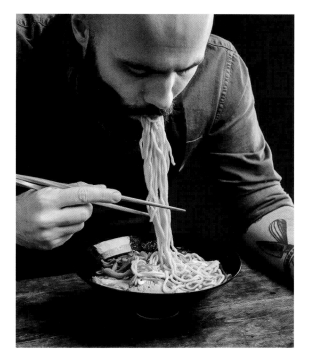

MR. AND MRS. TENORMAN CHILI

SERVES 10 TO 12

South Park's dalliances with food might be best remembered when Randy became borderline sexually obsessed with his frittata, but it's far from the first time the series has focused on cuisine. Chef's Chocolate Salty Balls were one of the gags that helped put the show on the map, and the episode featuring Scott Tenorman's Parent's Chili is considered by many to be the greatest episode of all time. The former was easiest to create, as Randy's put-on sophistication prompted him to list all the artisanal ingredients gracing his frittata, but the latter presented other challenges. Chef might have sung the precise recipe for his balls, but the actualization of that recipe turned out boozy and sickly sweet. Then there's the matter of the key ingredient in Cartman's chili . . . best approximated with pork, the meat largely agreed upon as that most closely resembling human flesh.

VERDICT: The combination of "pork" and chorizo make this a flavorful, spicy, bold chili, and a nice variation on the usual ground beef.

---

3 ounces cascabel chiles, stemmed, seeded, and cut into 1-inch pieces

3 ounces guajillo chiles, stemmed, seeded, and cut into 1-inch pieces

3 ounces ancho chiles, stemmed, seeded, and cut into 1-inch pieces

3 cups chicken stock

½ cup cornmeal

1 tablespoon dried oregano

2 tablespoons unsweetened cocoa powder

1 tablespoon ground cumin

1 pound fresh (Mexican) chorizo, casings removed

4 pounds boneless pork shoulder, trimmed and cut into 1-inch pieces

1 habanero pepper, seeded, deveined, and finely chopped

1 jalapeño, seeded if desired, finely chopped

1 onion, chopped

1 garlic clove, minced

1 (12-ounce) bottle Mexican beer

Two (14-ounce) cans chopped tomatoes, with their juices

Kosher salt and freshly ground black pepper

Cheddar cheese, shredded, for serving

Chopped fresh chives, for serving

IN A dry skillet, toast the chiles over medium-high heat until smoking slightly and fragrant, about 3 minutes. While the pan is still hot, add 1½ cups of the stock and bring to a bare simmer. Cover, remove from the heat, and let steep for about 30 minutes.

TRANSFER THE mixture to a food processor and pulse a few times. Add the cornmeal, oregano, cocoa powder, and cumin. Process until smooth, about 2 minutes. Set the spice paste aside.

HEAT A large heavy pot over medium-high heat. Add the chorizo and cook, breaking it up into small pieces as it cooks, until browned and all the fat has rendered out, about 5 minutes. Transfer the chorizo to a plate. Add the pork shoulder to the pan and cook it in the chorizo fat, stirring, until browned all over, about 5 minutes. Transfer the pork shoulder to the plate with the chorizo. Add the habanero, jalapeño, onion, and garlic to the pot and cook, stirring, until softened, about 3 minutes. Add the

beer and cook, stirring and scraping up all the browned bits from the bottom of the pot. Add the spice paste, the remaining 1½ cups stock, and the tomatoes and their juices. Return the chorizo and pork to the pot. Stir, reduce the heat to low, cover the pot with the lid ajar, and simmer for 3 to 4 hours, until the meat is fully cooked and the chili has thickened. Season with salt and pepper. Ladle into bowls, top with cheddar cheese and chives, and serve.

FUN FACT

If you look closely in the video, when I'm scraping up curls of chocolate for use as the surrogate ball hair, you can see that I'm accidentally shaving up bits of metal from the pan. Yeah, don't do that.

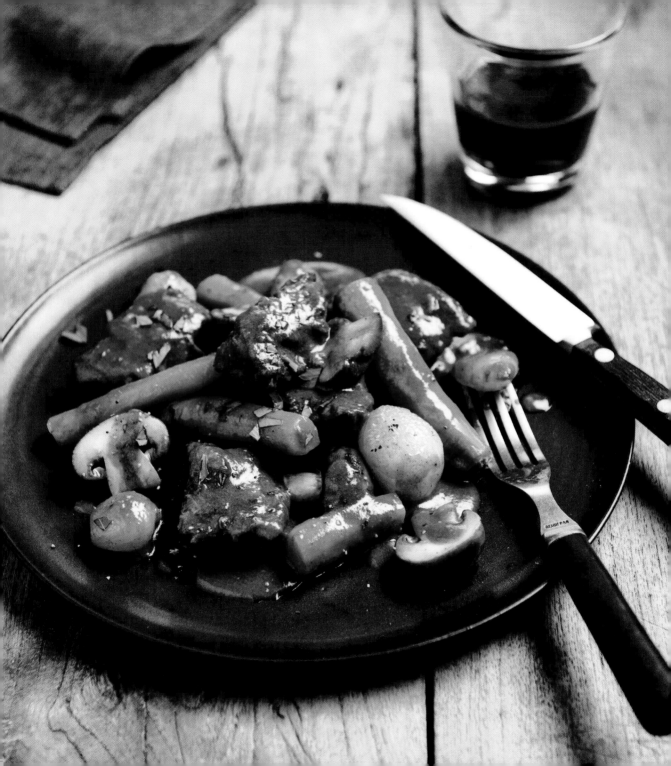

BEEF BURGUNDY

SERVES 6

Julie Powell issued herself an interesting challenge: cook every dish from Julia Child's *Mastering the Art of French Cooking* in one year. Her blog was a hit, her book was a success, the movie based on her life was a delight—and, gracefully, they included boeuf bourguignon in the film. Folks, this is my all-time favorite dish. It's what I'd choose for my last meal. It's what I've served to anyone I've ever cared deeply for. It is, I think, one of the greatest all-inclusive cooking lessons: you learn chopping, light butchery, searing, deglazing, braising, seasoning, and more. You learn how flavors develop over time. You learn how to take the bright, the harsh, the tough, and mellow each of them into something harmonious and beautiful. It's also an important part of food history: it was the very first dish cooked by Julia on the very first episode of her groundbreaking TV cooking show, *The French Chef*, a show that would define cooking shows as we know them today. It is pure cooking, and you owe it to yourself and those you care about to whip up a batch.

VERDICT: Beef Burgundy is a rich, comforting, relatively easy French classic, and Julia Child's version is its epitome. There are easier ways, faster ways, even arguably better ways to do it—but sometimes, there isn't anything quite like the genuine article.

3 pounds chuck roast, cut into 2-inch cubes

Kosher salt and freshly ground black pepper

6 slices thick-cut bacon, chopped

2 tablespoons vegetable oil

1 onion, sliced

4 or 5 carrots, chopped

3 cups red Burgundy wine

¼ cup all-purpose flour

2 cups beef stock, plus more as needed

3 garlic cloves, minced

1 tablespoon plus 1 teaspoon chopped fresh thyme leaves

1 bay leaf

2 tablespoons tomato paste

1 pound pearl onions, unpeeled

Boiling water, as needed

2 tablespoons unsalted butter

8 ounces cremini mushrooms, halved

Chopped fresh parsley, for garnish

(recipe continues)

SEASON THE beef with salt and pepper; set aside.

IN A large saucepan, bring 1½ quarts water to a simmer. Add the bacon and cook for 10 minutes. Drain and set aside to dry.

PREHEAT THE oven to 400°F.

IN A large skillet, heat 1 tablespoon of the oil over medium heat. Add the bacon and cook for 3 minutes, until browned and all the fat has rendered out. Transfer the bacon to a paper towel–lined plate, reserving the fat in the skillet.

ADD THE beef to the skillet—in batches, if necessary, to avoid crowding the pan. Cook until deeply browned on all sides, about 5 minutes, then transfer to a paper towel–lined plate.

ADD THE onion and carrots to the skillet. Cook in the remaining fat, stirring, until softened, 3 minutes. Transfer to a bowl and set aside. Add the wine to the skillet, stirring and scraping up all the browned bits from the bottom of the pan. Remove from the heat and set aside.

TRANSFER THE beef to a Dutch oven and toss with the flour. Bake for about 10 minutes, or until the flour is toasted. Remove from the oven, flip the beef, and bake for 10 minutes more.

REDUCE THE oven temperature to 325°F. Add the sliced onion, carrots, bacon, the wine from deglazing the skillet, and enough stock to barely cover the beef and vegetables in the Dutch oven (about 1 cup). Add the garlic, 1 tablespoon of the thyme, the bay leaf, and the tomato paste. Stir well to incorporate. Return to the oven and braise, stirring occasionally, for about 3 hours, or until the beef is very tender.

MEANWHILE, PLACE the pearl onions in a heatproof bowl. Fill a bowl with ice and water. Cover the onions with boiling water and let soak for 10 minutes. Using a slotted spoon, transfer the onions to the ice bath to stop the cooking, then drain. Pinch each onion at the stem to slip off the skin or peel with a paring knife.

IN A large skillet, heat the remaining 1 tablespoon oil over medium-high heat. Add the pearl onions and cook, tossing, until browned, 4 minutes. Add 1 cup of the stock, stirring and scraping up the browned bits from the bottom of the pan. Cover the skillet and simmer over low heat for 45 minutes, or until the onions are soft but still retain their shape.

IN ANOTHER skillet, melt the butter over high heat. Add the mushrooms and cook, tossing frequently, for about 5 minutes, or until the mushrooms have released most of their liquid. Add the remaining 1 teaspoon thyme and season with salt and pepper. Cook, stirring, for 10 minutes. Remove from the heat and set aside.

REMOVE THE Dutch oven from the oven. Transfer the beef to a plate and set aside. Strain the braising liquid into a large saucepan. Reserve the vegetables and discard the bay leaf. Over medium-high heat, reduce the liquid until thick enough to coat the back of a spoon, 10 minutes.

FOR EACH serving, place a few pieces of beef on a plate. Add a couple of carrots, a healthy pile of the sliced onions, and a little pile each of mushrooms and pearl onions. Top with extra sauce and garnish with parsley.

HOMER SIMPSON'S PATENTED SPACE-AGE OUT-OF-THIS-WORLD MOON WAFFLES

SERVES 4

The Simpsons changed television as we know it with its bold, surreal, and often daring comedy. Homer's Patented Space-Age Out-of-This-World Moon Waffles are a breakfast only the man himself could have dreamed up: caramels fried into waffle batter, wrapped around a stick of butter, impaled on a skewer, and consumed. Five tests and three waffle makers later, it was proven to be impossible outside the cartoon world. Caramel burns far more quickly than waffle batter cooks, and even if it didn't, there isn't a nonstick surface in the world slippery enough to repel the molten sugar-lava. Waffles with caramel sauce and brown butter? That sounds much more feasible (and delicious), while still staying true to Homer's original formula.

VERDICT: Homer's waffle is inedible. The Babish deconstruction is sweet, salty, and delicious—be sure not to skimp on the brown butter! As a matter of fact, keep chilled brown butter in your fridge (it'll keep for 1 to 2 weeks) or freezer (up to 3 months) at all times—you never know when it might come in handy.

½ cup (1 stick) unsalted butter

1 cup sugar

1 cup heavy cream

½ teaspoon pure vanilla extract (optional)

1¾ cups all-purpose flour

1 tablespoon cornmeal

1 teaspoon baking powder

1 teaspoon kosher salt

2 large eggs, separated

1¾ cups buttermilk

Nonstick cooking spray

Smoked sea salt

(recipe continues)

IN A small saucepan, melt the butter over medium-low heat. Swirl and shake the pan continuously until the milk fats begin to brown. You should see some little brown particles in the butter. Measure out ¼ cup of the brown butter and set aside for the batter. Pour the rest of the brown butter into a ramekin and reserve for serving. (The butter will solidify as it cools.)

IN A large saucepan, bring ½ cup water and the sugar to a boil over medium-high heat. Stir gently, making sure the sugar doesn't stick to the sides of the pan. Pour yourself a glass of Scotch for reference—that's the caramel color you're aiming for—and bring the mixture to 350°F. Meanwhile, in a small saucepan, heat the cream to almost boiling. Very carefully pour the cream into the sugar mixture, ¼ cup at a time—the caramel will bubble up and double in size. Whisk over low heat and add the vanilla, if desired. Remove from the heat, transfer to a heatproof bowl, and set aside to cool and thicken.

IN A medium bowl, whisk together the flour, cornmeal, baking powder, and salt until well combined. In another medium bowl, whisk together the egg yolks, buttermilk, and the reserved ¼ cup brown butter until well combined. Add the wet ingredients to the dry ingredients and whisk gently to combine.

IN A separate medium bowl, using a handheld mixer, whip the egg whites on medium-high speed until they hold stiff peaks. Carefully fold the egg whites into the batter until fully incorporated; do not overmix.

HEAT AN 8-inch round waffle iron and generously spray with cooking spray. Pour about ¾ cup of the batter into the waffle iron and spread it evenly. Cook according to the manufacturer's instructions until golden brown.

SLICE THE waffle into quarters and arrange it decoratively on a plate to impress any brunch guests (or just yourself). Hit it with a dollop of the reserved brown butter, a generous drizzle of the caramel sauce, and a sprinkle of smoked sea salt, then serve. Repeat with the remaining batter, brown butter, caramel, and smoked salt.

FUN FACT

I really did go through three waffle makers to film this episode. The guy at the hardware store where I bought them was very confused.

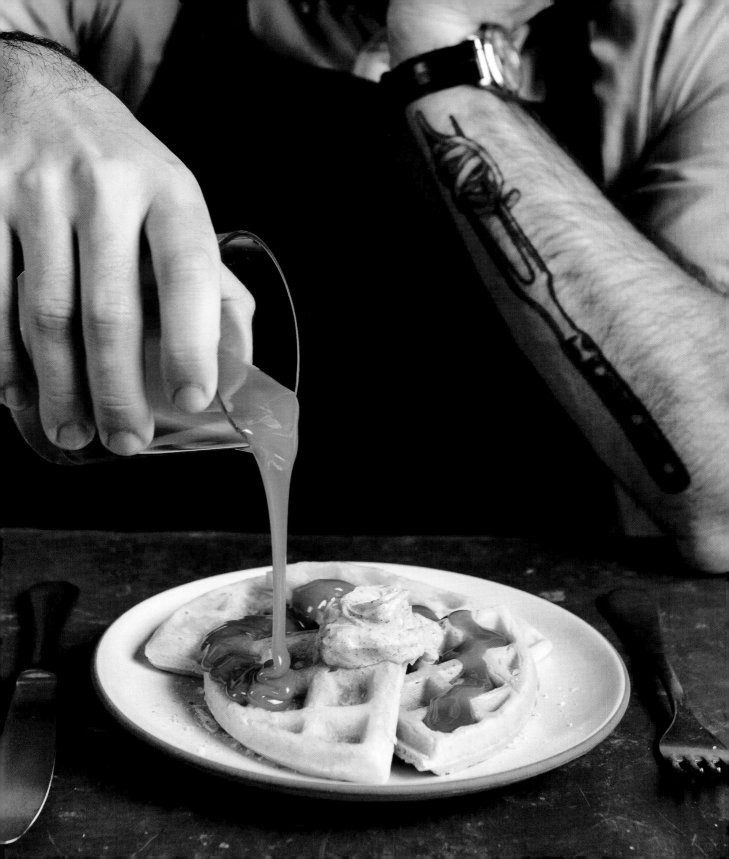

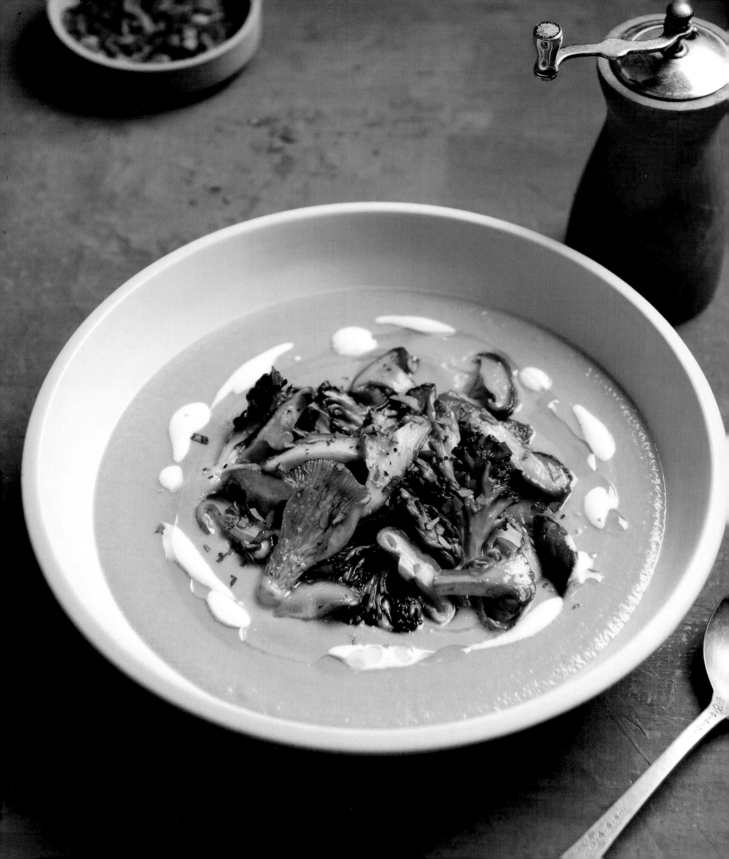

Seinfeld is, of course, a show about nothing. But if it had to be about something, it could very well be food. Food frequently plays a central role in the great undoing of our anti-heroes' best laid plans, from penile-peeping revenge tales to the thievery of a sixty-year-old royal wedding cake. Even when it's not compelling America's favorite foursome to commit unspeakable acts, it is near ever-present—consommé, marble rye, calzones, soup, lobster, big salads, Chinese takeout, salsa—even going so far as to introduce food into lovemaking. It was difficult to choose from such a wealth of options, but I really wanted to make babka, was really curious about muffin tops, and knew I simply had to address the soup Nazi. Each presented their own unique challenges: Do muffin tops really need the stump to taste great? How does one go about making a fictional wild mushroom soup so delicious, the eater is compelled to sit down? How the hell do you make babka?

WILD MUSHROOM SOUP

SERVES 4

VERDICT: This is the very apex of any mushroom soup
I've ever had, and it's well worth the time and effort.

3 ounces dried porcini mushrooms

6 cups homemade chicken stock, plus more
as needed

¾ cup extra-virgin olive oil, plus more
for drizzling

2 pounds assorted fresh wild mushrooms,
chopped

3 garlic cloves, chopped

4 celery stalks, chopped

1 medium onion, diced

½ cup dry sherry

Leaves from 5 sprigs fresh parsley, some
chopped and reserved for garnish

1 teaspoon chopped fresh thyme leaves

Kosher salt and freshly ground black pepper

2 slices white bread, crusts removed, bread
torn into pieces

2 lemons

½ cup crème fraîche

(recipe continues)

PLACE THE porcini mushrooms in a large heat-proof bowl. Bring 4 cups of the stock to a boil in a medium saucepan. Pour the stock over the mushrooms. Let soak, stirring occasionally, for 30 minutes.

MEANWHILE, HEAT ¼ cup of the olive oil in a large stockpot over medium heat until shimmering. Add the fresh mushrooms and cook, stirring, until soft and well browned, about 10 minutes. Transfer to a bowl and set aside.

IN THE same pot, heat ¼ cup of the olive oil over medium heat. Add the garlic and cook, stirring, until fragrant, about 30 seconds. Add the celery and onion and cook, stirring, until a dark fond (layer of cooked-on browned bits) forms on the bottom of the pot, 7 to 10 minutes. Increase the heat to medium-high and add the sherry, stirring and scraping up all the browned bits from the bottom of the pot. Add the whole parsley leaves, thyme, and the porcini mushrooms and their soaking liquid (stop pouring before you reach the grit at the bottom of the bowl; discard the grit) and simmer for 30 minutes. Add the remaining stock and taste; add more stock, if desired, if the porcini flavor is too strong.

LET COOL for 5 minutes, then carefully transfer the soup to a high-powered blender, taste, and season with salt and pepper. Blend until nearly smooth. Add the torn bread. With the machine running on high speed, slowly stream in the remaining ¼ cup olive oil through the feed hole and blend until the soup is creamy and emulsified.

PILE A handful of the sautéed mushrooms in the center of each of four warmed shallow soup bowls. Pour the soup around the mushrooms until it comes halfway up their sides. Grate lemon zest over the top of each bowl, sprinkle with a bit of chopped fresh parsley, drizzle with olive oil and crème fraîche, and serve.

BABKA

MAKES ONE 9-INCH CHOCOLATE BABKA AND ONE 9-INCH CINNAMON BABKA

VERDICT: Babka is an intermediate baking challenge, but a
rewarding one—both the cinnamon and chocolate iterations are to die
for, not to mention highly Instagrammable.

BABKA DOUGH

½ cup whole milk

1 (¼-ounce) packet active dry yeast

2½ ounces granulated sugar (about ⅓ cup),
plus a pinch

18 ounces all-purpose flour (about 4¼ cups),
plus more for dusting

1 teaspoon kosher salt

½ teaspoon freshly grated nutmeg, plus more
to taste

4 large eggs, lightly beaten

¾ cup (1½ sticks) unsalted butter, cut into
tablespoons, plus more for greasing

SIMPLE SYRUP

1 cup granulated sugar

CHOCOLATE FILLING

½ cup (1 stick) unsalted butter

9 ounces dark chocolate, chopped

2 teaspoons espresso powder

⅔ cup unsweetened cocoa powder

⅔ cup confectioners' sugar

CINNAMON FILLING

4 tablespoons ground cinnamon

1 cup packed dark brown sugar

1 cup (2 sticks) unsalted butter, melted

BABKA DOUGH

IN A small saucepan, heat the milk over low
heat to 110°F. Remove from the heat and stir in
the yeast and a pinch of granulated sugar. Let
stand at room temperature for 10 to 15 minutes, until foaming.

MEANWHILE, IN the bowl of a stand mixer fitted with the paddle attachment, mix the flour,
granulated sugar, salt, and nutmeg on medium

speed just until combined. Replace the paddle
attachment with the dough hook. Add the yeast
mixture and knead on medium speed for 1 minute, or until barely combined. Add the eggs and
knead on medium speed for about 5 minutes,
or until the dough pulls away from the sides of
the bowl and forms a cohesive ball. Add 6 tablespoons of the butter and knead on medium
speed for 5 to 7 minutes, until incorporated.

(recipe continues)

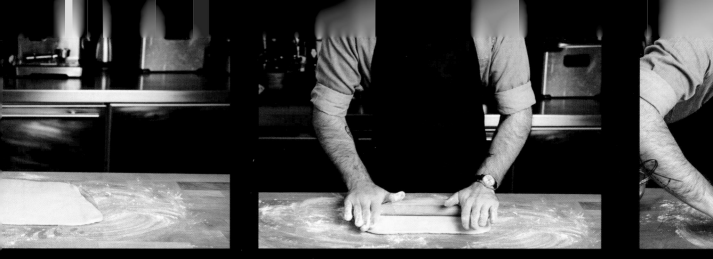
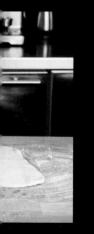
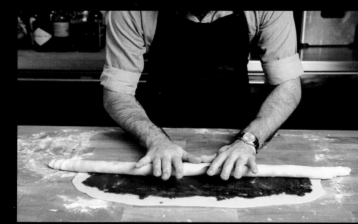
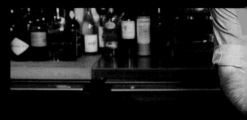
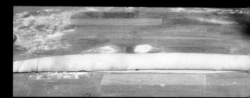
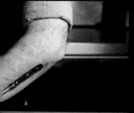
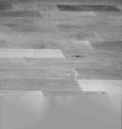
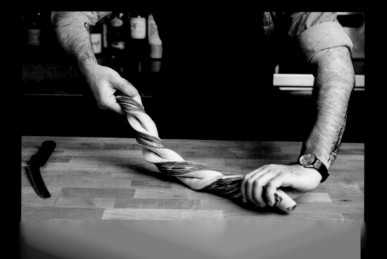
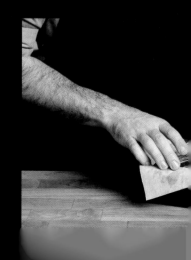

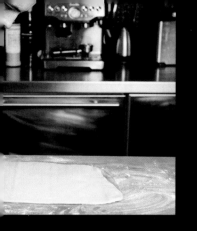
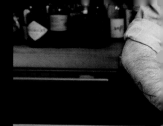
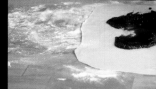
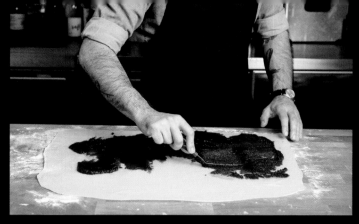
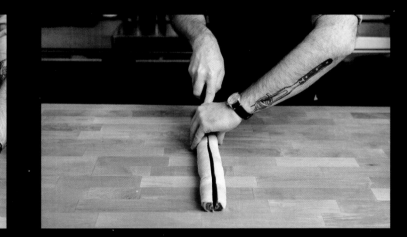
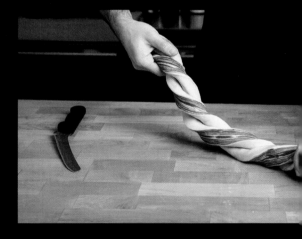
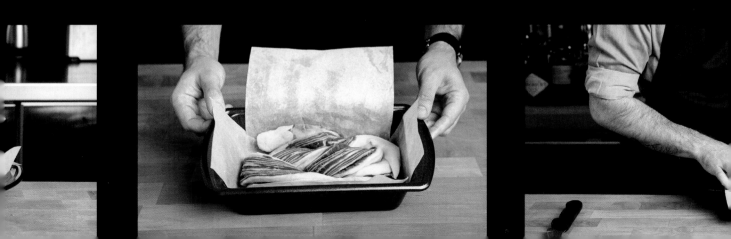

Add the remaining 6 tablespoons butter and knead for 5 to 7 minutes. If the dough is still sticking to the sides of the bowl, add more flour, 1 tablespoon at a time, until the dough is smooth and supple.

BUTTER A large bowl. Pull the dough off the dough hook, roll and stretch it into a smooth ball, and transfer it to the prepared bowl. Roll the dough around in the bowl to coat it with butter. Cover with a clean kitchen towel and place the bowl in the oven (the oven should be off). Let rise for 1½ hours. Remove the dough from the oven, punch it down in the bowl, cover with plastic wrap, and refrigerate overnight or for at least 4 hours.

SIMPLE SYRUP

IN A small saucepan, combine the granulated sugar and 1 cup water. Bring to a simmer over medium heat, stirring, and cook until the sugar has dissolved and the mixture is syrupy, about 15 minutes. Remove from the heat and let cool completely.

CHOCOLATE FILLING

IN A medium microwavable bowl, combine the butter and chocolate. Microwave on medium power for 2 minutes, or until completely smooth, stopping to stir every 30 seconds. Whisk in the espresso powder, cocoa powder, and confectioners' sugar until a spreadable paste forms.

CINNAMON FILLING

IN A medium bowl, combine the cinnamon, brown sugar, and melted butter. Stir well until a spreadable paste forms.

ASSEMBLY

LINE TWO baking sheets with parchment paper.

TRANSFER THE chilled dough to a lightly floured work surface, divide it in half, and roll out each half to a 24 x 18-inch rectangle. Spread one rectangle evenly with the chocolate filling to within 1 inch of the edges. Starting from one long side, roll the dough into a log and transfer it to one of the prepared baking sheets. Repeat with the remaining dough rectangle and the cinnamon filling. Freeze for 15 to 20 minutes, until the dough is firm.

BUTTER TWO 9-inch loaf pans and line them with parchment paper. Transfer the chocolate log to a work surface. Using a serrated knife, halve the log lengthwise. Hold the two halves of dough against each other so the cut sides are facing out, then twist into a decorative loaf. (Watch my video to see it done!) Transfer to one of the prepared loaf pans, cover with a damp kitchen towel, and put the pan in the oven (the oven should be off). Repeat with the cinnamon log. Let the dough rise for 1½ hours.

REMOVE THE dough from the oven and set aside. Preheat the oven to 375°F.

BAKE BOTH babkas for 30 to 40 minutes, until a tester inserted into the thickest part of the loaf comes out clean. Remove from the oven, place the pans on wire racks, and immediately brush the tops of the babkas with the simple syrup. Let cool in the pans for at least 2 hours.

TURN THE babkas out of the pans, slice, and serve.

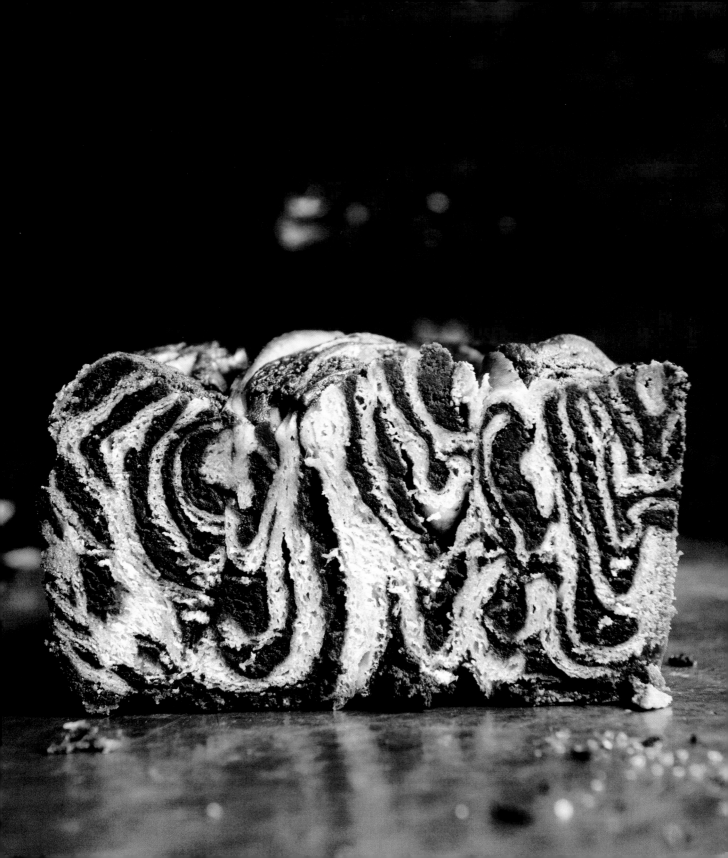

LEMON–POPPY SEED MUFFIN TOPS

MAKES 12 TO 16 MUFFIN TOPS

VERDICT: Separately baked muffin tops are far superior to traditional muffins, as they allow for much more surface area to become browned and flavorful— and these are bright, zesty, lemony little muffin tops.

12 ounces all-purpose flour (about 2¾ cups)

3 tablespoons poppy seeds

1 tablespoon baking powder

½ teaspoon baking soda

¼ teaspoon fine salt

7 ounces granulated sugar (about 1 cup)

10 tablespoons unsalted butter, melted, plus more for brushing

2 large eggs

Zest and juice of 2 lemons

¾ cup buttermilk

2¼ ounces confectioners' sugar (about ½ cup), sifted

PREHEAT THE oven to 375°F. Line 2 baking sheets with parchment paper.

IN A medium bowl, whisk together the flour, poppy seeds, baking powder, baking soda, and salt. In a large bowl using a handheld mixer, beat together the granulated sugar and melted butter until light and fluffy, about 3 minutes. Add the eggs, half the lemon zest, and half the lemon juice and beat on low speed until just combined. Add half the flour mixture and beat on low speed until barely incorporated. Add half the buttermilk, mix to combine, then add the remaining flour mixture, followed by the remaining buttermilk, gently whisking to combine after each addition, until all the ingredients are incorporated.

USING A small (¼-cup) ice cream scoop, portion the batter onto the prepared baking sheets. Bake the muffin tops for 20 to 25 minutes, until a toothpick inserted into the muffins comes out with a few crumbs clinging to it. Let cool completely.

IN A small bowl, whisk together the remaining lemon zest and lemon juice and the confectioners' sugar to make a glaze.

POUR THE glaze over the muffin tops and let set for 30 minutes before serving.

KEVIN'S FAMOUS CHILI

SERVES 8

The first of a great many episodes about chili, re-creating Kevin Malone's was no mean feat, as it required trips to two specialty stores: Kalustyan's spice shop and Home Depot. First, dried ancho (and cascabel) chiles to build the toasty spices and rich sauce for Kevin's painstaking family recipe. Second, a sizeable bolt of poly-fiber carpet upon which to dump it and eat it. Despite that commitment to accuracy, once I laid eyes on some beautiful short ribs in the butcher case, I decided to abandon all reason and make the chili con carne–style. Don't ask me why—I don't know. This was my first time making the dish from whole dried chiles, and I can tell you that it makes all the difference in the world. I cannot, in good conscience, recommend that you eat it off the floor, however.

VERDICT: This chili has a deep and complex flavor thanks to a homemade chile paste, and the chili con carne–style preparation gives it a rich body and steak-y bite. Far and away the finest chili made on the show—but don't be afraid to make it your own! Try other chiles, add more habanero for heat, add or omit beans . . .

3 ounces ancho chiles, stemmed, seeded, and cut into ½-inch pieces

1 ounce cascabel chiles, stemmed, seeded, and cut into ½-inch pieces

3 tablespoons cornmeal

1 tablespoon unsweetened cocoa powder

1 tablespoon freshly ground toasted cumin seeds

1 tablespoon dried oregano

4 cups chicken stock

2 tablespoons vegetable oil

3 pounds chuck steak, trimmed and diced into very small cubes

1 large Spanish onion, chopped

4 large garlic cloves, minced

2 jalapeños, seeded and chopped

1 habanero pepper, seeded and chopped (optional)

1 (12-ounce) bottle Mexican lager

6 plum tomatoes, cored and chopped

1 (12-ounce) can red kidney beans, drained and rinsed

2 tablespoons light brown sugar

Kosher salt and freshly ground black pepper

1 (3-foot) square low-quality poly-fiber carpet (optional)

(ingredients continue)

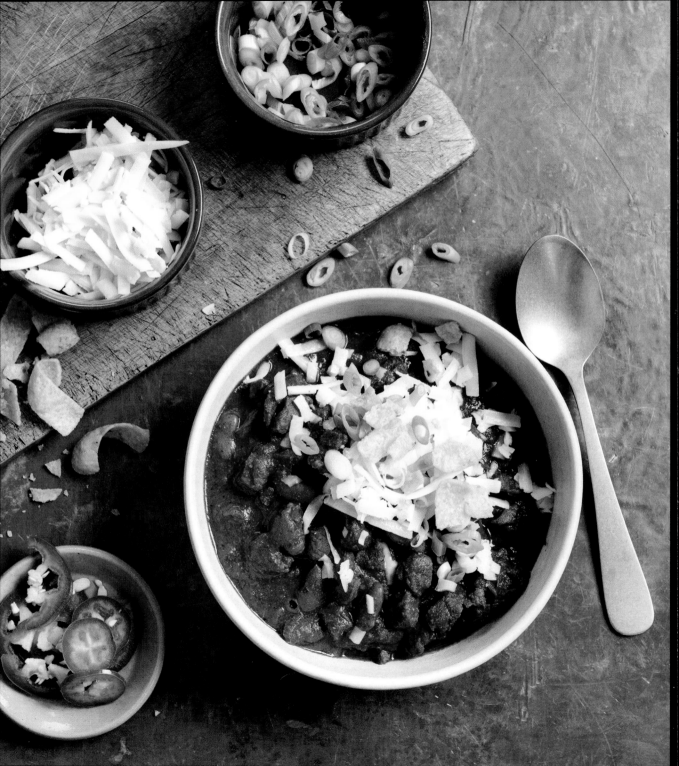

Shredded white cheddar cheese, for serving (optional)

Optional garnishes: chopped parsley, sliced scallions, corn kernels, sliced jalapeños, corn chips, and sour cream

---

IN A dry pan, toast the ancho and cascabel chiles until fragrant and barely smoking, about 2 minutes. Transfer to a food processor and process until ground to a fine powder, about 3 minutes. Add the cornmeal, cocoa powder, cumin, and oregano and pulse to combine. Add ¾ cup of the stock and process until a paste forms. Set the spice paste aside.

IN A large stockpot, heat the vegetable oil over medium-high heat until shimmering. Add the beef in batches to avoid crowding the pan and sear until browned on all sides, about 5 minutes. Transfer to a bowl and set aside. Add the onion, garlic, jalapeños, and habanero to the pot and sweat briefly, about 1 minute. Pour in the beer and cook, stirring and scraping up all the browned bits from the bottom of the pot. Add the tomatoes, kidney beans, and brown sugar and return the beef to the pan. Stir in the spice paste and the remaining 3¼ cups stock until combined. Bring to a bare simmer. Simmer for 2 to 3 hours, until the beef is tender and the chili has thickened. Season with salt and pepper.

POUR THE chili onto a square of poly-fiber carpet* or ladle into bowls, then top with shredded cheese and garnish as desired.

*Don't actually do this.

FUN FACT
This episode features the first-ever outtake, wherein I inhale a lungful of freshly ground spices, *The West Wing* theme song blaring proudly in the background. 0/10 do not recommend.

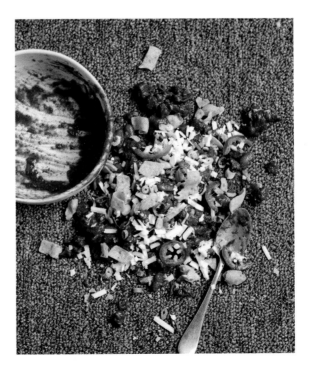

SPAGHETTI CARBONARA

SERVES 4

Master of None is another show so passionate about food, it often plays a pivotal role in the progression of the story. Pasta becomes the new focus of Dev's entire life in the beginning of the second season as he learns to make delicate tortellini guided by the expert hand of an Italian octogenarian. Before that, however, he takes his first steps toward proper foodie status by shelving Yelp in search of the best homemade pasta, opting instead to dust off the stand mixer extruder attachment given to him by his girlfriend. After making his first-ever batch of creamy, chewy carbonara, he can't help but exclaim, "I DID IT!" upon taking his first bite. His reaction alone is enough to prompt a first-time cook to experiment in the kitchen—this sentiment of excited accomplishment is an accessible, tangible sensation that we can manifest from our favorite pieces of fiction. All you've got to do is try.

VERDICT: Dev's first steps in pasta-making aren't totally stable, as he makes a few beginner's mistakes, but with some minor revisions produces an impossibly delicious bowl of pasta.

---

7 ounces semolina flour (about 1¾ cups)

7 ounces all-purpose flour (about 1¾ cups), plus more for dusting

6 large eggs

1 teaspoon kosher salt, plus more if needed

1 tablespoon vegetable oil

½ pound guanciale, pancetta, or bacon, cut into ¼-inch dice

2 or 3 garlic cloves, minced

1 cup freshly grated Parmesan cheese, plus more for serving

Freshly ground black pepper

IN A large bowl, whisk together the semolina flour and 7 ounces of the all-purpose flour. Create a well in the center large enough to contain 4 eggs. Crack 4 eggs into the well, add the salt, and beat with a fork. Slowly add more and more of the flour, until a thick slurry forms. Work in the flour with your hands to form a shaggy dough. Turn the dough out onto a floured work surface and knead for 5 minutes, or until smooth and not tacky, adding more flour as necessary. Wrap the dough in plastic wrap and let rest at room temperature for

(recipe continues)

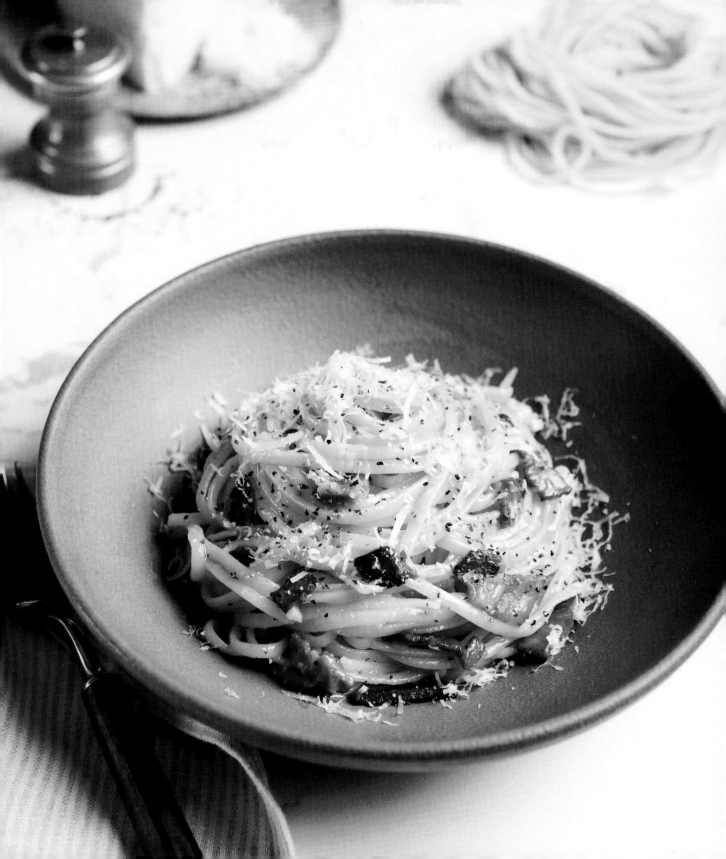

30 minutes. (Note: If you're using a pasta extruder like I do in the video, you want a particularly dry dough that's slightly rough to the touch—the hopper will knead it further.)

DUST A baking sheet with flour. Using a spaghetti extruder fitted to a stand mixer, feed golf ball–size pieces of the dough into the hopper with the machine running on high speed. Use the cutter to cut the spaghetti to the desired length. Toss the pasta with flour, then arrange it into nests on a floured baking sheet. Cover with plastic wrap and refrigerate until ready to use. (This pasta also freezes very well.)

BRING A large pot of salted water to a boil.

BEAT THE remaining 2 eggs in a small bowl and set aside.

IN A large skillet, heat the vegetable oil over medium heat. Add the guanciale and fry, stirring occasionally, until crisp, about 7 minutes. As the guanciale finishes cooking, add the pasta to the boiling water and cook for 2 to 3 minutes, until al dente. Add the garlic to the guanciale and cook, stirring, until fragrant, about 30 seconds. Remove the pan from the heat and, using tongs, transfer the pasta from the pot to the hot skillet. (Make sure you don't drain the spaghetti too well—you want about ¼ cup of the cooking water still clinging to the spaghetti to end up in the skillet). Toss the spaghetti with the guanciale and, while stirring continuously, add the beaten eggs to the hot pasta and toss until thickened. Toss with the Parmesan and season with pepper (and salt, if necessary). Transfer to a plate, top with more cheese, and serve.

FUN FACT

This was another episode critiqued by a panel of real Italian chefs, whose chief complaint was the inclusion of garlic. Garlic in carbonara might not be traditional, but it'd be hard to try it and say with a straight face that it isn't a positive addition to the dish.

BUTTERMILK PANCAKES, HAM, AND COFFEE

SERVES 4

Agent Dale Cooper famously said, "Nothing beats the taste sensation when maple syrup *SMACK* collides with ham!" Truer words perhaps have never been said. *Twin Peaks* is not only a surrealist piece of performance art that somehow made its way onto network television and changed entertainment as we know it forever, it's also a show that cares a great deal about coffee (*especially* coffee), pie, pancakes, and ham. It was only fitting, then, that the first-ever guest on the show should be fellow YouTuber Nick Fisher of Cocktail Chemistry, showing us not only how to properly brew the best-possible coffee at home, but using that coffee to make the Black Yukon Sucker Punch, a cocktail as strange as its source material.

VERDICT: A simple but essential breakfast, a short stack of these pancakes and a ham steak should satisfy even the brunchiest of cravings. Make sure to serve them on the same plate so the maple syrup *SMACK* collides with the ham. Pour-over coffee is a revelation for those of us accustomed to the plasticky piss that comes out of drip machines.

---

7 ounces all-purpose flour (about 1¾ cups)

2 tablespoons sugar

2 teaspoons baking powder

1 teaspoon kosher salt

½ teaspoon baking soda

2 cups buttermilk

1 large egg

3 tablespoons unsalted butter, melted and cooled, plus more for serving

Nonstick cooking spray

1 tablespoon vegetable oil

4 large ham steaks, each about ½ inch thick

Pure maple syrup, warmed, for serving

Hot coffee, for serving

(recipe continues)

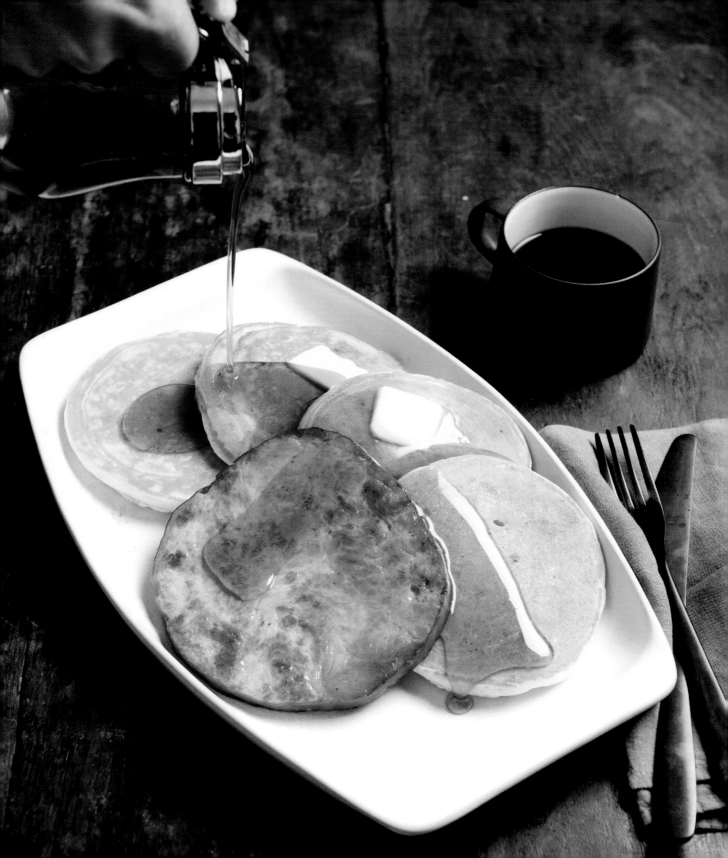

IN A large bowl, whisk together the flour, sugar, baking powder, salt, and baking soda. In a medium bowl, whisk together the buttermilk, egg, and melted butter. Make a well in the center of the dry ingredients, pour the buttermilk mixture into it, and gently whisk until just combined—the batter should still be lumpy. Cover and refrigerate for 30 minutes to 1 hour.

SPRAY A large cast-iron or nonstick skillet with cooking spray and heat over medium to low heat for 5 minutes. Increase the heat to medium and pour ⅛ to ¼ cup of the batter (depending on how large you want your pancakes) onto the skillet. Cook for 1 to 3 minutes, until the edges of the pancake become dull,

bubbles form on top of the pancake, and the bottom is brown. Flip the pancake and cook on the golden side for 1 to 2 minutes, until golden brown. Transfer to a plate. Repeat with the remaining batter. If desired, transfer the pancakes to a wire rack set on a rimmed baking sheet and keep them warm in a low oven (about 250°F).

MEANWHILE, IN a large nonstick skillet, heat the vegetable oil over medium heat. Add the ham steaks and fry until browned on both sides and heated through, about 3 minutes. Transfer to plates, add the pancakes, and serve with warm maple syrup and melted butter—and coffee, of course.

GIANT CHOCOLATE LAYER CAKE

SERVES 10

This was the first truly divisive episode of *Binging with Babish*, given its stomach-turning secret ingredients. I cannot, in good conscience, recommend that you add blood and sweat to this cake—not only do they not provide any flavor or nutritional value, they are potentially dangerous, and you just obviously shouldn't do that, okay? I, however, decided to eschew health and safety codes in favor of accuracy, wiping my sweat and shedding my blood with food podcaster Dan Pashman. The result is the sweet, moist, and absolutely gigantic chocolate layer cake of your childhood dreams. I also can't recommend that you eat the entire thing in one sitting, no matter what kind of pressure you're under from your tyrannical principal.

VERDICT: This is a gold-standard chocolate cake that, thanks to a couple of special ingredients, transcends the dry and flavorless out-of-a-box sponge we've grown accustomed to. Buttermilk in the batter and cream cheese in the frosting guarantee enhanced flavor, and baking the cakes until just barely cooked ensures a moist crumb.

CAKE

Butter, for greasing

3 cups all-purpose flour, plus more for dusting

3 cups granulated sugar

1½ cups unsweetened cocoa powder

1 tablespoon baking powder

2 teaspoons baking soda

1 teaspoon fine salt

1½ cups buttermilk

4 large eggs

½ cup vegetable oil

CHOCOLATE FROSTING

1½ cups (3 sticks) unsalted butter, at room temperature

1 (8-ounce) package cream cheese, at room temperature

1 cup unsweetened cocoa powder

1½ pounds confectioners' sugar (about 5⅓ cups), sifted

Whole milk, for thinning (optional)

CAKE

PREHEAT THE oven to 350°F. Liberally butter three 9-inch round cake pans and dust each evenly with about 1 tablespoon of flour, tapping out any excess. Line the bottom of each pan with parchment paper rounds.

IN A large bowl, whisk together the flour, granulated sugar, cocoa powder, baking powder, baking soda, and salt. In a medium bowl, whisk together the buttermilk, eggs, and vegetable oil. Add the wet ingredients to the dry ingredients and whisk until smooth. Divide the batter evenly among the prepared cake pans and bake for 30 to 35 minutes, until a tester inserted into the center of the cakes comes out clean. Let cool in the pans on wire racks for at least 30 minutes, then invert the cakes onto the racks, remove the parchment paper, and let cool completely, 30 minutes to 1 hour more.

CHOCOLATE FROSTING

WHILE THE cakes cool, in the bowl of a stand mixer fitted with the paddle attachment, beat together the butter and cream cheese on medium speed until fluffy, about 2 minutes. Add the cocoa powder and mix on medium-low speed until combined. Add the confectioners'

sugar a cup or two at a time, stopping and scraping down the sides occasionally, and beat on medium speed until the frosting is creamy and smooth, about 1 minute. Add a splash of milk, if desired, to thin out the frosting.

FLIP THE cakes right-side up and, using a serrated knife, gently trim off the domed top of each cake layer to completely level it. Place one cake layer on a platter and spread ¾ cup of the frosting on top. Top with a second cake layer, trimmed-side down, and spread ¾ cup of the frosting on top. Top with the third layer, trimmed-side down, and spread the remaining frosting over the top and sides of the entire layer cake. Slice into wedges and serve.

FUN FACT

For a Patreon-exclusive episode, Dan and I went on to make goose liver doughnuts that very same day. Which is grosser? Goose liver doughnuts, no question.

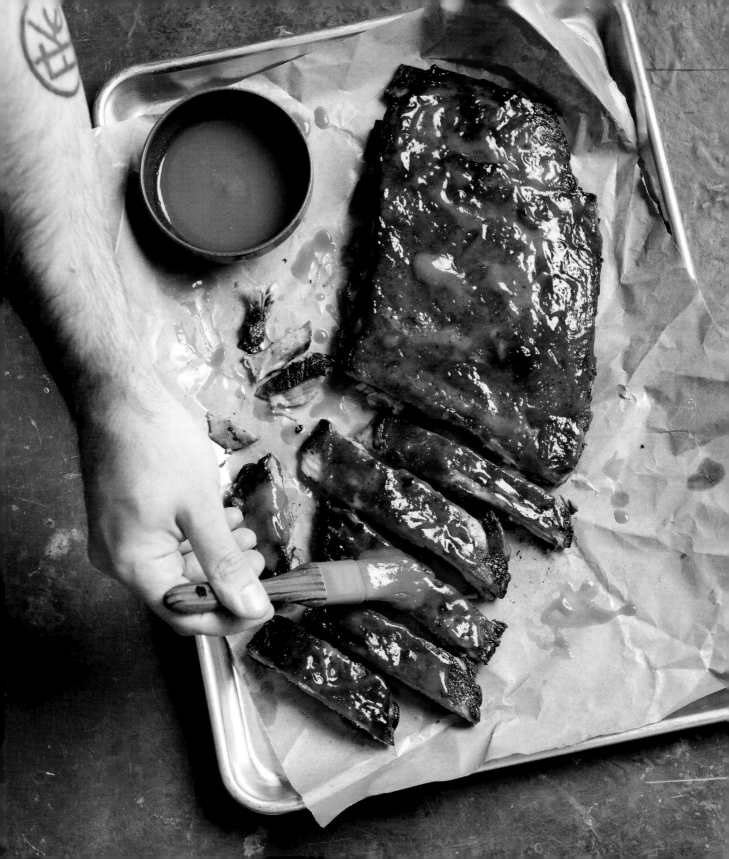

FREDDY'S RIBS

SERVES 8 TO 10

There's a reason barbecue is the go-to analogy for all things regional: barbecue varies wildly region by region. Since Frank Underwood would likely gravitate toward 'cue resembling that from his hometown of Gaffney, South Carolina, it made sense that Freddy's ribs would feature the spicy, tangy "Carolina Red" variation of the state's many barbecue sauces. Unlike the more famous "Carolina Gold," the red iteration adds tomato puree to its tangy, mustardy sauce base. That,

in concert with a relatively standard (but nonetheless delicious) dry rub, produces ribs that must be eaten to be believed.

VERDICT: While real barbecue can only be yielded by virtue of a real smoker, a delicious approximation can be achieved using either liquid smoke or an extremely complicated and fussy wok-smoking method. All three methods are listed here, and all three produce barbecue that's nothing short of exquisite.

3 full racks pork spareribs (about 10 pounds total)

DRY RUB

3 tablespoons chili powder

2 tablespoons ground mustard

1 tablespoon garlic powder

1 tablespoon onion powder

1 tablespoon paprika, or 1 tablespoon smoked paprika for oven methods

1 tablespoon dried oregano

1 tablespoon kosher salt

1 tablespoon freshly ground black pepper

1 tablespoon ground white pepper

1 tablespoon ground cumin (omit for oven methods)

1 teaspoon cayenne pepper (optional)

BARBECUE SAUCE

2 cups apple cider vinegar

2 cups tomato puree, or 1½ cups ketchup for oven methods

¼ cup packed dark brown sugar, or ¾ cup for oven methods

½ teaspoon paprika

2 teaspoons ground mustard, or ¼ cup yellow mustard for oven methods

2 teaspoons Worcestershire sauce

1 teaspoon garlic powder

1 teaspoon onion powder

1 teaspoon kosher salt

(ingredients continue)

PAT THE ribs dry and remove and discard the membrane. Put the ribs on a rimmed baking sheet.

DRY RUB

IN A medium bowl, whisk together all the dry rub ingredients.

COAT THE ribs liberally with the dry rub, making sure to cover every nook and cranny. Wrap tightly with plastic wrap and refrigerate for at least 4 hours, or ideally overnight.

BARBECUE SAUCE

IN A large saucepan, combine all the barbecue sauce ingredients and bring to a simmer over medium-high heat. Whisk to combine, reduce the heat, and cook at a bare simmer until thick and syrupy, about 1½ hours. The sauce can be made up to 3 days ahead; let cool and store in an airtight container in the refrigerator. Reheat before using.

SMOKER METHOD

PREPARE THE smoker with the wood chips according to the manufacturer's instructions (or your favorite time-honored family tradition). Stabilize the heat at 225°F. Arrange the ribs in the smoker as desired, close the lid, and smoke for 2 to 3 hours, or until the meat is tender but still holding on to the bones. Every 30 minutes, baste the ribs with the barbecue sauce and spray with the apple juice. Remove the ribs from the smoker, wrap in aluminum foil, and let rest for 10 minutes. Slice the ribs, transfer to a plate, top with more barbecue sauce, and serve.

OVEN METHOD: LIQUID SMOKE

PREHEAT THE oven to 250°F. Place an extra-long sheet of aluminum foil on a rimmed baking sheet and top with a wire rack.

PLACE THE ribs on the rack. Stir together the bourbon and liquid smoke in a small bowl and drizzle the mixture over the ribs. Top with another long sheet of foil and wrap the ribs and the rack, crimping the edges to create a tight seal. Bake for 2 to 2½ hours, until the ribs are tender but not falling apart. Unwrap, baste with the barbecue sauce, and bake, uncovered, for 1½ hours more, basting with more barbecue sauce every 20 to 30 minutes, or every time the ribs look sticky and lose their sheen. During the last 10 minutes of cooking, increase the oven temperature to 500°F and bake until a crust forms on the ribs. Remove the ribs from the oven, brush with more barbecue sauce, slice, and serve.

OVEN METHOD: WOK SMOKE

NOTE: *Only attempt this method with proper ventilation in your kitchen.*

PREHEAT THE oven to 250°F.

LINE A deep wok with four sheets of aluminum foil, leaving a 6-inch overhang all around the edge. Add the wood chips and heat over medium-high heat until just starting to smoke, about 5 minutes. Set a rack on the wok, place the ribs on top, and cover with another sheet of foil, crimping the edges tightly with the overhanging foil so no smoke escapes. Reduce the heat to medium and smoke the ribs for 10 minutes. Remove the wok from the heat and let the ribs smoke for another 20 minutes.

PLACE AN extra-long sheet of foil on a rimmed baking sheet. Transfer the rack with the ribs to the foil. Drizzle the ribs with the bourbon and continue the recipe as instructed in the Liquid Smoke method.

FUN FACT

This was the very first episode to take *Binging with Babish* into the great outdoors. Returning to my dear buddy Steve's house in Delaware, he was kind enough to let me use his egg-style smoker, a cookery tool that makes me often contemplate moving to the suburbs just so I can have one.

TOMATE DU SALTAMBIQUE

SERVES 4

Here's an example of an episode that exactly zero people were asking for: a furiously fussy, overly obscure, only-discussed-but-never-seen dish from *The West Wing*. Seemingly included in the script only to establish our heroes' sophisticated palates, the very concept of a dessert tomato sounds like a reality-show cooking challenge. Stuffed with exotic fruit and stewed in "crème de caramel" (an incorrectly used alternate name for flan), the literal interpretation of Jed and Leo's description of the dish leads to something rather unpalatable, but a few tweaks turn this tomato into a dessert worth devouring.

VERDICT: Strange but impressive, *tomate du saltambique* is the successful rendering of a tomato in dessert form. There's room for interpretation and experimentation in the filling, but this baseline recipe will yield a dish to wow (and initially disgust) your dinner guests.

STUFFING

1 tablespoon unsalted butter

1 Honeycrisp apple, peeled, cored, and minced

1 Bartlett pear, peeled, cored, and minced

¼ pineapple, cored and minced

¼ cup roasted pistachios, finely chopped

¼ cup halved walnuts, toasted and finely chopped

Zest of 1 lemon

Zest of 1 orange

1 tablespoon sugar

1 tablespoon grated fresh ginger

1 star anise pod

Pinch of ground cinnamon

Pinch of ground cloves

"CRÈME DE CARAMEL"

2 cups heavy cream

½ cup (1 stick) unsalted butter

1 cup sugar

TOMATOES

4 Campari tomatoes with stems attached, tops sliced off and reserved, cored, and seeded

Peel of 1 orange, thinly julienned

Flaky sea salt, for serving

Candied orange peel, very thinly sliced, for garnish

Vanilla ice cream, for serving (optional)

(recipe continues)

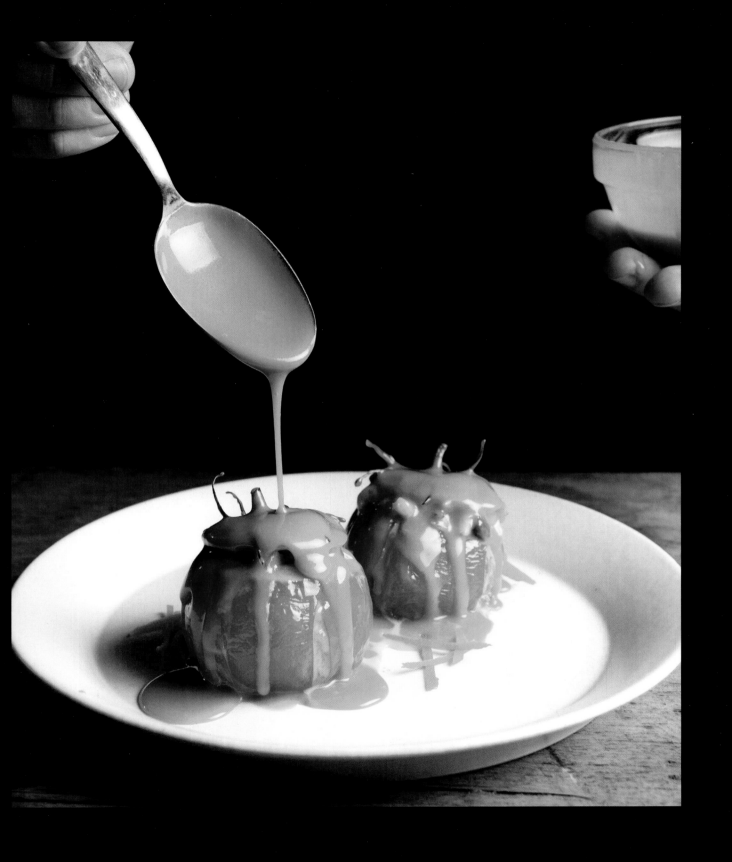

STUFFING

IN A large sauté pan, melt the butter over medium heat until foaming. In a large bowl, stir together the apple, pear, pineapple, nuts, lemon zest, orange zest, sugar, ginger, star anise, cinnamon, and cloves until well combined. Transfer to the pan and cook, stirring, for 5 minutes, or until the apple and pear are softened and fragrant. Remove from the heat, pick out and discard the star anise, and set aside.

"CRÈME DE CARAMEL"

IN A medium saucepan, heat the cream and butter over medium-low heat until steaming. In a large heavy pot, heat the sugar over medium heat, occasionally stirring gently, until completely melted and amber in color, about 10 minutes. While whisking continuously, slowly add the hot cream mixture and whisk vigorously until completely incorporated.

TOMATOES AND ASSEMBLY

PLACE THE tomatoes in a small sauté pan, leaning them against each other so they stay upright. Fill each tomato with the stuffing and top with the tomato top. Pour the caramel into the pan until it comes halfway up the sides of the tomatoes. Add the sliced orange peel to the caramel and heat over the lowest possible heat just until the caramel steams and occasionally bubbles. Cook, spooning the caramel over the tomatoes every few minutes, until the tomatoes are very tender but not falling apart, 1½ to 2 hours.

FOR EACH serving, spoon some caramel into a shallow bowl and place one tomato on top. Sprinkle with sea salt and candied orange peel and serve with a scoop of ice cream, if desired.

FUN FACT

Oliver Babish, my almost arbitrarily chosen pseudonym, is a name taken from *The West Wing*. Portrayed by Oliver Platt, the Bartlet administration's legal counsel is perhaps best known for a famous scene in which he smashes a tape recorder with a gavel.

FRIED CHICKEN BREAKFAST "LASAGNA"

SERVES 12

Fried chicken breakfast lasagna is one of the many so-unhealthy-it's-gross menu items dreamed up by contrarian patriarch Robert Freeman for his fantasy restaurant. It's lucky that Riley didn't sample this calorie bomb; if he was sent into sugar shock by the so-called "Luther Burger," this abomination would likely land him in a coma. An (admittedly ingenious) amalgam of Southern breakfast mainstays, the breakfast lasagna is not for the faint of heart—literally, if you have a faint heart, don't eat this, or you'll likely die.

VERDICT: A prime candidate for a stock photo about trans fats, Fried Chicken Breakfast Lasagna is everything wonderful about both breakfast and lunch, layered and cemented together by sausage gravy. Exercise extreme caution.

Butter or nonstick cooking spray, for greasing
Fried Chicken (recipe follows)
Sausage Gravy (recipe follows)
2 cups shredded cheddar cheese

Waffles (recipe follows)
4 large eggs, soft scrambled
Pure maple syrup, warmed, for serving

PREHEAT THE oven to 375°F. Grease a deep 9 x 13-inch baking pan.

ASSEMBLE THE lasagna in the pan as desired—I recommend starting with a layer of fried chicken thighs, top with some of the gravy and cheese, then a layer of waffles. Next up, the fried chicken breasts, more cheese, gravy, scrambled eggs, another layer of waffles, then finish with even more cheese. Bake for 15 to 20 minutes, until the cheese has melted.

REMOVE FROM the oven, slice, and serve with warm maple syrup—only to those with excellent health insurance.

(recipe continues)

FRIED CHICKEN

MAKES 8 PIECES OF FRIED CHICKEN

2 boneless, skinless chicken breasts

6 boneless, skinless chicken thighs

2 cups buttermilk

3 tablespoons kosher salt

2 teaspoons hot sauce

1 teaspoon paprika

1 teaspoon garlic powder

1 teaspoon onion powder

3 cups vegetable oil

3 cups peanut oil

4 large eggs, beaten

4 cups all-purpose flour

2 teaspoons baking soda

2 teaspoons baking powder

BUTTERFLY THE chicken breasts and pound them between two sheets of plastic wrap until ½ inch thick. Butterfly the thick parts of the chicken thighs until they are a uniform thickness.

IN A large bowl, whisk together the buttermilk, salt, hot sauce, paprika, garlic powder, and onion powder. Add the chicken and toss to evenly coat. Cover and refrigerate for at least 4 hours, or ideally overnight.

IN A large Dutch oven, combine the vegetable oil and peanut oil and heat over medium-high heat to 375°F. Set a wire rack over paper towels or a brown paper bag.

PLACE THE eggs in a pie pan. In another pie pan, whisk together the flour, baking soda, and baking powder. Remove the chicken pieces from the buttermilk mixture, letting any excess drip back into the bowl. Dredge each piece in the flour mixture until evenly coated, then dip in the eggs until evenly coated, letting any excess drip back into the pie pan. Dredge once more in the flour, then, working in batches, transfer immediately to the hot oil and fry, flipping as necessary to brown the chicken evenly, for 6 to 10 minutes, until the internal temperature registers 155°F for the breasts and 175°F for the thighs. Transfer the fried chicken to the wire rack to drain.

SAUSAGE GRAVY

MAKES ABOUT 1¼ CUPS

1 pound plain pork sausage, casings removed

3 tablespoons all-purpose flour

¾ cup whole milk, plus more as needed

Kosher salt and freshly ground black pepper

HEAT A large saucepan over medium heat for 1 minute. Add the sausage and cook, breaking it up into small chunks with a wooden spoon as it cooks, until browned and plenty of fond (the layer of cooked-on browned bits) has formed on the bottom of the pan, about 4 minutes. Add the flour and cook, stirring, for 2 minutes more. Slowly add the milk, stirring and scraping up all the browned bits from the bottom of the pan, and simmer gently until thickened, about

5 minutes. Add more milk to the gravy as necessary to reach your desired consistency. Season liberally with pepper and season with salt, if necessary.

WAFFLES

MAKES 6 WAFFLES

1 cup cornmeal

1 cup all-purpose flour

2 teaspoons baking soda

3 large eggs, separated

½ cup buttermilk, plus more as necessary

½ cup (1 stick) unsalted butter, melted and cooled

Nonstick cooking spray

IN A large bowl, whisk together the cornmeal, flour, and baking soda. In a medium bowl, using a handheld mixer, whip the egg whites on medium-high speed until they hold stiff peaks; set aside.

IN A separate medium bowl, whisk together the egg yolks, buttermilk, and melted butter to combine, then gently whisk the egg mixture into the dry ingredients until a mostly smooth batter forms, adding more buttermilk if necessary. Gently fold in the egg whites until just barely combined.

SPRAY A waffle iron with cooking spray. Cook the waffles according to the manufacturer's instructions. As they are done, transfer the waffles to a wire rack.

FUN FACT
This whole lasagna rings in at over 5,000 calories, before syrup is even added. I cannot, in good conscience, recommend that you actually make one of these.

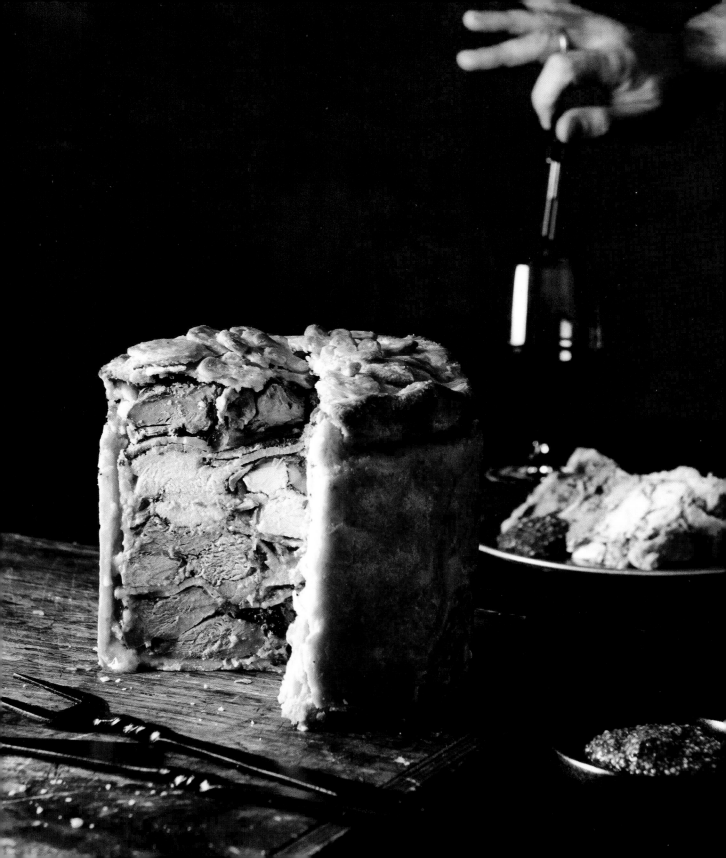

Game of Thrones is home to some of the most sumptuous (and sometimes deadly) feasts in all of fiction, taking full advantage of its antiquated-fantasy world to dream up dishes every bit as imaginative and sprawling as its cast of characters—and that's just from the show. The books describe a litany of regionally unique dishes, ranging from the nomadic offal of the Dothraki to the unrestrained opulence of King's Landing. In the first of what I am sure will be several *GoT*-themed episodes, I tried to run the gamut of Seven Kingdoms' cuisine. I was particularly intimidated by raised game pie, a notoriously difficult dish with difficult-to-source ingredients, but my patience (and investment) eventually paid off. Pro tip: Don't drink the wine.

PIGEON PIE WITH WILD GAME

SERVES 8

VERDICT: Dripping with regality (and meat juices), raised game pie is a dastardly difficult but ultimately rewarding challenge for the home cook.

---

6 ounces lard (about ¾ cup), plus more
　　for greasing

¼ cup dried cherries

½ cup Madeira wine

1 tablespoon vegetable oil

½ Vidalia onion, diced (about 4 tablespoons)

2 tablespoons unsalted butter

¼ cup finely chopped apple

½ cup sliced cremini mushrooms

2 pounds squab breasts, sliced

3 teaspoons finely chopped fresh rosemary

5 teaspoons finely chopped fresh thyme leaves

5 teaspoons kosher salt

3 teaspoons freshly ground black pepper

1 pound boneless wild boar, cut into
　　2-inch pieces

1 garlic clove, minced

2 teaspoons finely chopped fresh sage

1 pound boneless rabbit, cut into 2-inch pieces

16 ounces all-purpose flour (about 3¾ cups),
　　plus more for dusting

3½ ounces bread flour (about ¾ cup plus
　　2 tablespoons)

6 slices bacon, halved crosswise

1 large egg, beaten

Whole-grain mustard, for serving (optional)

(recipe continues)

PREHEAT THE oven to 400°F. Liberally grease a tall 6¼-inch-diameter springform pan with lard.

IN A small bowl, combine the dried cherries and Madeira. Let soak for 1 hour or until the cherries are rehydrated. Drain the cherries and discard the soaking liquid.

MEANWHILE, HEAT the oil in a small sauté pan over medium heat. Add the onion and cook, stirring, for 5 minutes or until lightly browned and translucent. Transfer the onion to a small bowl and wipe out the pan.

MELT 1 tablespoon of the butter in the pan over medium heat until foaming. Add the apple and cook, stirring, for 5 minutes or until softened. Transfer the apple to a small bowl and wipe out the pan.

MELT THE remaining 1 tablespoon of butter in the pan over medium heat until foaming. Add the mushrooms and cook, stirring, for 5 to 7 minutes or until their moisture has evaporated. Transfer the mushrooms to a small bowl.

IN A medium bowl, combine 1 pound of the squab, 2 tablespoons of the onion, the cherries, 1 teaspoon of the rosemary, 1 teaspoon of the thyme, 1 teaspoon of the salt, and 1 teaspoon of the pepper.

IN ANOTHER medium bowl, combine the wild boar, garlic, remaining 2 tablespoons onion, 1 teaspoon of the rosemary, 1 teaspoon of the thyme, 1 teaspoon of the salt, and 1 teaspoon of the pepper.

IN A third medium bowl, combine the remaining 1 pound squab, the apple, sage, 1 teaspoon of the thyme, 1 teaspoon of the salt, and 1 teaspoon of the pepper.

IN A fourth medium bowl, combine the rabbit, mushrooms, 2 teaspoons of the thyme, the remaining 1 teaspoon rosemary, and 1 teaspoon of the salt. Keep all the meats separate.

WHISK TOGETHER the flours and remaining 1 teaspoon salt in a large heatproof bowl.

IN A small saucepan, combine the lard and ¾ cup plus 2 tablespoons water and bring to a bare simmer over medium heat. Pour the lard mixture into the flour and stir with a wooden spoon until a shaggy dough forms. Once it's cool enough to handle, knead the dough until smooth and tacky.

RESERVE A third of the dough and cover with a warm, damp towel. Roll out the remaining dough to a 24-inch round. Roll the round onto your rolling pin and unroll it over the prepared pan. Gently coax the dough down into the pan and press it into the corners, patching as necessary to seal it, leaving a 1-inch overhang. Fill the pastry as follows: the cherry squab, a layer of bacon (about 4 pieces), the wild boar, another layer of bacon, the apple squab, the remaining bacon, and finally the rabbit. Make sure the meat is packed tightly and fills every crevice. Roll out some of the reserved dough into a round large enough to cover the pan and place it over the filling. Crimp the edges, as you would with a piecrust, to create a tight seal. Cut a small hole in the center of the top crust to allow steam to escape and decorate as desired with the remaining dough. Brush the top with the beaten egg.

BAKE THE pie for 30 minutes, then reduce the oven temperature to 325°F and bake for 1½ hours more, or until the pastry is browned and the internal temperature of the pie registers 165°F. Remove from the oven and trim the crust as necessary to ease the eventual release of the pie from the springform pan, but do not remove it from the pan. Let the pie cool in the pan for at least 2 hours, or ideally refrigerate it overnight.

RELEASE AND remove the springform ring from the pan. Slice the pie and serve with whole-grain mustard.

FUN FACT

This was, at the time, the most expensive *Binging with Babish* episode ever produced, with ingredients and tools clocking in at around $400. Exotic game, pints of blood, and specialized equipment tend to add up!

DOTHRAKI BLOOD PIE

SERVES 8

VERDICT: Dothraki Blood Pie is pretty gross.

CRUST

7 ounces all-purpose flour (about 1¾ cups)

1 teaspoon kosher salt

¾ cup (1½ sticks) unsalted butter, cut into 1-inch pieces and chilled, plus more for greasing

2 to 3 tablespoons ice water

FILLING

1 pound pork fat, finely diced

1 medium Spanish onion, diced

2 tablespoons rolled oats

1 tablespoon smoked paprika

1 teaspoon paprika

1 teaspoon ground allspice

1 teaspoon freshly grated nutmeg

2 cups pig's blood (available at specialty butcher shops)

1 cup heavy cream

Kosher salt and freshly ground black pepper

1 (4-ounce) log fresh goat cheese, cut into 5 rounds

2 large figs, quartered

CRUST

PLACE THE flour and salt in a food processor and pulse to combine. Add the butter and pulse until the mixture resembles bread crumbs. Transfer to a large bowl. Sprinkle in the ice water, folding it in with a rubber spatula until a shaggy dough forms. Turn the dough out onto a floured work surface and pat it into a 5-inch disc. Wrap the dough in plastic wrap and refrigerate for at least an hour or up to overnight.

PREHEAT THE oven to 350°F. Liberally butter a 9-inch pie plate.

TRANSFER THE dough to a floured work surface and pound it with a rolling pin until doubled in width. Roll out the dough to a round about ⅛ inch thick, making sure not to overwork it. Roll the round onto your rolling pin and unroll it over the prepared pie plate. Trim the edges of the dough as desired. Line the dough with parchment paper and fill with pie weights or dried beans. Bake for 10 minutes, or until the crust turns golden. Remove the weights and parchment paper, transfer the pie pan to a wire rack, and let cool for 20 minutes. Keep the oven on.

FILLING

HEAT A high-walled skillet over medium heat. Add the pork fat and cook, stirring, until translucent, about 5 minutes. Add the onion and cook, stirring occasionally, until soft, about 10 minutes. Remove from the heat and let cool completely.

STIR IN the oats, smoked paprika, paprika, allspice, and nutmeg and then add the blood and cream to the onion mixture. Season with salt and pepper. Stir well to combine and pour into the parbaked piecrust. Bake for 20 minutes, or until the filling just begins to set. Top with the goat cheese and figs and bake for 10 minutes more. Remove from the oven, let cool for 1 hour, then slice into wedges and serve.

FUN FACT

This would not be the last time I would eat blood, as I elected to eat a coagulated blood cube on *Good Mythical Morning* some months later. There's probably more blood in my future.

LEMON CAKES

MAKES 9 INDIVIDUAL CAKES

VERDICT: Sansa's Lemon Cakes are a simple, elegant teatime pleasure.

CAKE

½ cup (1 stick) unsalted butter, at room temperature, plus more for greasing

8½ ounces all-purpose flour (about 2 cups), plus more for dusting

1 teaspoon baking powder

1 teaspoon baking soda

1 teaspoon fine salt

1 cup sugar

3 large eggs

1 cup buttermilk

Zest and juice of 2 lemons

CANDIED LEMON SLICES

1 cup sugar

2 lemons, sliced ⅛ inch thick and seeded

LEMON CURD

1 cup fresh lemon juice

½ cup sugar

3 large eggs

6 tablespoons (¾ stick) unsalted butter, cut into pieces

Whipped Cream (see page 186), for serving (optional)

CAKE

PREHEAT THE oven to 350°F. Butter a 9 x 13-inch baking pan and dust it with flour, tapping out any excess. Line the bottom of the pan with parchment paper rounds cut to fit.

IN A medium bowl, whisk together the flour, baking powder, baking soda, and salt.

IN THE bowl of a stand mixer fitted with the paddle attachment, cream together the butter and sugar on medium-high speed. With the mixer on medium-low speed, beat in 1 egg at a time, then increase the speed to medium and beat for 1 minute more, or until light and ribbony. Add the dry ingredients and mix on low speed until combined. Add the buttermilk, lemon zest, and lemon juice and beat on medium-high speed until the batter is light and fluffy, about 3 minutes.

POUR THE batter into the prepared pan and bake for 25 to 30 minutes, until a tester inserted into the cake comes out clean.

(recipe continues)

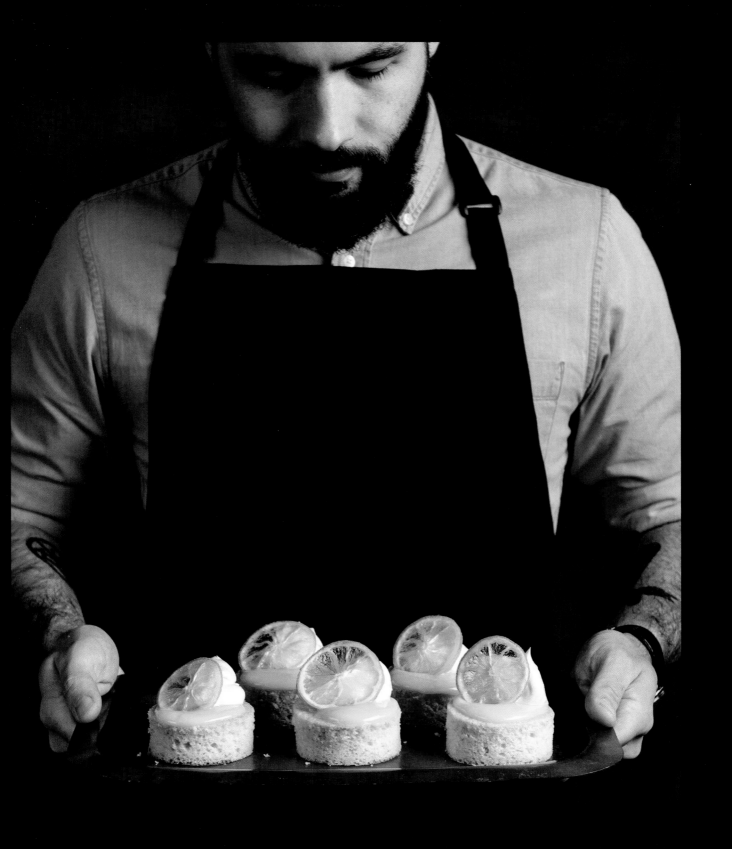

Remove from the oven and let cool in the pan for 30 minutes. Invert the cake onto a wire rack, remove the parchment paper, and let cool for 30 minutes more.

CANDIED LEMON SLICES

WHILE THE cake bakes, line a baking sheet with parchment paper. In a medium saucepan, combine the sugar and ½ cup water and bring to a simmer over medium heat. Add the lemon slices and cook for 15 minutes, or until soft and translucent. Using tongs, transfer the lemon slices to the lined baking sheet and let cool.

LEMON CURD

IN A wide saucepan, whisk together the lemon juice, sugar, and eggs over medium-low heat. Add the butter and cook, whisking continuously, until thick and pudding-like. Transfer the lemon curd to a bowl and refrigerate for at least 1 hour before using.

ASSEMBLY

FLIP THE cake right-side up onto a work surface. Using a biscuit cutter, stamp out 9 rounds from the cake. For each serving, dollop a round of cake with lemon curd, top with a candied lemon slice, and serve with whipped cream, if desired.

TACO TOWN TACO

MAKES 1 TACO, LARGE ENOUGH TO SERVE 8

In this first subscriber-milestone episode, I decided to try to tackle something ridiculous, something so obviously fictional that no one in their right mind would try to make it at home. Doing so yielded a fourteen-inch-long, fifteen-layer-thick deep-fried monstrosity, just barely resembling an actual taco in form. Mixing competing flavors and textures with wild abandon, the Taco Town Taco ended up being consumed almost entirely, with my "dinner" guests describing it as "not as bad" as they thought it would be. Remarkably, there's only one unfeasible aspect to the cartoonish dish: its inclusion of an inedible corn husk as one of its layers. For shame, *SNL* staff writers.

VERDICT: The Taco Town Taco is a parody for a reason: this Russian doll of a taco is not worth the time, effort, or money spent to create it at home. A few key substitutions (swap merguez and Gruyère for chorizo and cheddar) can make it more palatable, but you're better off stopping several steps prior to wrapping it up in a blueberry pancake.

CREPE

2 large eggs

1 cup whole milk

1 cup all-purpose flour

2 tablespoons vegetable oil

1 teaspoon kosher salt

Unsalted butter, for greasing

BLUEBERRY PANCAKE

1 cup all-purpose flour

1 tablespoon sugar

1 teaspoon baking powder

½ teaspoon baking soda

¾ cup whole milk

1 large egg

2 tablespoons unsalted butter, melted and cooled, plus more for greasing

½ cup frozen blueberries, thawed

PICO DE GALLO

¼ cup chopped tomato

¼ cup chopped onion

½ teaspoon kosher salt

1 teaspoon fresh lime juice

1 tablespoon chopped fresh cilantro

BEER BATTER

3 cups all-purpose flour

3 cups cornstarch

3 (12-ounce) cans lager

3 tablespoons kosher salt

4 large eggs

(ingredients continue)

SOUTHWESTERN SAUCE

1 tablespoon sour cream

1 tablespoon mayonnaise

1 teaspoon paprika

1 teaspoon cayenne pepper

1 teaspoon chili powder

GUACAMOLITO SAUCE

¼ cup smooth guacamole

¼ cup sour cream

REMAINING WRAPS AND TOPPINGS

1 tablespoon unsalted butter

4 ounces cremini mushrooms, sliced

2 ounces ground beef

2 teaspoons taco seasoning

1½ to 2 gallons vegetable oil, for frying

1 hard taco shell

1 tablespoon nacho cheese, warmed

1 ounce shredded lettuce

1 ounce chopped tomatoes

2 tablespoons refried beans

1 small flour tortilla

2 ounces shredded Monterey Jack cheese

1 medium corn tortilla, toasted

1 chalupa shell (I got mine from Taco Bell)

1 large corn husk

1 large egg, scrambled

1 merguez sausage, cooked and sliced

3 ounces Gruyère cheese, shredded

1 (12-inch) frozen meat lover's pizza, baked according to the package directions

6 (15-ounce) cans vegetarian chili, heated

NOTE: *I strayed from the original recipe to discard the corn husk from the taco (because corn husks are inedible), and I recommend omitting the blueberry pancake altogether. To improve on the original further, substitute fresh pork chorizo for the merguez, and Monterey Jack for the Gruyère cheese, then hold the pico de gallo and skip the baking step. Frying this taco is dangerous—make sure to use extra-long/wide tongs, protective gloves, and extreme caution when lowering it into the hot oil. Better yet, just don't make this thing at all, please.*

CREPE

COMBINE THE eggs, milk, flour, vegetable oil, and salt in a blender. Blend on high speed until completely smooth, 1 to 2 minutes. Butter and heat a 13-inch crepe griddle, add ½ cup of the batter, and use a wooden dowel to spread the batter into a thin layer. Cook according to the manufacturer's instructions and transfer to a plate. Wrap with aluminum foil to keep warm. Reserve the remaining batter to make more crepes another time.

BLUEBERRY PANCAKE

IN A large bowl, whisk together the flour, sugar, baking powder, and baking soda. Add the milk, egg, and butter and whisk until a slightly lumpy batter forms. Butter and heat a 13-inch crepe griddle, add about ¾ cup of the batter, and spread it to the edges of the griddle. Scatter some of the blueberries over the top and cook until bubbles begin forming all over the pancake, the edges turn glossy, and the bottom has browned. Flip and cook until the pancake is fluffy and thick. Transfer to a plate and cover with aluminum foil to make the pancake as flexible as possible. Reserve the remaining batter and blueberries to make more pancakes another time.

PICO DE GALLO

PLACE ALL the ingredients in a small bowl and toss well to combine.

BEER BATTER

IN A large bowl, combine all the ingredients and whisk until smooth. Transfer the batter to a 9 x 13-inch baking dish and set aside.

SOUTHWESTERN SAUCE

IN A small bowl, whisk together all the ingredients until incorporated. Set aside until ready to serve.

GUACAMOLITO SAUCE

IN A small bowl, stir together the guacamole and sour cream. Set aside until ready to serve.

REMAINING WRAPS AND TOPPINGS

PREHEAT THE oven to 350°F.

MELT THE butter in a small skillet over medium heat until foaming. Add the mushrooms and cook, stirring, for 5 to 7 minutes or until their moisture has evaporated and the mushrooms are browned. Transfer to a small bowl and wipe out the pan.

HEAT THE skillet over medium-high heat. Add the beef and cook, stirring, until browned all over, about 5 minutes. Add the taco seasoning and 2 to 3 tablespoons water (or as directed on

FUN FACT
Deep-frying this thing was the single most frightening experience of my life. Almost two gallons of hot oil and about ten pounds worth of taco are a "recipe for disaster," you might say. Exercise extreme caution if attempting this one!

the package) and cook until thick, about 2 minutes. Fill a very large pot (at least 15 inches in diameter) with vegetable oil to a depth of 3 inches, being sure to leave 6 inches of headroom so the oil doesn't overflow when you add the taco. Heat the oil over medium-high heat to 350°F. Set a wire rack on a rimmed baking sheet.

MEANWHILE, BEGIN assembling the Taco Town Taco: Fill the hard taco shell with ground beef, then top with the nacho cheese, lettuce, tomatoes, and southwestern sauce. Spread the refried beans on the flour tortilla and wrap that around the taco shell. Scatter the Monterey Jack cheese on the toasted corn tortilla and wrap that around the flour tortilla. Fill the chalupa shell with the guacamolito sauce and place the multilayered taco inside. Transfer the chalupa taco to the corn husk, top with the pico de gallo, and bake for 5 minutes on a baking sheet, or until warmed through.

(recipe continues)

MEANWHILE, SCATTER the scrambled egg, merguez, Gruyère, and mushrooms on the crepe. Remove the taco from the oven, pull out and discard the corn husk, and wrap the crepe around the taco. Wrap the meat lover's pizza around the crepe-taco, then wrap the blueberry pancake around the pizza. Press together as tightly as possible without breaking any of the layers and secure with long wooden skewers. Dip the entire taco in the beer batter, letting any excess drip off. Very carefully lower the battered taco into the hot oil, using a metal ladle to baste it with oil if it's not completely submerged. Fry for about 10 minutes on each side, until golden brown and crispy all over. Remove from the oil and let cool for 5 to 10 minutes on the rack.

FILL A canvas tote bag with the chili and place the taco inside. Enjoy?

LEMON PEPPER WET

SERVES 8

Donald Glover's Hotlanta-based dramedy doesn't feature a whole lot of food, but it managed to get the whole world crazy curious about the storied Lemon Pepper Wet wings. It goes so far as to treat them like the MacGuffin briefcase in *Pulp Fiction*, letting them cast their saucy glow on the faces of their beholders, never actually showing them outright. There seem to be two major styles: lemon-pepper seasoning mixed with either clarified butter or traditional Buffalo wing sauce. The latter, popularized by J. R. Crickets (and the version portrayed in the show), were originally named "fester" wings by their own chef, who reportedly despised them. The sour-and-spicy mix is certainly a strange one, but a tasty and unique combination best enjoyed while binging the acclaimed series.

VERDICT: Strange but tasty, Lemon Pepper Wet wings are a regional delight worth trying at home. Both traditional deep-frying and the oven-frying method outlined below yield perfectly crispy, juicy wings.

DEEP-FRIED OR OVEN-FRIED WINGS

2 pounds chicken wings

Vegetable oil, for frying

2 teaspoons kosher salt (optional, for oven-frying)

2 teaspoons baking powder (optional, for oven-frying)

J. R. CRICKETS FESTER WINGS

1 tablespoon lemon-pepper seasoning

¼ cup Buffalo sauce

AMERICAN DELI LEMON PEPPER WINGS

1 tablespoon lemon-pepper seasoning

¼ cup clarified butter or ghee, melted

Blue cheese dressing, for serving

(recipe continues)

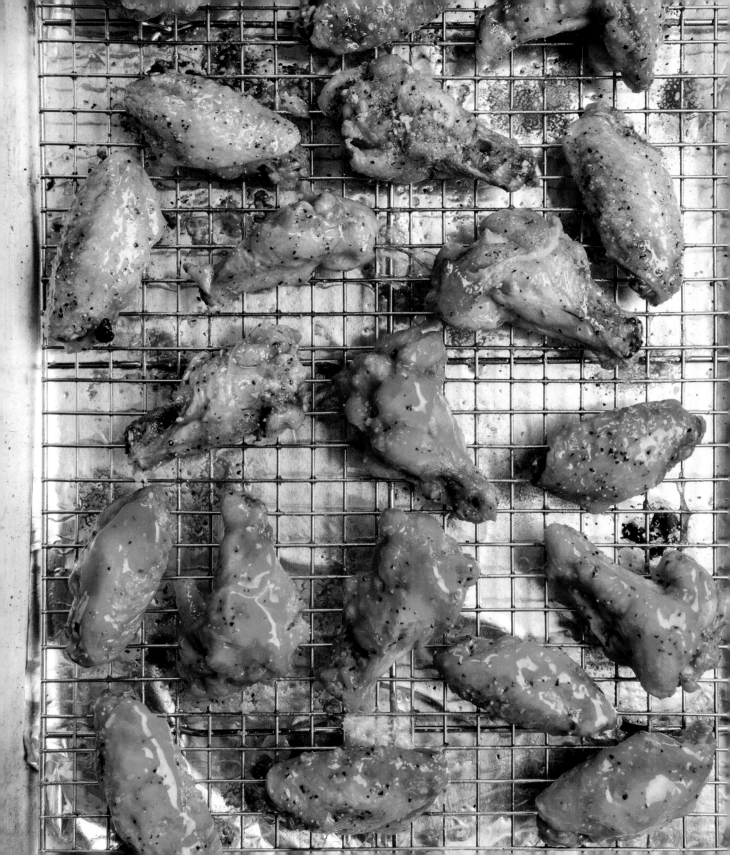

WINGS

SEPARATE THE wings at the joints into flats and drumettes.

TO DEEP–FRY the wings, fill a large heavy pot with vegetable oil to a depth of 2 inches. Heat the oil over medium-high heat to 350°F. Add the wings in batches to avoid overcrowding the pot and fry until golden brown and crisp, 7 to 10 minutes. Transfer to a wire rack set over paper towels to drain.

TO OVEN–FRY the wings, line a rimmed baking sheet with a wire rack. Place the kosher salt and baking powder in a small bowl and stir to combine. Put the wings in a large bowl, sprinkle the salt mixture over the wings, and toss until thoroughly coated. Transfer the wings to the rack set on the baking sheet, spacing them apart so they're not touching. Refrigerate overnight, uncovered.

WHEN READY to cook the wings, preheat the oven to 450°F.

REMOVE THE wings from the refrigerator and let stand at room temperature for 30 minutes. Bake on the rack for 35 to 45 minutes, until brown and crisp. Remove from the oven.

J. R. CRICKETS FESTER WINGS

PLACE THE wings in a large bowl. Toss them with the lemon-pepper seasoning, followed by the Buffalo sauce. Transfer to a plate and serve with blue cheese dressing.

AMERICAN DELI LEMON PEPPER WINGS

PLACE THE wings in a large bowl. Toss them with the lemon pepper seasoning, followed by the clarified butter. Transfer to a plate and serve with blue cheese dressing.

FUN FACT

This episode was the first time I had prepared the make-ahead element of the recipe prior to shooting, so I was able to immediately show the results of air-drying in the refrigerator overnight. A small detail, but important to the evolution of the show.

MONSTER CAKE

SERVES 6

Ah, *Binging with Babish*'s first-ever foray into video game foods. *Breath of the Wild* spoiled me rotten with cooking playing an integral role in its gameplay, whipping up and discovering different dishes by tossing together ingredients in a wood-fired wok. Some were familiar (risottos, stir-fries, salmon meunière), while others were tinged with fantasy-meets-reality strangeness (spicy simmered fruit, meat-stuffed pumpkins, sautéed rocks). I was keen to dig into some of the more familiar dishes, but having recently acquired a small dram of ube (purple yam) extract, I was most curious how I could pull off the otherworldly purple "monster" dishes made with a similar-looking extract. I decided to use the famously funky durian (also available in-game) to give the cake a monstrous edge, something I recommend omitting if you are at all averse to sweet-garlicky-garbage fruit smells.

VERDICT: Monster cake, challenging to a home cook's skills and palate alike, also has a number of difficult-to-source ingredients. Ube extract has a lovely flavor and would make a positive addition to any pantry, but purple food coloring and vanilla would make acceptable substitutes.

WHITE CHOCOLATE HORNS

6 ounces white chocolate

¼ cup light corn syrup

Ube extract or purple food coloring

Cornstarch, sifted, for dusting

CAKE

½ cup vegetable oil, plus more for greasing

2½ cups all-purpose flour

1 tablespoon baking powder

1½ cups granulated sugar

1 teaspoon fine salt

7 large eggs, separated

¾ cup whole milk

4 ounces grated ube or other purple or white yam

Ube extract or purple food coloring

FROSTING

1 (8-ounce) package cream cheese, at room temperature

4 ounces goat butter or unsalted cow butter, at room temperature

(ingredients continue)

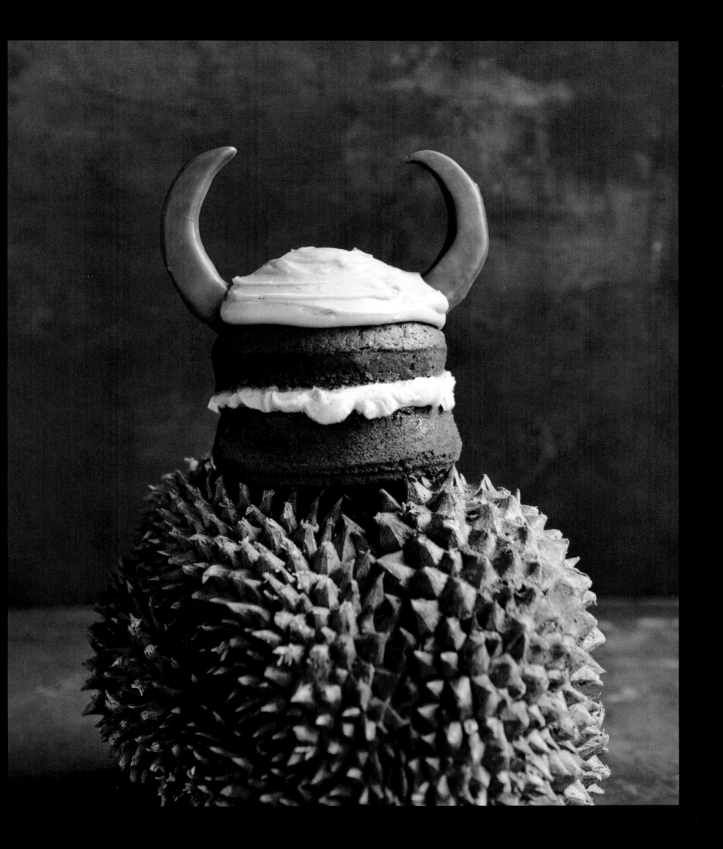

4 cups confectioners' sugar, sifted

Ube extract or purple food coloring

4 ounces durian flesh or other tropical fruit, such as coconut; pineapple, pureed; or mango, pureed

Brown food coloring

WHITE CHOCOLATE HORNS

FILL A pot about one-quarter full with water and bring to a simmer. Place a heatproof bowl on top so that the water is not touching the bottom of the bowl. Place the white chocolate in the bowl above the simmering water. Stir until completely melted and remove from the heat. Fold in the corn syrup and stir until well incorporated and a thick paste forms. Transfer the chocolate to a sheet of plastic wrap and wrap tightly. Let stand in a cool place for 24 hours. Remove from the plastic wrap and, using gloved hands, massage a few drops of ube extract into the chocolate until the desired color is achieved. If the chocolate starts to become oily, dust it with a bit of cornstarch. Shape the chocolate into twelve horns and set aside or refrigerate them if the chocolate needs to firm up.

CAKE

PREHEAT THE oven to 350°F. Lightly oil six 4-inch mini springform pans (or six wells of a muffin pan or one 9 x 13-inch baking pan).

INTO A large bowl, sift together the flour, baking powder, ¾ cup of the granulated sugar, and the salt. Whisk to combine. In a medium bowl, whisk together the egg yolks, vegetable oil, milk, and grated ube. Whisk in ube extract until the

mixture is deep purple, then whisk the ube mixture into the dry ingredients.

IN THE bowl of a stand mixer fitted with the whisk attachment, beat the egg whites on medium speed until light and frothy, about 2 minutes. Add the remaining ¾ cup granulated sugar and beat on medium-high speed until stiff, glossy peaks form, about 3 minutes. Gently fold the egg whites into the cake batter, taking care not to deflate them.

FILL THE prepared cake pan(s) three-quarters full with batter. Bake for 35 to 40 minutes, until a tester inserted into the center of the cakes comes out clean and the exterior of the cakes is golden brown. Let cool in the pans for 10 minutes, then remove the cakes from the pans and let cool completely on a wire rack.

FROSTING

IN THE bowl of a stand mixer fitted with the paddle attachment, beat the cream cheese with the butter on medium speed until incorporated. Add the confectioners' sugar and mix on low speed, gradually increasing the speed as the sugar is incorporated, until thick, about 1 minute. Transfer half the frosting to a medium bowl and reserve the rest in the stand mixer bowl. Stir the ube extract into the frosting in the medium bowl until the frosting is light purple and set aside. Add the durian to the frosting in the stand mixer bowl and beat on medium speed until incorporated. Beat in brown food coloring until the desired color is achieved. Transfer the durian frosting to a pastry bag fitted with a decorative tip.

ASSEMBLY

SLICE EACH cake in half horizontally to create two even layers. (If using a 9 x 13-inch pan, use a biscuit cutter to stamp out 12 rounds of cake.) Spread a generous layer of light-purple frosting on the bottom halves and close with the top halves. Pipe a cone of durian frosting onto each cake, press a white chocolate horn into each side of the cone, and serve.

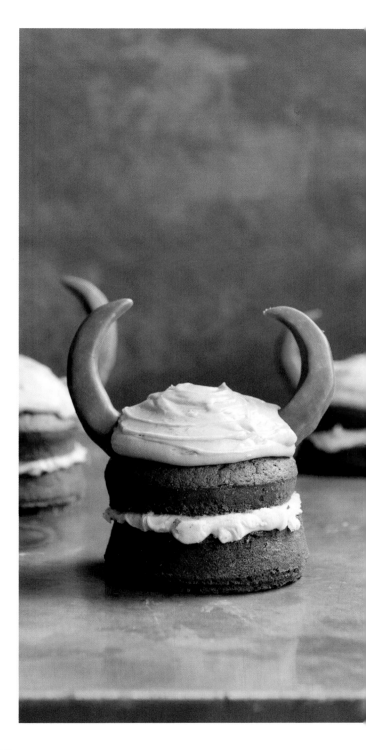

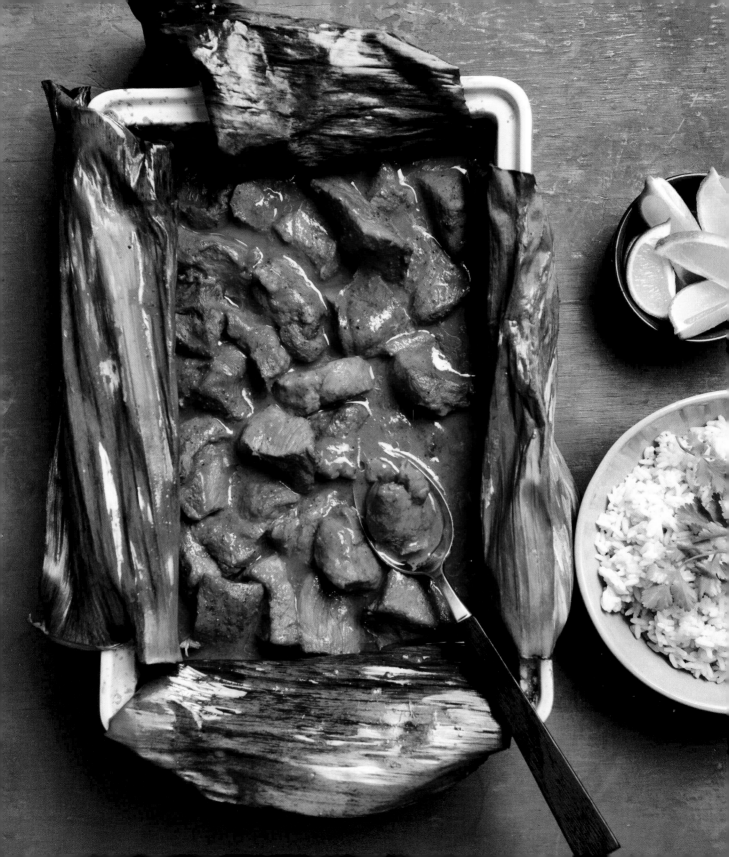

PUERCO PIBIL

SERVES 8 TO 10

Is pork ever worth killing over? This is the question posed to us by Hollywood's own guerrilla filmmaker, Robert Rodriguez, in his strange-but-pretty 2003 shoot-'em-up, *Once Upon a Time in Mexico*. Rodriguez is an established foodie himself, going so far as to have a "menu" of his specialties laminated for all to see in his home kitchen and including cooking tutorials in his films' special features. In the continuing efforts to make *Binging with Babish* as rigorously accurate as possible, this recipe proved to be a bit of a challenge: in its most authentic form, *puerco pibil* is slowly stewed in banana leaves. While widely available in New York City, it's one of those things you happen across and say, "huh!" but can never find when you have an episode to release the next day.

VERDICT: While not worth icing the cook over (I hope), *puerco pibil* is relatively easy, completely delicious, and an excellent introduction to some more authentic Mexican cuisine for those of us accustomed to the crumbled beef/refried beans/yellow cheese now endemic north of the border.

5 tablespoons annatto seeds

1 tablespoon whole black peppercorns

1 teaspoon whole cloves

2 teaspoons cumin seeds

8 allspice berries

½ cup orange juice

½ cup distilled white vinegar

Juice of 5 lemons

8 garlic cloves

2 habanero chiles, seeded, deveined, and chopped

2 tablespoons kosher salt

Splash of high-quality añejo tequila

5 pound bone-in pork shoulder, trimmed and cut into 2-inch cubes, bone discarded

2 banana leaves, cut into 16-inch lengths

4 cups apple cider vinegar

1 red onion, sliced

1 tablespoon mustard seeds

Corn tortillas, store-bought or homemade (see page 63), toasted, for serving

Cotija cheese, crumbled, for serving

(recipe continues)

IN A small dry skillet, combine the annatto seeds, peppercorns, cloves, cumin, and allspice and toast over medium heat for 3 to 5 minutes, until fragrant. Transfer to a spice grinder and process until ground into a fine powder, 2 to 3 minutes. Transfer to a blender and add the orange juice, white vinegar, lemon juice, garlic, habaneros, salt, and tequila. Blend on high speed until the marinade is well combined, 30 to 60 seconds.

PLACE THE pork in a large resealable plastic bag, pour in the marinade, seal, and massage until the pork is evenly coated. Let marinate at room temperature for 30 minutes or in the refrigerator for up to 4 hours.

PREHEAT THE oven to 325°F.

LINE A 9 x 13-inch baking dish with the banana leaves and pour the pork and the marinade into the center. Wrap the leaves around the pork, then wrap the baking dish tightly in aluminum foil to trap in the steam. Roast for 4 hours, or until the pork is fork-tender. Remove from the oven and unwrap the foil and banana leaves.

MEANWHILE, IN a medium saucepan, bring the apple cider vinegar to a boil over medium heat. In a large heatproof bowl, combine the red onion and mustard seeds and pour over the boiling vinegar. Let steep for 30 minutes.

TO SERVE, make tacos with the pork and tortillas, and top with cotija cheese and the pickled red onion.

VARIATION

Instead of making tacos, serve the *pibil* with rice, lime wedges, and chopped fresh cilantro.

FUN FACT

I can't say I'm as big a fan of this film as I was in high school, but back then, I was pretty obsessed. I watched the DVD and its special features relentlessly, getting inspired not only to cook, but to get into film. Rodriguez's "get out there and make it yourself" mentality was way ahead of its time, and resonates with me to this day.

COURTESAN AU CHOCOLAT

MAKES 12 PASTRY TOWERS

Like so many dishes featured on the show, I put off making *courtesan au chocolat* out of pure fear. The pastry is not unlike the film from which it hails: a delicate, meticulously constructed, filigree embodiment of fussiness itself. Done right, it's a thing of beauty—done wrong, it's a pretentious waste of time and energy. Wes Anderson decided to dish out his magnum opus with *The Grand Budapest Hotel*, so I wasn't about to serve up some saggy leaning tower of failure; so, after a few practice rounds with the notoriously difficult choux pastry, I finally took a crack at the dish I had wanted to try since before even starting the show.

VERDICT: Is this fastidious and fussy confection really "out of this world"? No, not really—the chocolate *crème pâtissière* dominates, and the icing makes the whole affair almost sickly sweet. Don't get me wrong—it's good, but it sure ain't worth the effort.

PÂTE À CHOUX

1 cup all-purpose flour

Pinch of salt

Pinch of granulated sugar

1 stick (½ cup) unsalted butter

4 large eggs, beaten

CHOCOLATE CRÈME PÂTISSIÈRE

¼ cup granulated sugar

1 tablespoon all-purpose flour

1½ teaspoons cornstarch

3 large egg yolks

2 cups whole milk

8 ounces dark chocolate, chopped

ICINGS

1 cup confectioners' sugar

¼ cup whole milk

Pink, green, and purple food coloring

STRUCTURAL FROSTING

2 cups confectioners' sugar

4 tablespoons (½ stick) unsalted butter, melted

1 tablespoon whole milk, plus more

Blue food coloring

FILIGREE AND ASSEMBLY

4 ounces white chocolate, chopped

Yellow food coloring

12 cocoa beans

(recipe continues)

PÂTE À CHOUX

PREHEAT THE oven to 400°F. Line two baking sheets with silicone baking mats or parchment paper.

IN A small bowl, whisk together the flour, salt, and granulated sugar and set aside.

IN A medium saucepan, combine 1 cup water and the butter and heat over medium heat, stirring, until the butter has melted. Add the dry ingredients and stir with a wooden spoon over medium-low heat until the dough pulls away from the sides of the pan and forms a ball. Remove from the heat and let cool for 1 minute. Add the eggs and stir until well incorporated.

TRANSFER THE dough to a pastry bag fitted with a wide tip. Pipe 12 rounds of dough onto the prepared baking sheets in three sizes: ½ inch, 1 inch, and 1½ inches. Bake for 15 to 20 minutes, or until the choux puffs have risen and are golden. Remove from the oven. Using a small knife, cut a hole in the bottom of each choux puff and let cool completely.

CHOCOLATE CRÈME PÂTISSIÈRE

IN A large bowl, whisk together the granulated sugar, flour, cornstarch, and egg yolks.

IN A medium saucepan, heat the milk over medium-low heat until steaming. Add the chocolate and whisk until completely incorporated—do not let boil. While whisking continuously, pour half the chocolate milk into the egg mixture and whisk until fully incorporated. Return the mixture to the chocolate milk remaining in the saucepan and cook over low heat, stirring

continuously, until thick enough to coat the back of a spoon, about 3 minutes. Transfer to a heatproof bowl and cover with plastic wrap, pressing the plastic directly against the surface of the pastry cream to prevent a skin from forming. Refrigerate until completely cool, at least 2 hours. Transfer the pastry cream to a pastry bag fitted with a narrow tip.

ICINGS

PLACE THE confectioners' sugar in a medium bowl and slowly whisk in the milk until a thin glaze forms. Divide the glaze among three ramekins and stir a different color food coloring into each, using just enough to tint the icing pink, pale green, and lavender.

STRUCTURAL FROSTING

IN A medium bowl, combine the confectioners' sugar, melted butter, and milk. Using a handheld mixer on medium speed, slowly beat in more milk until a thick frosting forms. Beat in just enough blue food coloring to tint the frosting pale blue.

PIPE THE pastry cream into the hole in the bottom of each choux puff, then dip the tops into one of the three glazes as follows: lavender for the largest, pale green for the medium, and pink for the smallest. Transfer to plates and let the glaze harden.

FILIGREE

MEANWHILE, FILL a pot about one-quarter full of water and bring to a simmer. Place a heatproof bowl on top so that the water is not touching the bottom of the bowl. Place the white chocolate in the bowl above the simmering water. Stir until completely melted, remove from the heat, and let cool until pipeable. Stir in just enough yellow food coloring to tint the chocolate pale yellow. Transfer to a pastry bag fitted with a very small tip and pipe a filigree (lacelike design) of white chocolate onto each choux puff.

ASSEMBLY

FOR EACH pastry tower, stack three choux puffs on a plate in decreasing size order, starting with the largest puff on the bottom and securing each puff to the one below with a dollop of structural frosting. Dab the top of the smallest puff with structural frosting, garnish with a cocoa bean, and serve.

FITZ'S SANDWICH

MAKES 2 SANDWICHES, PLUS AN EXTRA LOAF OF CIABATTA

I honestly have never seen this show. Solid sandwich, though.

VERDICT: Prosciutto and mozzarella are as classic a sandwich combo as can be imagined, and it's only elevated by homemade ciabatta and pesto aioli. Ciabatta can be a finicky bread due to its high hydration, but your effort is rewarded with a light, airy, chewy interior and a shatteringly crisp crust.

CIABATTA

¾ teaspoon active dry yeast

1¼ cups room-temperature water

15 ounces all-purpose flour (about 3¼ cups), plus more for dusting

1½ teaspoons kosher salt

¼ cup milk, at room temperature

Vegetable oil, for greasing

PESTO AIOLI

¼ cup pine nuts, toasted and cooled

1 cup packed fresh basil leaves

4 garlic cloves: 1 left whole, 3 grated

½ to ¾ cup extra-virgin olive oil, plus more for drizzling

1 large egg yolk

Kosher salt and freshly ground black pepper

SANDWICH

1 pound thinly sliced San Daniele prosciutto

2 (6-ounce) balls buffalo mozzarella, sliced

1 beefsteak tomato, sliced

4 ounces baby arugula

CIABATTA

MAKE THE biga: In a small bowl, combine ¼ teaspoon of the yeast, ¾ cup of the water, and 5 ounces of the flour. Stir until a sticky paste forms. Scrape down the sides of the bowl, cover with plastic wrap, and let ferment at room temperature for 8 to 24 hours (a longer ferment will yield more flavorful bread).

TRANSFER THE biga to the bowl of a stand mixer fitted with the paddle attachment. Add the remaining 10 ounces flour, ½ teaspoon yeast, and ¾ cup water, the salt, and the milk. Mix for 1 to 2 minutes on medium speed, until the ingredients are well incorporated. Replace the paddle attachment with the dough hook and knead on medium to high speed for

(recipe continues)

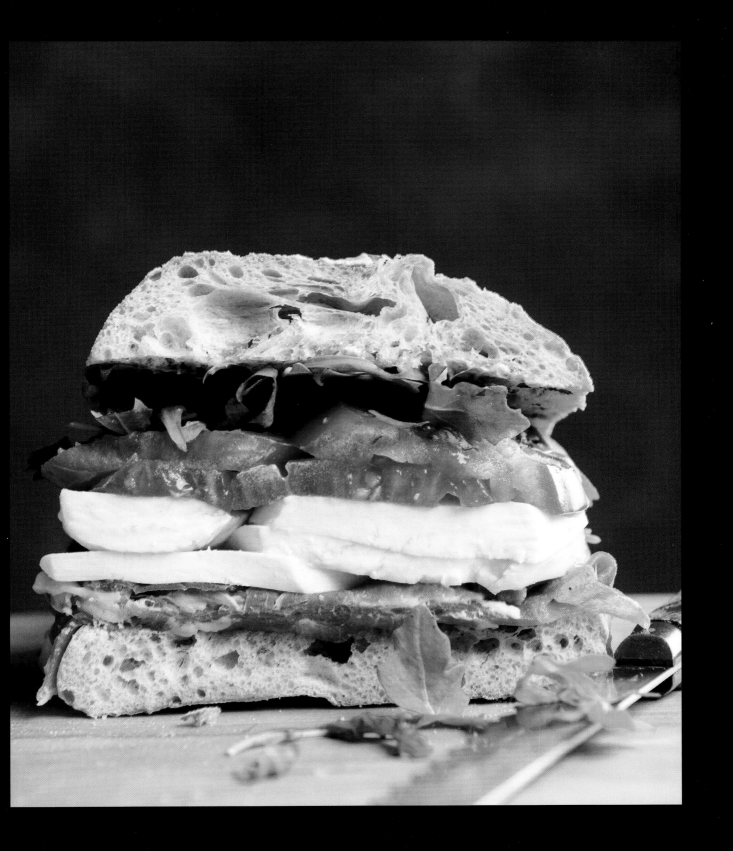

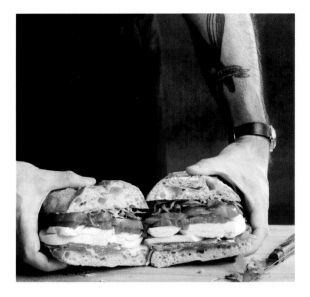

10 minutes, or until the dough is shiny and smooth. Pull the dough off the hook and transfer it to a large oiled bowl. Cover with plastic wrap and let rest for 30 minutes, or until doubled in volume.

OIL A rubber spatula and use it to fold the dough onto itself eight times, rotating the bowl so every part of the dough gets turned. Wrap the bowl again and let the dough rest for 30 minutes more. Repeat the process twice more.

PREHEAT THE oven to 450°F and place a pizza stone on the center rack to preheat.

TURN THE dough out onto a very well-floured work surface. Divide it into 3 equal pieces, and roughly shape each into a 9 x 12-inch rectangle, dusting the work surface with more flour if the dough sticks. Fold one dough rectangle in thirds lengthwise, like a letter, to create a 3 x 12-inch loaf. Repeat with the remaining

dough. Transfer each loaf, seam-side down, to a sheet of parchment paper cut just larger than the size of the loaf. Dust the loaves with flour, cover with plastic wrap, and let rest for 20 minutes.

REMOVE THE plastic wrap and spray the loaves with water from a spray bottle. Transfer the loaves on their parchment to the heated pizza stone. Bake for 22 to 30 minutes, until the ciabatta are deeply golden brown on the outside and the internal temperature registers 210°F. Remove from the oven and let cool completely on a wire rack.

PESTO AIOLI

IN A small food processor or blender, combine the pine nuts, basil, whole garlic clove, and 3 tablespoons of the olive oil. Process until smooth, adding more olive oil as necessary.

IN A medium bowl, combine the egg yolk and grated garlic. While whisking vigorously and continuously, slowly stream in ¼ to ½ cup of the olive oil down the side of the bowl until a thick aioli forms. Whisk in the pesto, then season with salt and pepper.

SANDWICH

SLICE TWO of the ciabatta loaves in half lengthwise. (Reserve the third ciabatta for another use.) Spread a generous amount of pesto aioli on the top halves. Fold the slices of prosciutto in half and shingle them on the bottom halves of the ciabatta to create at least two layers of prosciutto. Top with the mozzarella, tomato, then arugula. Close the sandwiches, slice in half, and serve.

THE ULTIMEATUM

MAKES 1 BURGER, LARGE ENOUGH TO SERVE 4

Regular Show has been, and continues to be, a source of culinary inspiration. Its blue-collar creature characters go to extreme lengths, often risking life and limb, in the pursuit of great (or absurd) foods. From hallucinatory Bloody Marys to sandwiches that will kill you when eaten without the proper accouterments (a mullet and jorts), there are few items that can accurately be re-created, but the Ultimeatum is often the first to come to mind. A send-up of modern "burgercraft," a field plagued by over-the-top grossness and unnecessary haute-cuisine flair, a few tweaks make this celebration of meatiness something worth trying at home.

VERDICT: The Ultimeatum, in its original form, has one fatal flaw: its burger-within-a-burger. There is no way to cook a burger bun within an actual burger patty without absolutely ruining it, so by nixing the burger-ception and upping the meat-and-cheese quotient, we can achieve a burger worthy of its title.

HIMALAYAN KETCHUP

1 tablespoon extra-virgin olive oil

1 (2-inch) knob fresh ginger, peeled and grated

1 (3-inch) knob fresh turmeric, peeled and grated

1 Thai bird's-eye chile, chopped

3 garlic cloves, grated

2 teaspoons chili powder

½ teaspoon mustard seeds

½ teaspoon ground cumin

½ teaspoon ground coriander

½ teaspoon nigella seeds

¼ teaspoon ground cinnamon

½ cup malt vinegar

1 (28-ounce) can crushed tomatoes

⅓ cup packed brown sugar

1 teaspoon Himalayan pink salt

ULTIMEATUM

2 pounds ground beef

4 slices American cheese

4 slices bacon, cooked

Kosher salt and freshly ground black pepper

6 slices pastrami

1 tablespoon vegetable oil

2 slices pepper Jack cheese

2 hamburger buns, toasted

(recipe continues)

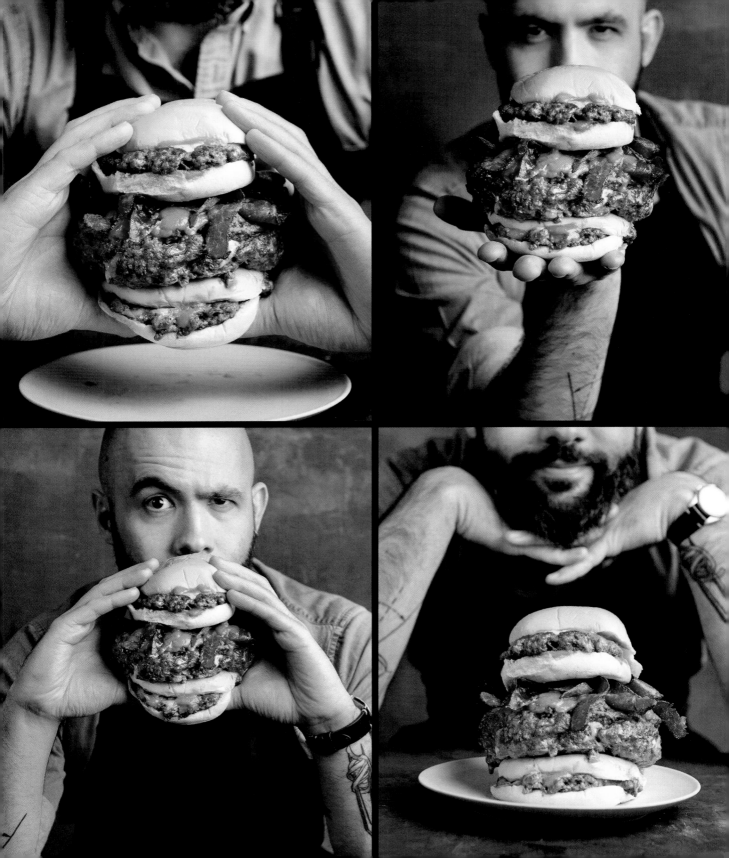

HIMALAYAN KETCHUP

IN A large saucepan, heat the olive oil over medium heat until shimmering. Add the ginger, turmeric, chile, garlic, chili powder, mustard seeds, cumin, coriander, nigella seeds, and cinnamon and cook, stirring, until fragrant, 1 to 2 minutes. Pour in the vinegar and stir to form a paste. Add the crushed tomatoes and brown sugar and stir until well combined. Reduce the heat and cook, uncovered, at a bare simmer for 1 hour, or until thickened.

TRANSFER THE mixture to a high-powered blender and blend on high speed for 3 minutes, or until completely smooth. Strain through a fine-mesh sieve, pressing down on the solids. Whisk in the salt and let cool.

ULTIMEATUM

MAKE THE stuffed patty: Form the ground beef into two 5-inch patties and two 2-ounce balls. Top one of the beef patties with the American cheese and bacon. Cover with the other patty and seal the edges. Season with salt and pepper.

HEAT A skillet over medium-high heat until nearly smoking. Cook the stuffed patty for about 5 minutes on each side, or to your desired doneness. Transfer to a plate. Fry up the pastrami in the meat fat until crisp. Remove from the heat and set aside.

MAKE TWO smash burgers: In a large cast-iron skillet, heat the vegetable oil over high heat until smoking. Place the beef balls several inches apart in the skillet and smash them using a large spatula. Press down firmly on the spatula with a rolling pin or the handle of another spatula until the patties are thin and craggy. Cook for about 1 minute, until the bottom is charred and crispy. Flip and immediately top each patty with the pepper Jack cheese. Remove from the heat, but leave the patties in the pan while you assemble the rest of the dish so the cheese can melt completely.

TOP THE stuffed patty with some Himalayan ketchup and the fried pastrami. Enclose each smashed patty in a hamburger bun, then sandwich the stuffed patty between the smash burgers and serve.

FUN FACT

I had an impromptu Meetup in my apartment with ten complete strangers to help me finish this meatstrosity. We got drunk, it was a good time, and I'm still friends with a few of 'em today.

In a rare instance dry of booze and unclouded by cigarette smoke, Roger Sterling extols a very 1950s room service spread that can't help but make one's mouth water. A celebration of butter, sugar, and beef, this puff-pastry-based feast of Beef Wellington and Napoleons is the perfect postcoital fuel for adulterers everywhere. I knew that any YouTube Wellington video would essentially go head-to-head with Gordon Ramsay's rightfully famous videos, so I had to find a way to set mine apart. The answer was simple: make puff pastry, a process no one in their right mind should undertake, as store-bought puff pastry is a near-perfect invention. If you find that you have just too much time on your hands over the holiday season (as we all do), by all means, bust out the butter square—otherwise, these decadent dishes are best wrapped up in the stuff from the freezer aisle.

BEEF WELLINGTON

SERVES 8

VERDICT: Homemade puff pastry is an experience worth having, but your time is better spent enjoying your life. Beef Wellington is an internet sensation for a reason: it's a feast for both the eyes and the . . . mouth.

10 button mushrooms, washed and trimmed

2 tablespoons unsalted butter

1 tablespoon fresh thyme leaves, chopped

1 garlic clove, minced

¼ cup Cognac

¼ cup heavy cream

Kosher salt and freshly ground black pepper

1 center-cut beef tenderloin (about 4 pounds), trimmed

1 tablespoon vegetable oil

¼ pound thinly sliced prosciutto

3 tablespoons English mustard

Puff Pastry (recipe follows)

1 large egg, beaten

Flaky sea salt

Whole-grain mustard, for serving (optional)

(recipe continues)

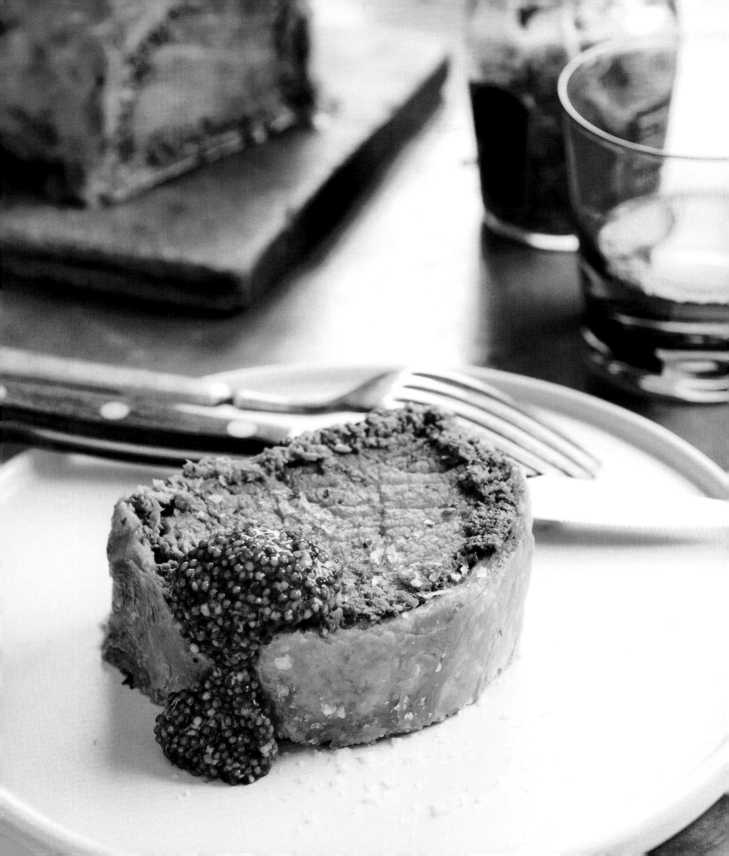

PLACE THE mushrooms in a food processor and pulse until finely chopped. In a large sauté pan, melt the butter over medium heat until the bubbling subsides. Add the mushrooms and thyme and cook, stirring, until the liquid released by the mushrooms has mostly evaporated, about 5 minutes. Add the garlic and cook, stirring, for 1 minute more. Increase the heat to high, add the Cognac, and cook until the smell of alcohol dissipates, 1 to 2 minutes. Add the cream, reduce the heat to medium, and cook until you have a thick, pâté-like mixture, 2 minutes more. Season the mushroom duxelles with salt and pepper. Remove from the heat and set aside.

SEASON THE tenderloin liberally with salt and pepper. In a large sauté pan, heat the vegetable oil over medium-high heat until nearly smoking. Add the beef and sear on all sides, including the ends. Remove from the heat and set aside.

LAY DOWN a layer of plastic wrap large enough to wrap twice around the tenderloin. Shingle the prosciutto over the plastic wrap, with each piece slightly overlapping the last, to form a rectangle large enough to wrap around the tenderloin. Spread the mushroom duxelles over the prosciutto in a thin, even layer. Brush the tenderloin liberally with the mustard and place it along one long edge of the prosciutto rectangle. Using the plastic wrap, roll the duxelles/prosciutto tightly around the roast, then wrap tightly in the plastic wrap. Refrigerate until firm, about 20 minutes.

MEANWHILE, ON a generously floured work surface, roll out the chilled puff pastry to a rectangle about 3 inches wider and 12 inches longer than the roast, large enough to generously encase it. Lay down a layer of plastic wrap large enough to wrap twice around the tenderloin and place the puff pastry on top. Remove the roast from the refrigerator, take off the plastic wrap, and place it at the bottom of the puff pastry. Use the plastic wrap to encase the roast in the puff pastry. Trim off any excess puff pastry, pinch the seam shut, and press the ends closed. Wrap tightly in the plastic wrap, as before, twisting to create tension and remove any air. Refrigerate for at least 20 minutes or up to overnight.

WHEN READY to roast the Wellington, preheat the oven to 450°F. Line a baking sheet with parchment paper.

UNWRAP THE Wellington and place it on the lined baking sheet. Brush liberally with the beaten egg, making sure to coat any exposed pastry. If desired, use the back of a paring knife to make indentations (not cuts) in the top of the pastry for decoration. Sprinkle with flaky salt and insert a temperature probe into the side of the roast so the tip of the probe is in the thickest part of the meat. Roast for about 20 minutes, until the center of the roast registers 125°F. Remove from the oven and let rest for 15 minutes before slicing and serving.

PUFF PASTRY

YIELDS 1 POUND OF PUFF PASTRY

---

2 cups all-purpose flour, plus more for dusting

1 teaspoon kosher salt

1 cup ice water

8 ounces (2 sticks) unsalted butter, cubed and chilled

MAKE THE lean dough: Mound the flour onto a work surface. Sprinkle with salt. Create a well in the center of the flour and pour in a few tablespoons of the ice water; using your fingers, carefully toss together. Re-form the well and repeat the process. Once the mixture becomes chunky, use a bench scraper to help combine the water and flour. Repeat and keep mixing more of the ice water into the flour until the dough holds its shape. Using the bench scraper, nudge the dough into a square, wrap in plastic wrap, and refrigerate for 30 minutes.

PLACE THE butter on a floured work surface, then sprinkle flour on top of the butter. Flour a rolling pin and pound the butter together into one mass. Flour the rolling pin and work surface again as necessary and pound the butter until pliable and foldable. Using the bench scraper, nudge the butter into a square, wrap with plastic wrap, and refrigerate for 10 minutes.

TRANSFER THE chilled lean dough to a generously floured work surface. Roll it out into a 12-inch square.

POUND THE butter square out to a 6-inch square. Place the butter square in the middle of the dough square and fold the corners of the dough over the butter so they meet in the middle. Seal the edges of the dough and roll the block out to a 5 x 12-inch rectangle.

FOLD THE rectangle in thirds, like a letter, and rotate it 90 degrees. Roll it out again to a 5 x 12-inch rectangle and repeat the folding, rotating, and rolling once more. Fold the dough in thirds, wrap with plastic wrap, and refrigerate for 30 minutes to let the gluten relax.

RETURN THE dough to your work surface and repeat the rolling, folding, and rotating twice more. Fold the dough in thirds once more, wrap in plastic wrap, and refrigerate for 30 minutes. Repeat this whole process of rolling, folding, and rotating once more to create 6 total folds and 720 layers of butter.

FOLD THE dough into thirds one final time and wrap in plastic wrap. Refrigerate for at least 1 hour or up to 24 hours before using.

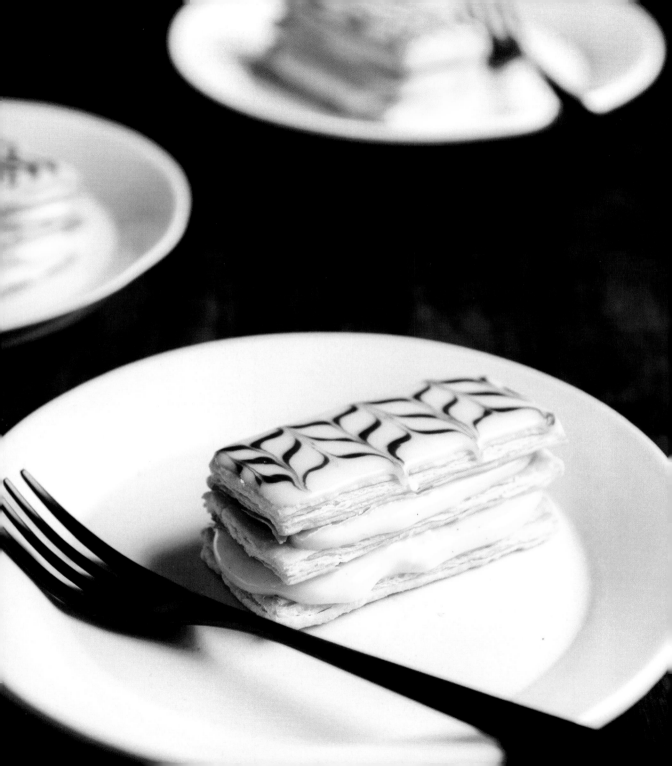

NAPOLEONS

SERVES 8

VERDICT: A napoleon is a fine thing to look at, but its flavors might be starting to show their age; any creative spins you can put on the crème pâtissière would be a welcome addition.

---

4 large egg yolks

½ cup cornstarch

2 cups plus 2 tablespoons whole milk

½ cup granulated sugar

2 teaspoons vanilla paste (or extract)

4 tablespoons (½ stick) unsalted butter:
  2 tablespoons cut into small pieces,
  2 tablespoons melted

1 cup confectioners' sugar, sifted

2 teaspoons light corn syrup

2 ounces milk chocolate, melted

1 (8-ounce) sheet puff pastry, thawed,
  or ½ recipe homemade puff pastry
  (see page 153)

IN A medium bowl, whisk together the egg yolks and cornstarch until light and ribbony.

IN A large saucepan, whisk together 2 cups of the milk, the granulated sugar, and the vanilla and bring to a bare simmer over medium heat. While whisking continuously, slowly add half the milk mixture, ½ cup at a time, to the egg mixture to temper the eggs. Whisk in the remaining milk mixture all at once until completely combined. Return the mixture to the saucepan. Cook over medium heat, whisking continuously, until a thick custard forms. Remove from the heat and, while whisking, add the butter pieces and whisk until melted and incorporated. Pour the custard into a bowl and cover with plastic wrap, pressing it directly against the surface of the custard to prevent a skin from forming. Refrigerate until completely cool, about 4 hours.

IN A large bowl, whisk together the confectioners' sugar, corn syrup, the remaining 2 tablespoons milk, and the melted butter until completely combined. Pour a few tablespoons of the icing into a small bowl and stir in the melted chocolate. Transfer the chocolate icing to a pastry bag fitted with a fine tip.

PREHEAT THE oven to 450°F. Line a baking sheet with parchment paper.

(recipe continues)

ROLL OUT the puff pastry and cut it into 3 equal-size rectangles. Transfer to the lined baking sheet and bake for about 6 minutes, or until puffed and blonde. Remove from the oven and place another baking sheet directly on top of the pastries to keep them flat. Bake for 4 to 6 minutes more, until crisp. Remove from the oven, lift off the second baking sheet, and let the pastries cool completely.

SPREAD ⅓ cup of the custard evenly over one of the pastries. Top the custard with another pastry, then add another layer of custard. Using an offset spatula, spread a thin layer of white icing evenly over the remaining pastry. Pipe 5 lines of the chocolate icing across the layer of white icing. Finally, drag a toothpick or skewer across the icing perpendicular to the chocolate lines, going back and forth to create a feathered pattern. Place this decorated pastry on top of the assembled napoleon and refrigerate for at least 30 minutes, then slice and serve.

Larry David is, no doubt, a big fan of food—though I'm sure he'd abhor being called a "foodie." Like *Seinfeld, Curb Your Enthusiasm* treats food like another member of the cast: as a constant source of conflict and annoyance for our contrarian hero. And, like *Seinfeld*, there were nearly too many options to choose from: frozen yogurt, kung pao shrimp, appetizers on sticks, vanilla bullshit latte cappa things, and even the opening of a restaurant as the central plot of an entire season. I decided that some easily replicable dishes, along with one curveball, would be the way to go. Palestinian chicken, simply praised by Larry and Jeff as the best chicken they'd ever had, was reportedly inspired by Zankou Chicken in LA. While Zankou is famous for their *toum* sauce, their chicken seems pretty generic; so I decided to draw inspiration from regional flavors by using yogurt, cardamom, and sumac. The result, I think you'll agree, is a bird that lives up to its reputation.

THE LARRY DAVID SANDWICH

SERVES 1

VERDICT: The Larry David Sandwich is surprisingly good, despite its gross-out intentions. The Ted Danson Sandwich, however, is clearly superior.

---

1 bagel, split in half
⅓ cup whitefish salad
3 or 4 slices smoked sable

4 slices white onion
1 tablespoon capers, drained
3 tablespoons cream cheese

TOAST THE bagel and scoop it out, if desired. Spread the whitefish salad on the bottom half of the bagel and top with the sable, onion, and capers. Spread cream cheese on the other half of the bagel, close the sandwich, and enjoy.

THE TED DANSON SANDWICH

MAKES 1 SANDWICH

Mayonnaise

2 slices rye bread

4 ounces sliced turkey

1 ounce sliced Swiss cheese

Coleslaw (recipe follows)

Russian Dressing (recipe follows)

SPREAD MAYO on both slices of the bread. In a large skillet, toast the bread over medium heat, mayo-side down, until golden brown, about 2 minutes. Remove from the pan and set aside.

MOUND THE turkey in the same pan and top with the Swiss cheese. Cover and heat over low heat until the cheese has completely melted. Transfer to the untoasted side of one slice of bread and top with some of the coleslaw. Spread Russian dressing on the untoasted side of the other slice of bread. Close the sandwich, cut in half, and serve.

COLESLAW

MAKES ABOUT 2 CUPS

½ cup mayonnaise

3 tablespoons white wine vinegar

2 tablespoons sour cream

2 tablespoons Greek yogurt

1 tablespoon fresh lemon juice

1 garlic clove, minced

1 teaspoon sugar

1 teaspoon celery seeds

½ teaspoon paprika

½ teaspoon mustard powder

Kosher salt and freshly ground black pepper

8 ounces shredded cabbage

IN A large bowl, whisk together the mayo, vinegar, sour cream, yogurt, lemon juice, garlic, sugar, celery seeds, paprika, and mustard powder until well combined. Season with salt and pepper. Fold in the cabbage with a rubber spatula until evenly coated, then refrigerate until ready to assemble the sandwich.

RUSSIAN DRESSING

MAKES ABOUT 1½ CUPS

½ cup bottled horseradish sauce (available in the salad dressing aisle at most supermarkets)

½ cup mayonnaise

¼ cup ketchup

1 teaspoon hot sauce

1 teaspoon Worcestershire sauce

½ teaspoon paprika

½ small white onion, finely chopped

IN A medium bowl, whisk together all the ingredients until well combined, then cover and refrigerate until ready to assemble the sandwich.

FUN FACT
This is the only instance thus far of an intentionally disgusting dish turning out delicious. Not holding my breath for that to happen again.

COBB SALAD

SERVES 2

VERDICT: A Cobb salad, no matter who invented it, is a classic for a reason: it's delicious.

SALAD

1 pound chicken breast

1 tablespoon salt

½ head iceberg lettuce, chopped

½ bunch watercress, chopped

1 head endive, sliced crosswise

6 slices bacon, cooked and chopped

2 hard-boiled large eggs, sliced

1 small tomato, cored and diced

½ cup crumbled Roquefort cheese

½ avocado, diced

Dressing (recipe follows)

Handful of fresh chives, minced, for garnish

SALAD

IN A medium saucepan, cover the chicken with 4 cups water. Add the salt and bring to a simmer over moderate heat. Flip the chicken and gently simmer until cooked through, about 15 minutes. Remove the chicken from the poaching liquid and transfer to a plate. Let rest for 15 minutes, then cover and refrigerate until cool. Shred or chop the meat. Discard the chicken poaching liquid.

TOSS THE greens together and place on a large plate. Arrange the bacon, eggs, chicken, tomato, cheese, and avocado in decorative rows over the bed of greens. Drizzle as much of the dressing as you like over the top, garnish with the chives, and serve.

DRESSING

MAKES ABOUT 1 CUP

2 tablespoons red wine vinegar

Juice of 1 lemon

2 teaspoons sugar

1 teaspoon Worcestershire sauce

½ teaspoon ground mustard

1 garlic clove, minced

¾ cup canola oil

Kosher salt and freshly ground black pepper

IN A medium bowl, whisk together the vinegar, lemon juice, sugar, Worcestershire, mustard, garlic, and 2 tablespoons water. Whisk in the oil in a slow, steady stream until emulsified. Season with salt and pepper. Refrigerate until ready to use.

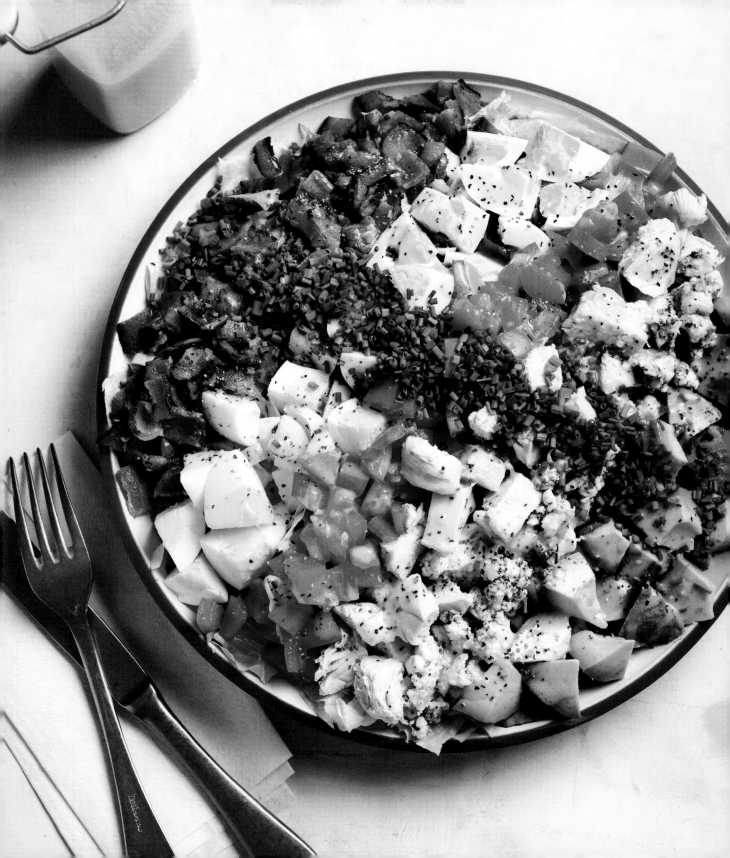

INGENUITY AND IDIOCY, IMMORTALIZED IN INK

KATRINA CODE

This was my first tattoo, gotten at some now closed shop in Plano, Texas. My girlfriend at the time lived there, and even though she was loudly opposed to me getting any tattoos, she wanted to be present for my first one. It was a simple design I had wanted to get for years, ever since I visited New Orleans in 2006 after Hurricane Katrina. The symbol is what's colloquially referred to as a "Katrina Code," a number spray-painted on houses after the storm by FEMA, each quadrant denoting different information about the house: the date it was inspected, hazards present, bodies or survivors found, and the organization that inspected it. In this case, going clockwise from the top, we have 5-25 (the date we left), 3 (there were three of us on the trip, or three hazards . . . bad joke), 0 (none of us died), and *DJR*, which stood for our last names: Duroseau, Jacobs, and Rea. Rashid and Sawyer, the other folks on the journey, can be frequently seen throughout the show.

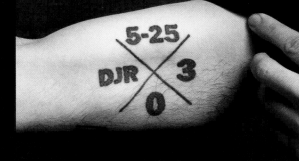

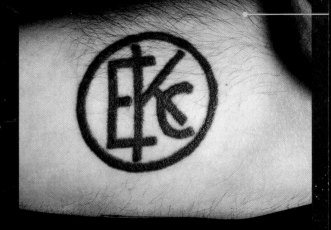

BORN & BREAD

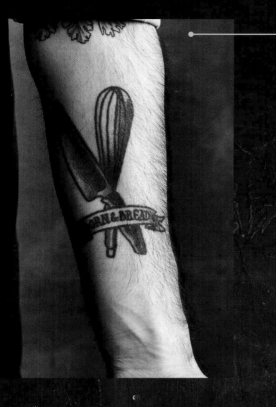

I knew I was going to get one of those stereo-typical knife-and-whisk tattoos, but I wanted at least a little something to set mine apart. I decided I'd allow myself to get this tattoo once I taught myself how to use Adobe Illustrator, the end result being my designing it from scratch with the program. Again, my desire to get this ink was hotly contested by those in my personal life—as a result, I got it from the first artist I laid eyes on, and the end product is sloppy. The lines on the whisk are shaky, the shading is heavy-handed and uneven, and the whole thing has an unintentionally "hand-drawn" vibe to it. I was initially horrified, finding myself wearing long sleeves more often than usual, but I've grown to love it. Like most tattoos, it's a reminder of a time and a place, and in this case, it's the haunting result of what happens when you let others dictate who you are.

KODAK LOGO

This is one of my favorite tattoos, not only because of its many mean-ings, but because it was a total impulse. I had the idea for it near the end of my workday, and after dinner (and a bit of wine), I decided to get it on my forearm. As we walked out of the restaurant, just down the block was the legendary Fun City Tattoo, and so my fate was sealed. This is the original Kodak logo from 1911 ("EKC" stands for Eastman Kodak Company), so it represents a few things: hometown pride, as Rochester is where Kodak was born (and died), my connection to film, and a reminder to never become complacent or stuck in the past, like some multinational corporations I could mention. I got this one without per-mission from my ex, and needless to say, there was hell to pay as a result.

SEATTLE SKYLINE

This tattoo has afforded me the opportunity to repeatedly make one of my favorite dad jokes: folks will approach me upon seeing it, exclaiming, "Oh, are you from Seattle?" to which I get to respond, "I've never been to Seattle, why do you ask? Oh, you mean FrasierTown?" Sometimes it's the simple things that get you through the day. I got this done in Lincoln, Nebraska, freshly divorced and newly falling in love. It went on to teach me another important lesson: love doesn't always last, but tattoos do. So get potentially hazardous ones where you can't see them.

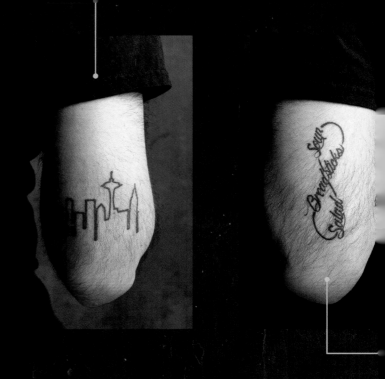

MOM'S RING

This was a ring that my mom made for my dad back in the early '80s, and when she passed away, he bequeathed it to me as a way to keep her nearby wherever I went. I wore it for a solid fourteen years, but when I got engaged, I realized I wasn't a two-ring kind of guy. So I took it off, put it in my travel toiletries kit, and there it lived for about three years. I knew for a long while that I wanted to replace wearing it with a tattoo facsimile, but was worried about how my (not-so-thrilled-about-tattoos) family would receive this tribute. Happily, once I summoned up the courage to show my father, he was touched by the gesture. Recently, he gave me his father's signet ring, which will be join-

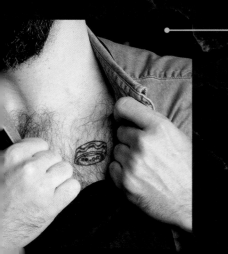

INFINITE SOUP, SALAD, AND BREADSTICKS

When you're here, you're family. I haven't come up with many jokes in my life, and this was a particularly odd one: it was timely, Olive Garden–oriented, and would really only work as a tattoo. A parody of the sorority-mandated "Live Laugh Love" tattoo, I decided to get this opposite my *Frasier* tribute, so they would both be on my "funny" bone. I flew out to Chicago to get this one, as one of my best friends was keen on getting his first-ever ink, and I had always wanted to get tattooed with a friend. After posting this tattoo on Instagram, I was delighted to see that some adventurous soul decided to get the same one on his chest. For the record, I'm no huge fan of the Olive Garden, but their salad and breadsticks are absolutely the shit.

LENS REFRACTION DIAGRAM

This one's pretty self-explanatory from its name: it's a diagram of how light enters a lens. I had an itch for some kind of geometric tattoo, but didn't want to get the random (but cool-looking) shapes that were becoming popular at the time. It was also around this time that I decided to start theming my arms—the left is reserved for food, the right for TV and film references—so I knew I wanted it to be something camera-related. I started looking at camera schematics and diagrams, but they were too complex and would have quickly turned into a sleeve, something I'm glad I didn't do. I was in Minneapolis for Halloween, we had a few hours to kill before a party, and I was drawn to the neon glow of the tattoo parlor like a moth to a flame. I ended up getting it much bigger than I had originally anticipated, but with the passing of time, I've grown very happy with the way it fits on my forearm.

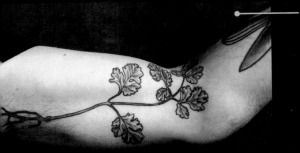

CILANTRO

Something you might not know about me is that up until recently, I hated seafood. All of it. Shellfish, sea bass, sea cucumber, sushi, salmon, shrimp—and those are just the S's. When I turned twenty-six, however, I decided I was going to learn to love seafood. After eating it repeatedly, trying everything I could get my hands and chopsticks on, I'm happy to say it worked. What fascinates me about cilantro is that no matter how hard I try to love the pervasive herb, I can't crack the code. That's because I'm part of a privileged few born with a certain genetic marker that predisposes me to think the green stuff tastes like soap. Well, for some people, it's soap—for me, it's more like burning tires. So I decided to celebrate the devil's lettuce by having it emblazoned on my skin, with its roots growing out of my armpit, of course.

P DIAMOND

his has got to be one of the stupidest things ve ever done, but it was appropriately punk-ock. One of my favorite bands to see live, the nfortunately named Diarrhea Planet, was play-g their final show in Nashville. I had an hour to ll before the show and decided that the most tting tribute for the occasion was an ill-advised, astelessly located tat. I went to dinner with ome friends and, after explaining my plans o them, actually got my friend's wife (whom I ad just met) to get the same piece. Dizzy from he adrenaline, we headed to the show, and I roceeded to have one of the greatest nights of hy life. I climbed up onstage during one of my avorite songs, the lead singer belted out the yrics with me, then I jumped backward into out-tretched hands and crowd surfed for the first and last) time. I got to meet the band afterward, ecause as it turned out, the drummer is a fan f the show; happily, I hadn't gotten my first-raft tattoo, a cartoon rendition of the name of heir most popular song: "Ghost with a Boner."

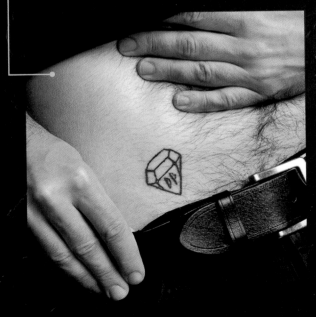

PASTA AGLIO E OLIO

There I was, newly single and heartbroken during my first visit to LA, when what should appear, but the renowned Honorable Society tattoo shop. I made an appointment, and was delighted to learn that my artist (Emily Effler) was a fan of the show. It was only fitting, then, that I get something meaningful from the show that had utterly changed my life. The carving fork featured in this early episode was a real symbolic turning point for me, as it represented a moment when I decided I would do virtually anything to make the show as accurate as possible. I was broke, exhausted, and just leaving work when I came up with the idea to re-create the sexy pasta, and I realized that I had no carving fork. I frantically tracked down the only kitchenware store still open, Whisk, and bought their least-expensive carving fork (which was still $65). Little did I know that this dedication would one day pay off, in the form of Jon Favreau himself inspecting my tattoo in person and giving me the actual fork from the film *Chef*. I still have to get it framed; I keep using it to plate up my *pasta aglio e olio*.

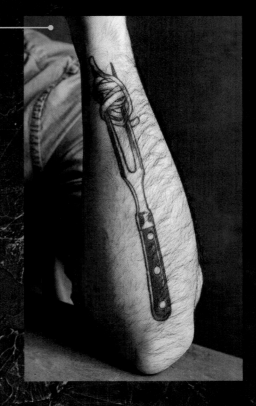

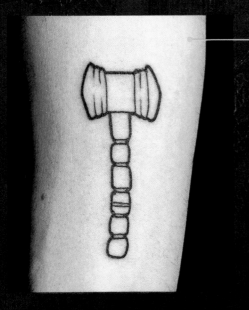

GAVEL

You might notice that this one is a little fresh—that's because I literally got it just, like, minutes before we photographed it. I thought that might be a fun little Easter egg for the book. This is the gavel wielded by none other than the real Oliver Babish, legal counsel to the Bartlet Administration in *The West Wing*. In the famous scene, Babish, after being confronted with the president's big secret, smashes a malfunctioning tape recorder using this very gavel. I figured that the silly-sounding name has given me so much, I ought to find some way to pay tribute to it. Its location was determined by a Twitter follower, who suggested I get it on my inner forearm. Next up: face tattoo?! . . . No, probably not. Hand tattoo maybe, though.

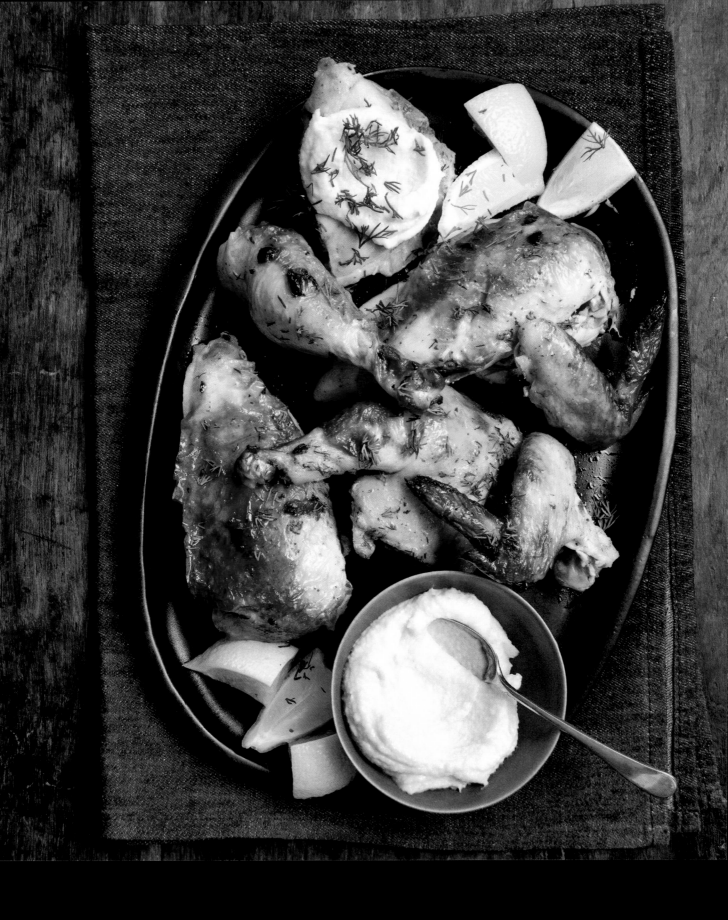

PALESTINIAN CHICKEN

SERVES 4

VERDICT: Yogurt-marinated chicken is a revelation, its spices are unique and balanced, and *toum* should be served at all restaurants alongside ketchup and mustard.

TOUM SAUCE

8 to 12 large garlic cloves

1 cup canola oil

Juice of 1 lemon

CHICKEN

1 whole chicken (about 5 pounds)

MARINADE

1 cup Greek yogurt

2 shallots, finely minced

Zest and juice of 1 lemon

1 bunch fresh dill, finely chopped

1 teaspoon ground sumac

½ teaspoon ground cardamom

2 tablespoons extra-virgin olive oil

Kosher salt and freshly ground black pepper

TOUM SAUCE

PLACE THE garlic in a food processor and process until a thick paste forms. With the machine running, slowly stream in ½ cup of the canola oil through the feed tube. Stop to add the lemon juice, then, with the machine running, slowly stream in the remaining ½ cup oil through the feed tube until a thick, spreadable paste forms. Refrigerate until ready to use.

CHICKEN

USING A sturdy pair of poultry shears, cut along each side of the chicken backbone and remove it (discard or reserve it for another use, such as making chicken stock). Press down firmly on the breastbone to flatten the chicken, then transfer the bird to a large resealable plastic bag.

MARINADE

IN A medium bowl, stir together the yogurt, shallots, lemon zest, lemon juice, dill, sumac, cardamom, and olive oil. Season with salt and

(recipe continues)

169

pepper. Stir well to combine, then add to the chicken in the bag. Press the air out of the bag, seal shut, and massage to evenly coat the chicken with the marinade. Place the bag in a bowl or on a rimmed baking sheet and refrigerate overnight.

WHEN READY to roast the chicken, preheat the oven to 450°F. Line a rimmed baking sheet with aluminum foil and set a rack over the foil.

REMOVE THE chicken from the bag and place it on the rack. Roast for 45 to 55 minutes, until the chicken is deeply browned and the internal temperature registers 165°F for the white meat and 180°F for the dark meat. Remove from the oven and let rest for 10 minutes, then carve and serve with the toum sauce.

THE MICHAEL SCOTT PRETZEL

MAKES 12 PRETZELS

It's Pretzel Day. With a ridiculous lineup of toppings (eighteen in total), the emphasis of this episode had to be on the pretzel itself, something I'd always been curious about: how does one re-create this soft, buttery, salty shopping-mall classic? While not as pretty as those crafted by Auntie Anne's expert pretzel-makers, it's a kitchen exercise more than worth trying. You can certainly be more judicious with the toppings, but when "sectioned off" into separate bites like my second attempt, it becomes an ill-advised delight to eat. Just be ready for the sugar crash.

VERDICT: This is an effective method for making shopping-mall-style pretzels—the number and volume of toppings should be deployed at your discretion.

PRETZELS

2 cups whole milk

2 (¼-ounce) packets active dry yeast

6 tablespoons light brown sugar

3¼ cups all-purpose flour, plus more as necessary

1 cup bread flour

1 teaspoon fine salt

4 tablespoons (½ stick) unsalted butter, melted and cooled, plus more melted butter for brushing

Vegetable oil, for greasing

Nonstick cooking spray

4 cups warm water (110°F)

½ cup baking soda

Pretzel salt, for sprinkling

Cinnamon sugar (granulated sugar mixed with an equal amount of ground cinnamon), for sprinkling

TOPPINGS

Sweet Glaze (recipe follows)

Cinnamon sugar

Melted milk chocolate

Melted white chocolate

Hot Fudge Sauce (recipe follows)

M&M's

Caramel Dip (recipe follows)

Mint chips

Chocolate chips

Miniature marshmallows

Nuts (peanuts for accuracy but use any nuts you like)

Toffee nuts (candied pecans for accuracy but use any nuts you like)

Sweetened shredded coconut

(ingredients continue)

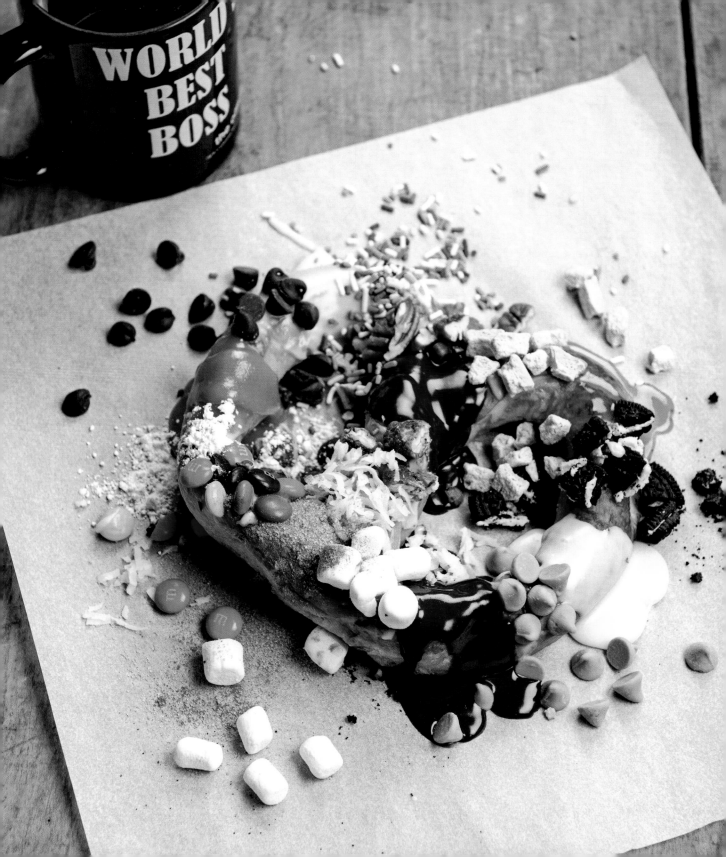

Peanut Butter Drizzle (recipe follows)
Crushed Oreos
Rainbow sprinkles

Cotton candy bits
Confectioners' sugar

PRETZELS

IN A small saucepan, heat the milk over medium-low heat to 110°F. Remove from the heat, stir in the yeast, and let sit for about 5 minutes, or until frothy and bubbling. Transfer the mixture to the bowl of a stand mixer fitted with the dough hook. Add the brown sugar, all-purpose flour, bread flour, salt, and melted butter. Knead on medium speed for 10 minutes, or until the dough is tacky but not sticky and pulls away from the sides of the bowl. If the dough is too sticky, knead in more all-purpose flour, a few tablespoons at a time, until the dough pulls away from the sides of the bowl. Transfer to a well-oiled bowl, cover with plastic wrap, and let the dough rise in a warm place (such as on top of or inside a turned-off oven) for 1 hour, or until doubled in size. (This a great time to make your toppings!)

PREHEAT THE oven to 450°F.

SPRAY A work surface with cooking spray, turn out the dough, and divide it into 12 equal pieces. Roll each piece into a 3-foot-long rope about the thickness of your finger. Grab each rope by the ends to form a U shape. Cross the ends over each other three times to form the twist. Then, bring the ends to the bottom of the U and press them on to form a classic pretzel shape. (Watch my video to see how it's done!) Transfer each pretzel to a baking sheet lined with parchment paper.

IN A large bowl, whisk together the warm water and baking soda. Dip each pretzel in the mixture, return it to the baking sheet, and sprinkle with pretzel salt or cinnamon sugar. Bake for 12 minutes, or until lightly browned, rotating the pan halfway through to ensure even cooking. Remove from the oven, let cool slightly, then brush the tops with melted butter.

FOR EACH serving, place a pretzel on a sheet of parchment paper and drizzle on the glaze, sprinkle with cinnamon sugar, then drizzle on each of the following: melted chocolate, white chocolate, and hot fudge sauce. Dot the top of the pretzel with some M&M's and drizzle generously with caramel dip to help secure a sprinkling of mint chips, chocolate chips, miniature marshmallows, nuts, toffee nuts, and shredded coconut. Top with peanut butter drizzle, crushed Oreos, rainbow sprinkles, cotton candy bits, and a gentle snowfall of confectioners' sugar and serve.

(recipe continues)

SWEET GLAZE

MAKES ABOUT 1¾ CUPS

1½ cups confectioners' sugar, sifted

3 to 4 tablespoons whole milk

1 teaspoon pure vanilla extract (optional)

PLACE THE sugar in a medium bowl and slowly whisk in the milk until a pourable glaze forms. Whisk in the vanilla, if desired, and set aside until ready to use.

HOT FUDGE SAUCE

MAKES ABOUT 2½ CUPS

2 cups sugar

1 (14-ounce) can sweetened condensed milk

½ cup unsweetened cocoa powder

4 ounces dark chocolate, chopped

4 tablespoons (½ stick) unsalted butter

IN A large saucepan, stir together the sugar, condensed milk, cocoa powder, chocolate, and butter and bring to a bare simmer over medium heat. Cook, stirring, for about 7 minutes, or until a beautiful chocolate fudge sauce forms. Pour the sauce into a microwavable container and set aside until ready to use. (The sauce will solidify as it cools. Rewarm in the microwave to make it pourable again.)

CARAMEL DIP

MAKES ABOUT 1½ CUPS

1 cup sugar

1 cup heavy cream

½ teaspoon pure vanilla extract (optional)

IN A large saucepan, bring the sugar and ½ cup water to a boil over medium-high heat. Stir gently, making sure the sugar doesn't stick to the sides of the pan. Pour yourself a glass of Scotch for color reference—that's the caramel color you're aiming for—and bring the sugar mixture to 350°F over medium-low heat. Meanwhile, in a small saucepan, heat the cream over medium heat to almost boiling. While whisking continuously, slowly pour the cream into the sugar mixture, ¼ cup at a time. Continue to whisk over low heat for 2 to 3 minutes, until thickened. Add the vanilla, if desired. Remove from the heat and set aside to cool and thicken.

PEANUT BUTTER DRIZZLE

MAKES ABOUT 1½ CUPS

½ cup heavy cream
¼ cup sugar
¼ cup light corn syrup
2 tablespoons unsalted butter
½ teaspoon pure vanilla extract (optional)
½ cup smooth peanut butter

IN A large saucepan, stir together the cream, sugar, corn syrup, butter, and vanilla (if using). Heat over medium heat, stirring, until just steaming and all the ingredients are incorporated. Remove from the heat and let cool slightly, then add the peanut butter. Stir until smooth and then pour into a heatproof container and set aside until ready to use.

FUN FACT

"Cotton candy bits" had to be one of the most difficult ingredients to source in the history of the show. I'm not entirely sure they're a thing. I ended up getting blue and pink sugar clusters, which I figured was close enough.

KRABBY PATTY—MSG VERSION

MAKES 4 BURGERS

THE KRABBY PATTY: the holy grail of fictional food. The internet was rabid for an answer: what is the secret formula to the creation of the notoriously cheap Mr. Krabs? Blogs and videos alike purporting to have the answer abound, but their connection to the cartoon is tenuous at best: make a burger, and assemble it roughly to specifications. As such, I wasn't going to even attempt this episode until I was damn sure I had something approaching a satisfying answer. I decided to offer three hypotheses: First, that the secret ingredient was nothing, making the Krabby Patty into its own viral marketing campaign. Second, that the secret ingredient (once referred to as King Neptune's Poseidon Powder) is MSG, a harmless but vilified umami enhancer. Third, that it contained some other umami-boosting ingredients, preferably from the sea: anchovies and kelp. At the very least, it was an opportunity to make a video defending MSG—which has hopefully made an impression on a few of its 20 million (at the time of this writing) combined Facebook and YouTube viewers.

VERDICT: MSG tastes good and doesn't hurt you, unless you have an intolerance, in which case it might give you a headache. The umami version is a bit funky, but definitely something worth experimenting with—you might find a component that becomes a standard in your burger repertoire.

BEEF PATTIES

1 pound boneless short ribs

1 pound chuck steak

2 teaspoons MSG (available at most grocery stores)

Kosher salt and freshly ground black pepper

2 tablespoons vegetable oil

TO ASSEMBLE

4 sesame seed hamburger buns

8 ounces shredded iceberg lettuce (about ¼ head)

4 slices yellow American cheese

1 small white onion, thinly sliced

1 beefsteak tomato, thinly sliced

Ketchup, for serving

Yellow mustard, for serving

1 large dill pickle, thinly sliced

(recipe continues)

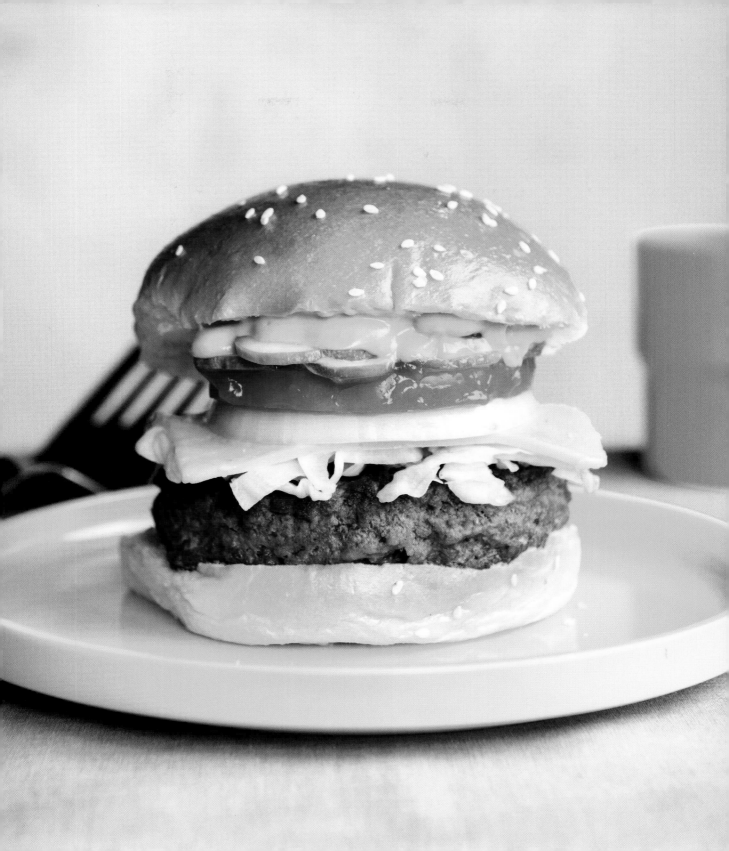

BEEF PATTIES

TRIM ALL the beef of connective tissue. Cut into 1-inch pieces, and place on a parchment paper–lined baking sheet. Freeze for 15 minutes, or until the beef is very firm. Freeze the blade of a food processor as well.

REMOVE THE beef and the blade from the freezer, transfer to the food processor, and pulse the beef until well ground and pebbly. Divide the beef into 4 portions, shape into patties, and season with the MSG, salt, and pepper.

IN A large cast-iron skillet, heat the vegetable oil over medium-high heat until barely smoking. Add the patties and reduce the heat to medium. Cook to your desired doneness, flipping once. Remove from the heat.

TO ASSEMBLE each burger the Mr. Krabs way, stack the following on the bottom bun in this order: patty, lettuce, cheese, onion, tomato, ketchup, mustard, pickles. The better (Babish) way is the following sequence: patty, cheese, onion, tomato, ketchup, pickles, lettuce. Either way, close the burgers and serve.

KRABBY PATTY—UMAMI VERSION

MAKES 4 BURGERS

1 beefsteak tomato, thinly sliced

1 tablespoon vegetable oil

1 white onion, thinly sliced

3 dried shiitake mushrooms

1 tablespoon bonito flakes (smoked dried tuna; available at Asian markets)

½ ounce kombu (dried kelp; available at Asian markets), broken into pieces

1 dried anchovy (available at Asian markets)

½ cup Dijon mustard

1 tablespoon yellow miso paste

2 or 3 large oil-packed sun-dried tomatoes, drained

½ cup ketchup

½ cup grated Parmesan cheese

Beef Patties (see page 176; omit the MSG)

4 sesame seed hamburger buns

PREHEAT THE oven to 200°F. Line a baking sheet with a silicone baking mat or other nonstick surface.

ARRANGE THE tomato slices on the baking sheet, spacing them apart. Bake for 1½ hours, or until dry and wrinkled. Remove from the oven and let cool. Increase the oven temperature to 375°F.

MEANWHILE, HEAT the oil over low heat in a large sauté pan. Add the onion and cook, stirring, until soft and deep caramel in color, about 45 minutes. Add a splash of water if the onion dries out and begins to brown too quickly. Remove from the heat and set aside.

IN A spice grinder, combine the shiitake mushrooms, bonito, kombu, and anchovy and grind to a fine dust. Set aside.

PROCESS THE mustard and miso in a food processor until well combined. Transfer to a bowl and set aside.

CLEAN THE food processor and combine the sun-dried tomatoes and the ketchup. Pulse until the tomatoes are pureed and well combined.

LINE A baking sheet with a silicone baking mat or other nonstick surface. Arrange the Parmesan into 4 round piles on the baking sheet. Bake for 15 minutes, or until lightly browned and crisp. Transfer the cheese crisps to a wire rack and let cool.

AFTER FLIPPING the beef patties, season them with the mushroom powder. Toast the buns in the burger fat remaining in the pan and let the patties rest for 2 minutes before assembling the burgers.

STACK THE toppings on the bottom buns in the following order: patty, caramelized onions, oven-dried tomato, miso mustard, sun-dried tomato ketchup, cheese crisp, lettuce. Close the burgers and serve.

FUN FACT

The fear of MSG stems from "Chinese restaurant syndrome," an entirely imagined (and pretty xenophobic) myth started in the late 1960s. MSG is found naturally in foods you already enjoy, like tomatoes, broccoli, soy sauce, seaweed, and Parmesan cheese.

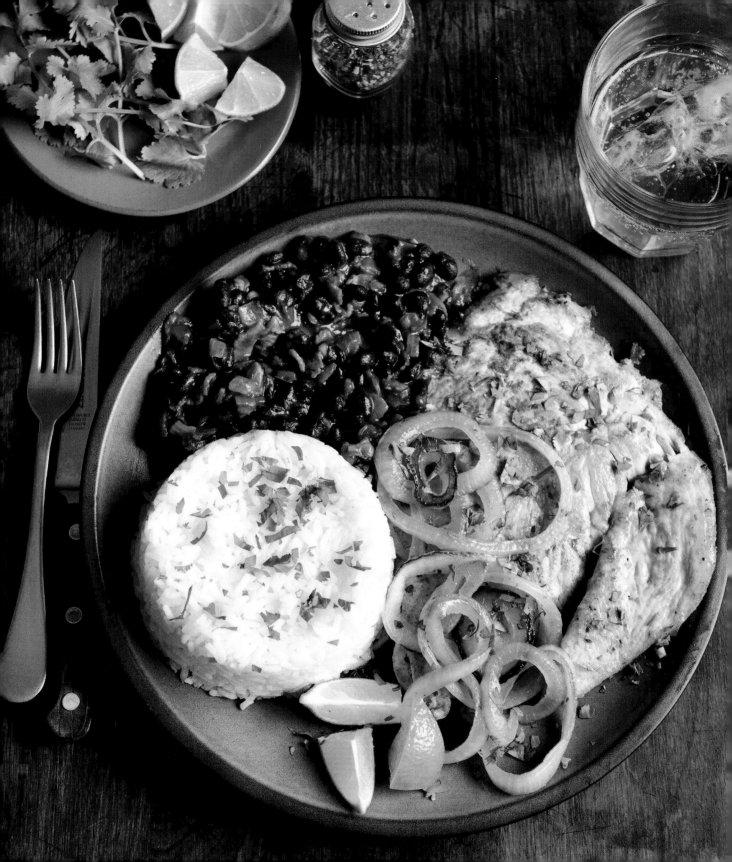

CHEF'S SPECIAL

SERVES 4

The show triumphantly returned to my buddy Steve's house as I commandeered his kitchen for my own nefarious purposes: re-creating *pollo a la plancha*, a popular Cuban dish lovingly prepared in the stunning film *Moonlight*. Oscar gag aside, this has been one of the most re-created dishes from the show, second only to Pasta Aglio e Olio (page 29), and with good reason: it's impressive, relatively easy, and delicious. It can be a huge confidence-booster to burgeoning home cooks grown accustomed to dry, stringy chicken, mushy rice, and boring beans.

VERDICT: Pounding chicken breasts flat and briefly marinating (with a hint of sugar) produces a flavorful, juicy, and caramelized paillard quickly and easily. Beans cooked with aromatics and bacon are just as good as you think they are. Add lightly seasoned rice and sautéed onions to the equation, and you've got a Cuban classic on your hands.

4 chicken breasts, butterflied and pounded thin

4 garlic cloves: 2 chopped, 1 left whole, and 1 minced

Juice of 2 limes

1 teaspoon ground cumin

1 teaspoon cayenne pepper

3 teaspoons kosher salt

1 teaspoon freshly ground black pepper

1 tablespoon extra-virgin olive oil

2 cups long-grain white rice

1 bay leaf

4 ounces fatty bacon, finely diced

2 Spanish onions: 1 minced, 1 sliced into rings

1 green bell pepper, minced

12 ounces dried black beans, soaked overnight, plus ½ cup of the soaking liquid, or 1 (15-ounce) can black beans, undrained

2 tablespoons vegetable oil

2 tablespoons fresh cilantro, chopped

1 lime, sliced thinly or into wedges, for serving

(recipe continues)

PLACE THE chicken in a large resealable plastic bag.

IN A small bowl, whisk together the chopped garlic, lime juice, cumin, cayenne, 1 teaspoon of the salt, the black pepper, and the olive oil. Pour the marinade over the chicken, seal the bag, and refrigerate for 30 minutes to 2 hours.

RINSE THE rice in a fine-mesh colander until the water runs clear. Drain and transfer to a large saucepan. Add 3½ cups water, the bay leaf, 1 teaspoon of the salt, and the whole garlic clove. Bring to a simmer over medium heat, then reduce the heat to low, cover, and cook until the water has been absorbed and the rice is tender, about 18 minutes. Remove from the heat and remove and discard the bay leaf. Fluff the rice with a fork and keep warm until ready to serve.

WHILE THE rice is cooking, combine the bacon and ¼ cup water in another large saucepan. Bring to a simmer over medium heat and cook, stirring occasionally, until the bacon is crisp and the fat has rendered completely, about 15 minutes. Using a slotted spoon, transfer the bacon to a bowl, reserving the rendered fat in the saucepan. Add the minced onion and bell pepper to the pan and cook over medium heat, stirring, until softened, about 3 minutes. Add the minced garlic clove to the pan and cook,

stirring, until fragrant, 30 seconds to 1 minute. Return the bacon to the pan and add the soaked beans and the reserved soaking liquid (or the entire contents of the can of beans). Simmer, uncovered, until the beans are tender and the liquid has thickened, about 30 minutes. Remove from the heat, season with the remaining 1 teaspoon salt (or to taste), cover, and keep warm until ready to serve.

ON A large cast-iron griddle, heat 1 tablespoon of the vegetable oil over medium-high heat until shimmering. Add the sliced onion and sear, flipping, until golden and lightly charred, about 5 minutes. Transfer to a bowl and cover with aluminum foil to keep warm.

HEAT THE remaining 1 tablespoon vegetable oil on the griddle. Remove the chicken from the marinade and shake off any excess. Sear on the griddle until well browned on one side, about 3 minutes. Flip and cook, flipping as necessary to prevent burning, until the internal temperature registers 165°F.

FOR EACH serving, pack cooked rice into a ½-pint takeout container and unmold it onto a plate. Arrange 1 chicken breast on one side of the rice and one-quarter of the beans on the other side. Top the chicken with one-quarter each of the seared onions and cilantro. Garnish with lime slices and serve.

STRUDEL

SERVES 6

Re-creating the infamous strudel from *Inglourious Basterds* probably took the most research of any episode at the time. I was determined to find a legit "*oma*" recipe, something handed down from a frail-handed but sure-fingered Austrian matriarch. I ended up reading several blog entries by internet chefs sharing their *großmama*'s secret recipe, comparing notes, and coming up with my own amalgam of the antiquated pastry. Most recipes call for phyllo as a shortcut—this one, instead, opts for a lean dough stretched paper-thin, drizzled with butter, stuffed with

apples and nuts, and rolled by virtue of a flour-dusted tablecloth. The resulting layers create a flaky, luxuriant dessert, elegant enough for even the fussiest of brunching war criminals. Be sure to "wait for the cream."

VERDICT: Exhausting, messy, and intimidating to make, strudel's bark is actually worse than its bite. Once you've beaten the dough into glutinous submission, it's a thrill to see it stretch until nearly transparent, and the end result is an impressive addition to any breakfast or dessert spread.

1½ cups bread flour, plus more as needed

¼ cup vegetable oil, plus more for greasing

2 large egg whites

¼ teaspoon fine salt

1½ teaspoons fresh lemon juice, plus more as needed

¼ cup warm water (110°F)

4 baking apples, such as Granny Smith

½ cup granulated sugar

1 tablespoon ground cinnamon

½ cup raisins

Zest of 1 lemon

2 tablespoons all-purpose flour

4 tablespoons (½ stick) unsalted butter, melted

½ cup finely chopped mixed hazelnuts and walnuts

1 large egg, beaten

Confectioners' sugar, for serving

Whipped Cream (recipe follows)

(recipe continues)

PLACE THE bread flour in a medium bowl and make a little well in the center. Pour the vegetable oil, egg whites, salt, and lemon juice into the well. Mix with your hands until everything just barely comes together. Add the warm water and mix with your hands until a rough dough forms. Mix in a little more flour if the dough is too sticky.

FLOUR A work surface and just knead the hell out of the dough. Seriously, pound it against the table. Take your frustrations out on the dough until you end up with a soft and supple mass. Place it in an oiled bowl, cover with plastic wrap, and let rest for 30 minutes.

MEANWHILE, PEEL, core, and thinly slice the apples. Transfer to a large bowl and toss with the granulated sugar, cinnamon, raisins, lemon zest, and up to 2 tablespoons lemon juice (to prevent the apples from browning). Stir in the all-purpose flour to soak up the moisture. Let stand for 30 minutes.

PREHEAT THE oven to 350°F. Line a baking sheet with parchment paper.

COVER A large work surface with a clean tablecloth and liberally dust it with flour. Flour a rolling pin and roll the dough out to an 18- to 24-inch round. Flour your knuckles and carefully pick up the round, carefully rotating it with your fists, like a fragile pizza dough. Continue to rotate the round, stretching it as much as you can without tearing, then set it down on the cloth. Gently tug at the edges, stretching the round into a rectangle, until the dough is

> **FUN FACT**
> If you want to be super accurate, you might consider making your strudel with lard, as butter would've likely been hard to come by in Nazi-occupied France. I opted to use butter, as the restaurant in question appeared to be uncompromising, despite the dire circumstances.

thin enough that you can see the pattern of the tablecloth through the dough. Trim off the rough edges.

USING A pastry brush, drizzle 2 tablespoons of the melted butter all over the dough. Gently brush the butter over the entire surface of the dough. Sprinkle the chopped nuts all over the buttered dough.

ARRANGE THE apples in a row along one short end of the dough rectangle. Using the tablecloth, tightly roll the dough one time over the apples to enclose them in the dough. Tuck in the long edges and brush the top with some of the melted butter. Repeat the rolling, tucking, and brushing until the strudel is all rolled up. Tuck the edges under to seal.

TRANSFER THE strudel to the lined baking sheet and brush all over with the beaten egg.

(recipe continues)

184

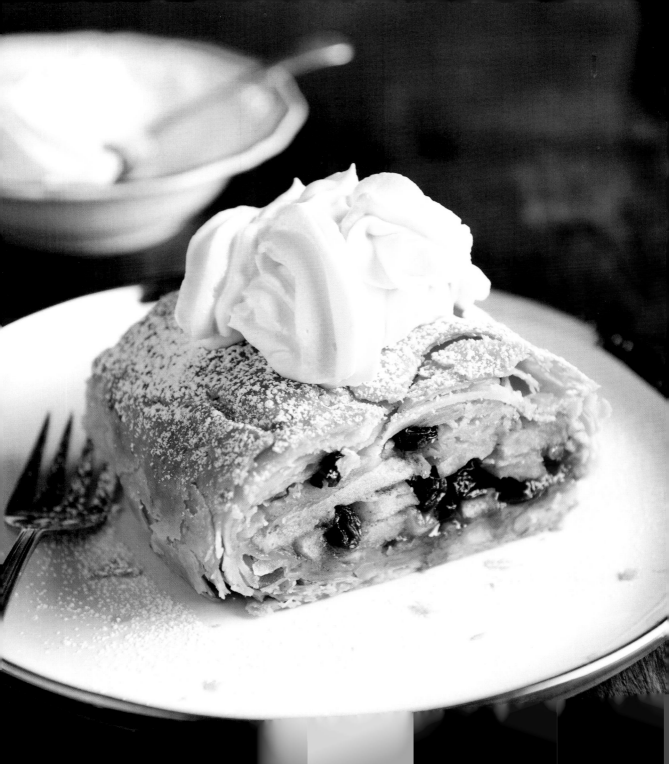

Bake for about 1 hour, or until golden brown, brushing the strudel with melted butter twice during baking. Remove from the oven and slide the parchment paper and strudel onto a wire rack to cool.

CUT THE strudel into about 4-inch pieces. Dust each piece with confectioners' sugar, and don't forget the whipped cream before serving. If desired, transfer the whipped cream to a pastry bag fitted with a decorative tip. Pipe into a bowl, making a nice little mountain of cream. Dollop some onto each serving of strudel. Otherwise, just heap on the whipped cream with a spoon.

WHIPPED CREAM
MAKES ABOUT 2 CUPS

1 cup heavy cream
1 tablespoon sugar

IN A medium bowl, combine the cream and sugar. Using a handheld mixer, beat on medium-high speed until soft peaks form. Refrigerate until ready to serve.

CONFIT BYALDI

CONFIT BYALDI

SERVES 4 TO 6

One of the greatest movies about the passion food inspires, *Ratatouille* has a surprisingly low number of replicable dishes. Remy's soup, for example, is something of a mystery—and it's difficult to imagine how a revolting stew can be saved by a few herbs, some wine, and heavy cream. Sweetbreads à la Gusteau, an intentional gross-out dish of calf's brains and cuttlefish, is somehow made sensational by the rodent puppeteer. The film's eponymous dish, however, is a real-life recipe developed by Thomas Keller, normally going by the fussier name *confit byaldi*. Reshaping the classic flavors of the Provençal peasant dish into an elegant tower of precision, the end result sends our restaurant critic antagonist on an acid flashback of childhood nostalgia. Manifested in the kitchen, the end result might not have the same effect, but seeing a cartoon masterpiece come to life is worth the time and effort alone.

VERDICT: *Confit byaldi* is as good as ratatouille can be—that is to say, simple, flavorful, simple, warm, and simple. You can only dress up a roasted vegetable medley so much.

---

6 large plum tomatoes

2 red bell peppers, stemmed and seeded

Leaves from 2 sprigs fresh rosemary, half left whole, half finely chopped

Leaves from 2 sprigs fresh thyme

1 garlic clove

½ small onion

½ cup vegetable stock

3 tablespoons extra-virgin olive oil

2 medium Japanese eggplants, sliced crosswise ⅛ inch thick on a mandoline

2 medium yellow squash, sliced crosswise ⅛ inch thick on a mandoline

2 medium zucchini, sliced crosswise ⅛ inch thick on a mandoline

1 teaspoon kosher salt

1 teaspoon freshly ground black pepper

5 fresh parsley leaves, torn

4 to 6 small fresh chives, for garnish

(recipe continues)

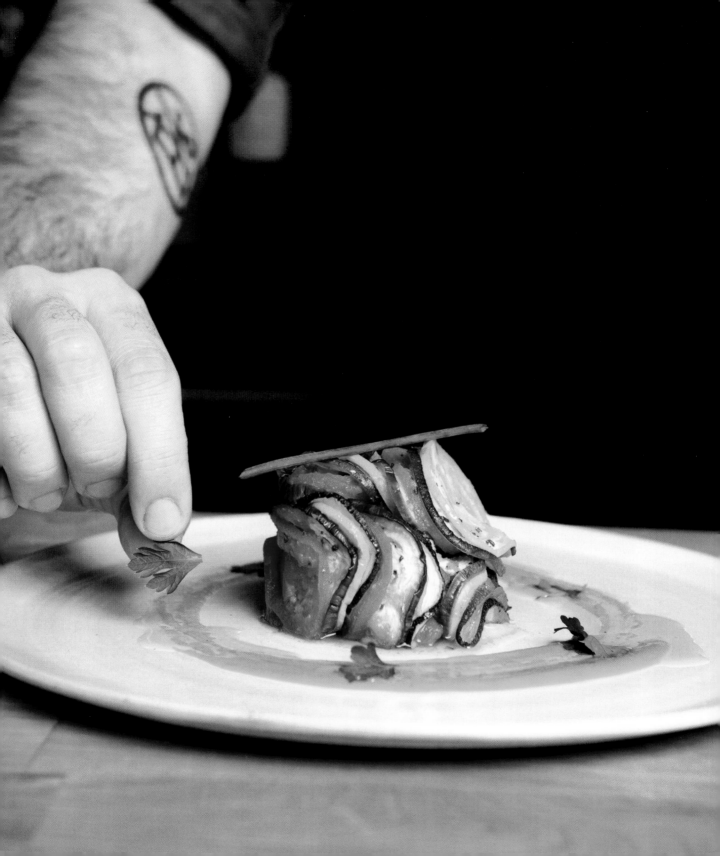

BRING A large pot of water to a boil. Fill a large bowl with ice and water. Score a small X into the bottom of 4 of the plum tomatoes and carefully lower them into the boiling water. Blanch for less than 1 minute, until the X just begins to split up the sides of the tomatoes. Using a slotted spoon, immediately transfer the tomatoes to the ice bath to stop the cooking. Drain, peel, and set aside.

CHAR THE bell peppers directly on the burner of a gas stovetop set to high, turning them frequently with the tongs, until blackened all over. Remove from the heat and cover with aluminum foil. Let the peppers steam and soften for about 5 minutes. Peel off and discard the skins and transfer the peppers to a high-powered blender or food processor. Add the 2 remaining tomatoes, the whole rosemary leaves, thyme leaves, garlic, onion, stock, ½ cup water, and 1 tablespoon of the olive oil. Blend on high speed until the roast pepper puree is completely smooth.

PREHEAT THE oven to 225°F. Line a baking sheet with parchment paper.

USING A very sharp knife, slice the blanched tomatoes ⅛ inch thick and transfer to the lined baking sheet. In a shallow roaster or 9 x 13-inch baking dish, pour a thin layer of the roast pepper puree and spread it evenly. Shingle the sliced vegetables on top of the puree, slightly overlapping 1 slice each of eggplant, tomato, yellow squash, and zucchini. Continue the pattern around the edge of the baking dish toward the center, packing the vegetables tightly until the dish is completely filled. Sprinkle the chopped rosemary leaves, 1 tablespoon of the olive oil, the salt, and the black pepper over the top. Cut a piece of parchment paper to the size of the baking dish and place it directly on top of the vegetables. Bake for 1 hour 10 minutes, remove the parchment paper, then bake for 20 minutes more, or until the vegetables are completely softened but still hold their shape. Remove the confit byaldi from the oven.

FOR EACH serving, place a 3-inch ring mold in the center of a large plate. Fill the ring mold with 1 layer of vegetables stacked vertically. Top that layer with another layer of vegetables fanned out horizontally. Carefully remove the ring mold to reveal a confit byaldi tower. Whisk together 1 tablespoon of the roasted pepper puree from the bottom of the baking dish with the remaining olive oil and drizzle it in a circle around the tower on each plate. Garnish with some torn parsley and a single chive, and serve.

FUN FACT

The "young Babish" featured in this episode is none other than my nephew, Christopher, who was kind enough to do his best impression of me using his play kitchen. I often wonder how he's going to feel as a teenager, seeing that 8 million people have heard him say, "I need to go to the bafroom."

SZECHUAN SAUCE AND NUGGETS

SERVES 4

I was excited to revisit the notorious 1998 McDonald's condiment, because due to its *Rick-and-Morty*-induced surge in popularity, the fast-food giant initially raffled off a few quarts of sauce to some lucky winners. Even luckier (for me), one of them was a fan of the show and was kind enough to send me a carefully wrapped Tupperware filled with his bounty. Later, McDonald's would go on to (disastrously) release the sauce for a single day, but at the time, this felt akin to corporate espionage. The sample of sauce and a photo of the ingredients list proved to be more than enough to reverse-engineer it, along with a batch of freshly fried nuggets. Both unfortunately turned out to be not quite worth making at home, but as always, the joy is in the journey.

VERDICT: Honest-to-god Szechuan sauce is decidedly underwhelming—maybe Rick was seeing the past through rose-colored glasses. Between that and the extremely difficult to make homemade McNuggets, both end up as recipes not worth the time or effort.

SZECHUAN SAUCE

½ cup distilled white vinegar

½ cup sugar

½ cup soy sauce

1 tablespoon apple cider vinegar

½ teaspoon sesame oil

¼ teaspoon garlic powder

¼ teaspoon onion powder

¼ teaspoon ground ginger

¼ teaspoon yeast extract (I used Marmite)

1 teaspoon dextrose (I used light corn syrup)

Ground black pepper

2 tablespoons cornstarch

CHICKEN NUGGETS

Nonstick cooking spray

Skin from 2 chicken breasts, frozen for 30 minutes

1 pound ground chicken

2 tablespoons kosher salt

2 tablespoons sugar

½ teaspoon garlic powder

½ teaspoon onion powder

½ teaspoon ground white pepper

Vegetable oil, for greasing

(ingredients continue)

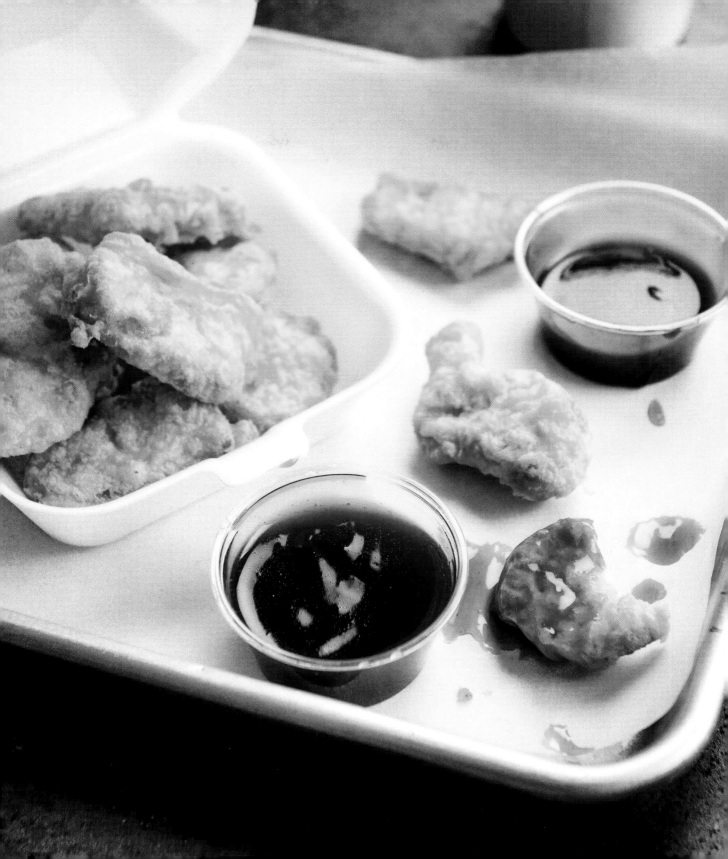

Canola oil, for frying

Vegetable oil, for frying

Beef tallow, for frying

1 cup all-purpose flour

½ cup cornstarch

½ cup cornmeal

1 cup vodka

1 large egg

Kosher salt and ground black pepper

SZECHUAN SAUCE

IN A medium bowl, whisk together ½ cup water, the white vinegar, sugar, soy sauce, apple cider vinegar, sesame oil, garlic powder, onion powder, ginger, yeast extract, and dextrose. Season with pepper. Pour ¼ cup of the Szechuan sauce into a liquid measuring cup and whisk in the cornstarch. Transfer to a medium saucepan and add the rest of the sauce. Cook over medium heat, whisking continuously, until the sauce is thickened, about 10 minutes. Remove from the heat and set aside.

CHICKEN NUGGETS

LINE A baking sheet with parchment paper. Line a cutting board with parchment paper as well and spray the parchment with cooking spray.

REMOVE THE chicken skin from the freezer and place in a food processor while still firm and cold. Process until a smooth paste forms. Transfer to a large bowl and add the ground chicken, salt, sugar, garlic powder, onion powder, and white pepper. Mix together well until a smooth paste forms. Using a rubber spatula, spread the chicken mixture over the lined baking sheet and smooth it out to ¼ inch thick. Press the lined cutting board down on the nugget mixture to flatten. Freeze for 15 minutes to firm up.

LINE A baking sheet with parchment paper and grease the parchment with vegetable oil.

USING CHICKEN nugget cutters (instructions follow) or nugget-sized cookie cutters, cut out as many nuggets as you can and transfer to the lined baking sheet. Transfer to the freezer for 10 minutes to firm up.

BATTER AND FRYING

FILL A large pot with equal parts canola oil, vegetable oil, and beef tallow to a depth of 2 inches. Heat the mixture over medium-high heat to 350°F. Line a large plate with paper towels.

IN A medium bowl, combine the flour, cornstarch, and cornmeal. Add 1 cup water, the vodka, and the egg and stir until smooth. Season the batter with pepper.

DIP THE nuggets in the batter, letting any excess drip back into the bowl, add them to the hot fat, and fry for 5 to 7 minutes or until golden brown, flipping as necessary. Transfer to the paper towels and immediately sprinkle with salt. Serve with the Szechuan sauce.

CHICKEN NUGGET CUTTERS

18 x 13-inch disposable aluminum baking sheet

A pair of sturdy scissors

Protective work gloves (very important; the cut edges of the aluminum are very sharp)

Super glue

Paper clips

CUT FOUR 3 x 12-inch strips from the baking sheet.

FOLD EACH strip in half lengthwise, leaving a little lip on one long edge. Fold the lip over to cover the razor-sharp edge that's exposed.

FORM EACH strip into one of the 4 Chicken McNugget shapes: bell, ball, bone, and boot.

SEAL EACH cutter with super glue and hold the seams shut with paper clips until the glue has dried completely.

FUN FACT

I made this episode almost immediately after an extremely painful breakup, as I was determined not to allow anything to interrupt my new career. As a result, this episode, about a dozen after, and my new *Basics* series were all made during one of the most difficult periods of my life. I didn't say all these facts would be fun. Oh wait, I did—never mind.

THEATER-STYLE POPCORN WITH CHOCOLATE-COVERED RAISINS

SERVES 4

I've written and rewritten this paragraph a few times because I realized I was fanboy-ing too hard about *Whiplash*. The fact is, I love this movie, and it's hard to hide it. Often, I use moments in film or TV as an excuse to make a dish I've wanted to try (see: cinnamon rolls from Jim Gaffigan's stand-up), but in this case, it was an excuse to make something from the source material. Happily, making movie-theater popcorn had also long been a dream of mine, and a little research yielded the answer: the otherworldly glow of an artificial butter–flavored seasoning salt known as Flavacol. A teaspoon of this stuff along with some coconut oil will make your house properly reek like a Regal Cinemas for your next movie night.

VERDICT: Even with this simple method, movie-theater-style popcorn is easily achievable at home. Chocolate-covered raisins, however, are better left to the pros: my homemade "gourmet" equivalents were way too sour and bitter to work in harmony with the popcorn.

---

8 ounces milk chocolate, chopped

4 ounces raisins or other dried fruit (such as cherries, cranberries, or blueberries)

3 tablespoons coconut oil

⅓ cup popcorn kernels

1 heaping teaspoon Flavacol (an alien-orange flavor additive; available on Amazon)

Melted butter, for topping (optional)

CHOCOLATE-COVERED RAISINS

LINE A baking sheet with parchment paper.

TEMPER THE chocolate: Bring 1 cup water to a simmer in a medium saucepan. Place two-thirds of the chocolate in a heatproof glass bowl—large enough so the bottom of the bowl does not touch the water when set over the saucepan of simmering water. Stir the chocolate continuously until it has melted and reaches 115°F. Remove the bowl from the saucepan and keep the water simmering. Add the remaining chocolate to the bowl and stir until fully melted and the chocolate reaches 82°F.

RETURN THE bowl to the saucepan and stir until the chocolate reaches 90°F. Remove the bowl from the heat. To check if the chocolate is tempered, dip a butter knife into it and refrigerate for 5 minutes. If the hardened chocolate is glossy, without noticeable streaks, it has been tempered properly.

ADD THE raisins (or other dried fruit) to the chocolate and stir until each raisin is completely coated in chocolate. Using chopsticks or two forks, remove each raisin, shake off the excess chocolate, and transfer to the lined baking sheet, spacing the chocolate-covered raisins apart. Let the chocolate cool and harden for 1 hour at room temperature.

POPCORN

IN A large stockpot, heat the coconut oil over medium-high heat. Add 2 or 3 popcorn kernels to the oil and heat until they pop. Remove the pot from the heat and add the remaining popcorn kernels and the Flavacol, shaking to coat evenly. Cover with the lid and remove from the heat for 30 seconds.

RETURN THE pot to medium heat and cook, shaking the pot gently and continuously, until all the kernels have popped, about 2 to 3 minutes.

POUR THE popcorn into a large bowl, add melted butter, if desired, and top with the chocolate-covered raisins.

FUN FACT
One of my first jobs was at a Regal Cinemas concession counter, making this very kind of popcorn. I couldn't eat the stuff for a solid year afterward.

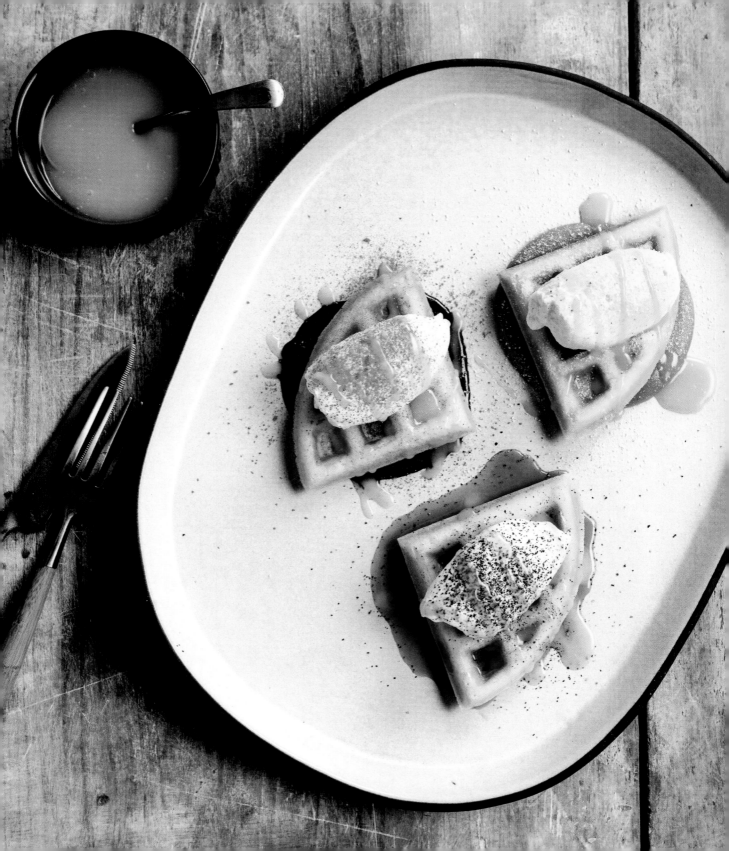

TRIPLE-DECKER EGGO EXTRAVAGANZA

SERVES 4, PLUS EXTRA BATTER FOR MORE WAFFLES

Much like the protagonist of *Stranger Things*, the Triple-Decker Eggo Extravaganza is a sci-fi sweet not to be trifled with. Following Eleven's culinary theme of only eating eclectic junk food, the towering pillar of sugar and carbs will not only upset your stomach, but your taste buds. The only way to make this monstrosity palatable was to really stretch its definitions, swapping jelly beans for freeze-dried fruit, Hershey's Kisses for rich sauces, and Eggos for some halfway decent waffles.

VERDICT: The updated TDEE is elegant, tasty, and extremely labor-intensive—you might want to cut it down to one sauce/topping for the waffles, which turn out incredibly light and lacy.

WAFFLES

2½ cups pastry flour

½ cup malt powder (available on Amazon)

2 tablespoons cornmeal

2 tablespoons buttermilk powder (available on Amazon and at Whole Foods)

1 teaspoon sugar

1 (¼-ounce) packet active dry yeast

½ teaspoon baking soda

¼ teaspoon fine salt

2⅔ cups whole milk

½ cup canola oil

2 large eggs

TOPPINGS

1 cup pure maple syrup

1 cup heavy cream

2 tablespoons unsalted butter

½ cup freeze-dried strawberries

½ cup freeze-dried bananas

½ cup freeze-dried blueberries

2 teaspoons sugar

1 teaspoon pure vanilla extract

Nonstick cooking spray

Hot Fudge Sauce (see page 174)

Peanut Butter Drizzle (see page 175)

(recipe continues)

WAFFLES

INTO A large bowl, sift together the pastry flour, malt powder, cornmeal, buttermilk powder, sugar, yeast, baking soda, and salt.

IN A medium saucepan, heat the milk and canola oil over medium-low heat to 110°F. Remove from the heat and, while whisking gently, slowly drizzle into the dry ingredients. Add the eggs and whisk gently until the batter barely comes together, taking care not to over-mix—it's okay if some lumps remain. Cover and let rest at room temperature for 2 hours.

TOPPINGS

WHILE THE batter rests, in a small saucepan, combine the maple syrup, ½ cup of the cream, and the butter and cook, whisking to combine, over medium heat for 3 to 5 minutes, until thickened. Let the maple sauce cool completely.

PLACE THE freeze-dried strawberries in a food processor and process until finely ground. Transfer to a small bowl. Repeat with the bananas and blueberries, keeping all the fruit powders separate.

IN A medium bowl, using a handheld mixer, beat the remaining ½ cup cream, the sugar, and the vanilla on medium-high speed to your desired consistency.

HEAT AN 8-inch Belgian waffle iron and generously spray with cooking spray. Pour about ⅔ cup of the batter into the waffle iron and spread it evenly. Cook according to the manufacturer's instructions until golden brown and crisp.

FOR EACH serving, pool each of the three sauces (fudge, peanut butter, and maple) into a 2-inch round on a wide plate. Cut the waffles into quarters, and place 1 quarter on each pool of sauce. Using a warmed spoon (dipped in hot water, then dried), roll quenelles of whipped cream and dollop onto each waffle. Sprinkle strawberry powder over the fudge waffle, banana over the peanut butter, and blueberry over the maple and serve.

Entering the world of Harry Potter was dangerous territory—fans of the behemoth series are the very definition of die-hard, some reportedly weeping upon taking their first sip of Butterbeer at the Orlando attraction. However, it ended up showing me how forgiving my audience is: criticism surrounding my pumpkin pasties was accurate, level-headed, and gave me a lot to consider for future episodes. While these mini pumpkin pies aren't accurate (the real version would've likely been savory), they're certainly tasty. In the words of another wildly popular series, may the force be with you.

PUMPKIN PASTIES

SERVES 6 TO 10

VERDICT: Pumpkin pasties, though inaccurate, are lovely little confections.

PASTIES

1 medium sugar pie pumpkin

½ cup heavy cream

½ teaspoon freshly grated nutmeg

¼ teaspoon ground cloves

1 teaspoon ground cinnamon

½ teaspoon ground allspice

1 teaspoon pure vanilla extract

½ cup packed light brown sugar

¼ cup pure maple syrup

1 large egg

½ teaspoon kosher salt

1 recipe Tart Dough (recipe follows)

1 large egg, beaten

Granulated sugar, for sprinkling

PREHEAT THE oven to 400°F. Line a baking sheet with parchment paper.

CUT THE pumpkin in half, scoop out the seeds, and place cut-side down on the lined baking sheet. Roast for 30 to 40 minutes, until a paring knife can cut into the pumpkin without resistance. Flip the pumpkin halves and let cool enough to handle.

SCOOP OUT the pumpkin flesh, transfer to a food processor, and puree until smooth. Add the cream, nutmeg, cloves, cinnamon, allspice,

(recipe continues)

vanilla, brown sugar, maple syrup, egg, and salt. Process until smooth, about 15 seconds. Cover and refrigerate until ready to use.

PREHEAT THE oven to 400°F. Line a baking sheet with parchment paper.

TRANSFER THE chilled tart dough to a floured work surface and roll out to about a ¼-inch thickness. Using a 4-inch round cutter, cut the dough into 6 rounds. (You can reroll the scraps and cut them into additional rounds, but they will be less tender.)

FOR EACH round of dough, brush half the outer edge with the beaten egg, fill with 1 to 2 tablespoons of pumpkin filling, fold the dough over to form half-moons, and seal shut with a fork or crimp decoratively. Transfer to the lined baking sheet. Brush the tops of the pasties with the beaten egg, sprinkle with sugar, and bake for 20 to 30 minutes, until golden brown and crisp. Remove from the oven, transfer the pasties to a wire rack, and let cool for 10 minutes, then serve.

TART DOUGH
MAKES ENOUGH DOUGH FOR ONE 9-INCH TART

¼ cup vodka

11½ ounces all-purpose flour (about 2⅔ cups)

1 ounce sugar (about 2 tablespoons)

1 teaspoon kosher salt

1¼ cups (2½ sticks) unsalted butter, cubed and frozen

IN A small bowl, combine ¼ cup water and the vodka and place in the freezer for 30 minutes.

IN A food processor, combine two-thirds of the flour and the sugar, salt, and butter. Pulse until the butter is the size of small peas. Transfer the mixture to a large bowl and sprinkle with the vodka mixture. Using a rubber spatula, gently fold the mixture together until a shaggy dough forms. Add the remaining flour. Knead gently until the dough comes together, taking care not to break up the dough or let the pieces of butter melt. Pat the dough into a disc, wrap tightly in plastic wrap, and refrigerate for at least 1 hour or up to overnight before using.

BABISH'S BUTTERBEER

MAKES 1 BUTTERBEER

VERDICT: Butterbeer is far too sweet for my taste but should satisfy younger readers, provided the butterscotch schnapps is swapped out for syrup to make them nonalcoholic.

½ cup cream soda, chilled

1 large egg white

2 ounces butterscotch schnapps

1 ounce heavy cream

⅛ teaspoon pure vanilla extract

½ ounce simple syrup (see page 91)

Ice

POUR THE cream soda into a pint glass. In a cocktail shaker, combine the egg white, schnapps, cream, vanilla, and simple syrup. Fill with ice and shake vigorously until thick and foamy. Strain into the pint glass and serve.

TREACLE TART

SERVES 8

VERDICT: Treacle tart is sticky, sweet, and totally delicious, especially with a generous dollop of soft-whipped cream.

All-purpose flour, for dusting

Tart Dough (see page 200)

16 ounces Lyle's Golden Syrup (available at specialty stores) or light molasses

2 tablespoons unsalted butter

3 tablespoons heavy cream

¼ cup plain bread crumbs

1 large egg

Whipped Cream (see page 186), for serving (optional)

PREHEAT THE oven to 400°F.

ON A floured work surface, roll out the tart dough to about a 12-inch round. Roll the round onto your rolling pin and unroll it over a 9-inch nonstick tart pan with a removable bottom. Without stretching the dough, ease it into the pan, pushing it into the corners. Trim the excess dough and prick the bottom with a fork about a dozen times. Line the tart pan with foil, fill with pie weights, and bake for 15 minutes, or until the tart shell is lightly browned. Remove from the oven and reduce the oven temperature to 350°F.

MEANWHILE, IN a medium saucepan, combine the golden syrup and butter and cook over low heat, whisking, just until the butter has melted. Remove from the heat and vigorously whisk in the cream until the mixture is smooth and has cooled slightly. Beat the bread crumbs and egg into the treacle until completely combined.

REMOVE THE foil and pie weights from the tart shell and fill the shell with the treacle. Bake for 45 to 50 minutes, until the pastry is a deep brown and the filling is caramelized and bubbling. Remove from the oven and let cool completely on a wire rack.

REMOVE THE tart from the pan, slice into wedges and serve, topped with whipped cream, if desired.

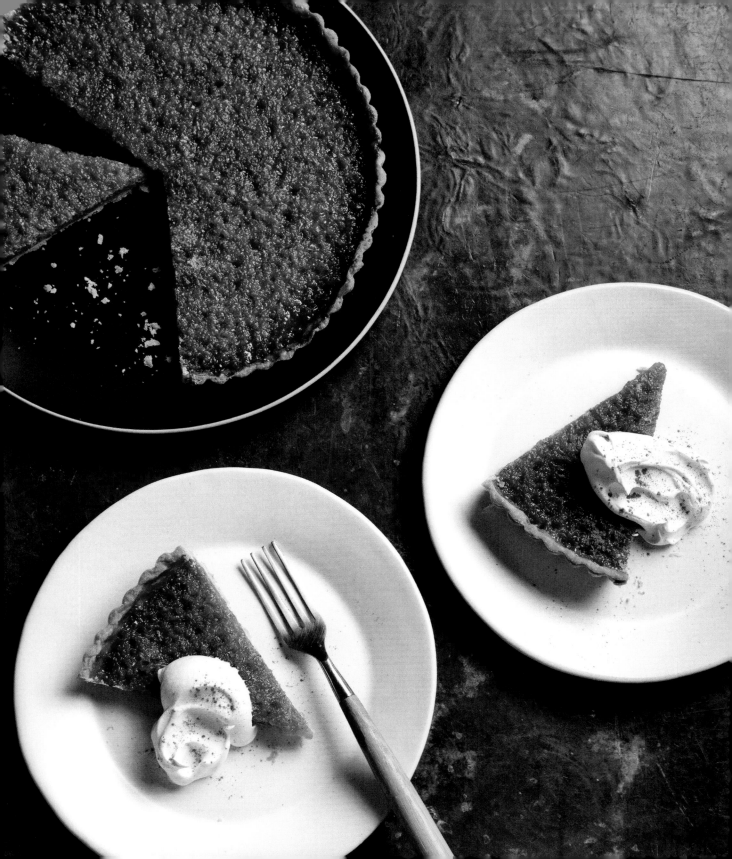

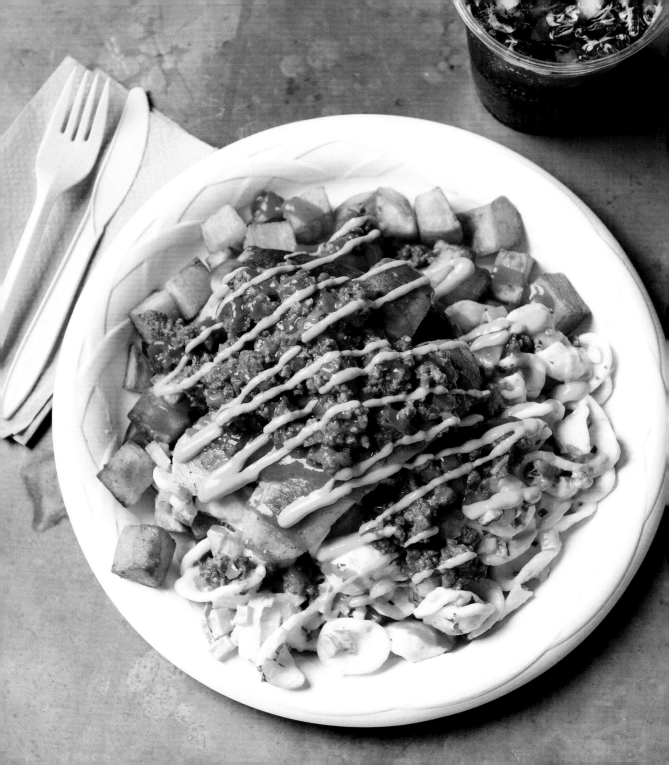

GARBAGE PLATES

SERVES 4

Probably the biggest stretch of the series, the mere off-camera mention of my hometown's official dish was excuse enough to whip one up. I grew up eating garbage plates (and having to explain them to outsiders) throughout Rochester, New York, so even when a political aide mentioned them in passing to a distracted Bradley Cooper in an arthouse cops-and-robbers film, I was thrilled. I could finally share the pride of western New York with the world. As luck would have it, fellow Rochesterian and YouTuber Jenna Marbles released a video in which she proclaimed plates as her favorite meal, and the internet "ate it up," so to speak. I can only hope I've done my part by, God willing, convincing you, dear reader, to take up the spatula and give it a try yourself.

VERDICT: The culinary zeitgeist of a generation, the humble garbage plate captures and inspires our collective consciousness, our imagination, and, dare I say, life itself. Sorry, I let this one go off the rails. In all seriousness, this recipe yields a delightful macaroni salad and crisp diner-style potatoes, and they come together to make something greater than the sum of their parts. Plus, it's awesome when you're drunk.

MACARONI SALAD

1 pound orecchiette or other short pasta, cooked according to the package directions, drained, rinsed, and cooled

3 small carrots, chopped

2 celery stalks, chopped

4 scallions, finely chopped

1 cup loosely packed fresh parsley, finely minced

½ cup Peppadew peppers, stemmed and chopped

½ teaspoon garlic powder

1 teaspoon kosher salt, plus more if needed

1 teaspoon freshly ground black pepper

¼ cup mayonnaise

2 tablespoons sour cream

1 tablespoon Dijon mustard

"HOT SAUCE"

3 teaspoons vegetable oil

1 small onion, diced

1 pound ground beef

4 ounces tomato paste

½ teaspoon kosher salt

½ teaspoon freshly ground black pepper

¼ teaspoon ground cloves

¼ teaspoon ground cinnamon

¼ teaspoon ground allspice

(ingredients continue)

¼ teaspoon cayenne pepper

¼ teaspoon ground cumin

¼ teaspoon paprika

¼ teaspoon garlic powder

DINER-STYLE HOME FRIES

3 medium russet potatoes, peeled and diced

3 tablespoons distilled white vinegar

1 tablespoon plus 1 teaspoon kosher salt

1 tablespoon vegetable oil

1 tablespoon unsalted butter

1 teaspoon paprika

1 teaspoon freshly ground black pepper

ASSEMBLY

8 white hots (veal-and-pork hot dogs) or weisswurst

1 tablespoon vegetable oil

Ketchup, for serving

Yellow mustard, for serving

MACARONI SALAD

IN A large bowl, combine all the ingredients. Taste and season with more salt, if necessary. Cover and refrigerate until ready to use.

"HOT SAUCE"

IN A large sauté pan, heat 1½ teaspoons of the vegetable oil over medium heat until shimmering. Add the onion and cook, stirring, until soft, about 3 minutes. Transfer to a bowl and set aside. Add the remaining 1½ teaspoons vegetable oil to the pan, increase the heat to medium-high, and heat until shimmering, 1 to 2 minutes. Add the beef and cook in a single layer until deeply browned, about 5 minutes. Using a wooden spoon, scrape the bottom of the pan, turn the beef over, and brown the other side, about 5 minutes. Repeat until the beef is browned and crisp all over. Reduce the heat to medium-low, add the tomato paste, and cook, stirring, for 1 minute. Add the salt, black pepper, cloves, cinnamon, allspice, cayenne, cumin, paprika, and garlic powder and cook, stirring, for 1 minute more. Return the onion to the pan.

Add ½ cup water and cook, stirring and scraping up all the browned bits from the bottom of the pan. Simmer until a thick meat sauce forms, adding more water if it gets too thick, about 5 minutes. Remove from the heat and keep warm until ready to use.

DINER-STYLE HOME FRIES

PLACE THE potatoes in a large saucepan and cover with cold water. Add the vinegar and 1 tablespoon of the salt. Cover and bring to a boil over medium-high heat. Cook for 5 minutes. Drain the potatoes and spread them out on a rimmed baking sheet. Let cool completely.

IN A large cast-iron pan, heat the vegetable oil and butter over medium heat until the butter's foaming subsides. Add the potatoes in batches to create a single, uncrowded layer. Cook, undisturbed, until golden brown on one side, about 4 minutes. Stir and flip the potatoes to brown another side. Repeat until the potatoes are brown and crisp all over, about 8 minutes total. Transfer to a large bowl. Repeat with the remaining potatoes. While the home fries are still warm, toss with the remaining 1 teaspoon salt, the paprika, and the pepper.

ASSEMBLY

WITHOUT CUTTING all the way through, split the hot dogs in half lengthwise and open them up like a book. In a cast-iron skillet, heat the vegetable oil over medium-high heat until shimmering. Place the hot dogs in the skillet, cut-side down, and weight them down with another pan to press them evenly against the heat. Cook until well browned, about 2 minutes, then flip and repeat on the other side.

FOR EACH serving, mound some of the potatoes and macaroni salad side-by-side on a large plate. Top with 2 hot dogs and some meat sauce. Drizzle with ketchup and mustard and serve.

FUN FACT
Jenna Marbles and I were in the same grades at nearby schools and, though we didn't know each other at the time, attended the same prom.

QUATRO QUESOS DOS FRITOS

SERVES 4

Four cheeses, twice fried: Sounds good in theory, right? In practice with Shawn and Gus, however, this artery-clogging decadence needs a bit of work. As is clearly visible in the *Psych* Slumber Party sketches, Shawn is constructing the QQDF out of whole skin-on Yukon Gold potatoes, unbreaded and secured with toothpicks. This is a recipe for disaster, unfortunately, as Yukon Golds (or any whole skin-on potato, for that matter) do not lend themselves to deep-frying, even twice. The result was a chewy, flabby potato bite with cheese spitting out the sides during both deep frying and consumption. The solution needed to be lighter, crisper, and better-designed to sop up the more brilliant bacon and ancho chile sour cream. Fried mashed potatoes, sort of like an all-American *arancini*, not only makes good use of leftovers, it makes for a genuinely delicious party snack.

VERDICT: Soft, melty, and crunchy (exactly how you imagined QQDF), this iteration of the *Psych* snack will satisfy the urges of any USA network fanatic.

---

3 large russet potatoes

1 tablespoon extra-virgin olive oil

1 tablespoon unsalted butter

2 teaspoons kosher salt, plus more for seasoning

1 teaspoon freshly ground black pepper

2 large eggs

½ cup mayonnaise

2 teaspoons ancho chile powder

Vegetable oil, for frying

1 cup all-purpose flour

1 cup panko bread crumbs

4 ounces sharp cheddar cheese, cut into 1-inch cubes

½ pound bacon, cooked until crisp and finely chopped

PREHEAT THE oven to 350°F. Line a baking sheet with aluminum foil.

PLACE THE potatoes on the lined baking sheet. Rub the potatoes with the olive oil, poke each four or five times with a fork, and bake until cooked through, about 45 minutes.

REMOVE FROM the oven and cut each potato in half lengthwise while hot to let the steam escape. Let stand for 15 minutes, until cool enough to handle but still warm.

SCOOP THE potato flesh into a potato ricer and press through the finest setting into a large bowl. Discard the potato skins. Add the butter, salt, pepper, and 1 egg and mix gently with a rubber spatula until combined. Cover with plastic wrap, pressing the plastic directly against the surface of the mashed potatoes, and refrigerate until chilled, about 1 hour.

MEANWHILE, IN a small bowl, whisk together the mayonnaise and ancho chile powder. Set aside.

FILL A large saucepan with vegetable oil to a depth of 3 inches. Heat over medium-high heat to 350°F. Line a large plate with paper towels.

PLACE THE flour, remaining egg, and bread crumbs in individual shallow bowls. Beat the egg. Wrap each cheese cube in about ⅓ cup of the mashed potatoes, forming the potato into a ball with your hands. Dredge each ball in the flour, dip in the egg, then dredge in the bread crumbs. Working in batches to avoid crowding the pan, add the balls to the hot oil and fry, flipping them as necessary, until golden brown, about 5 minutes. Transfer the fried potato balls to the paper towels. Season generously with salt.

SPREAD THE ancho mayo evenly over a large plate and stack the fried potato balls on top. Sprinkle the bacon over the top and serve hot.

FLANDERS'S HOT CHOCOLATE

SERVES 4

Some recipes in this book take a bit more conjecture and artistic license than others—Flanders's famed hot chocolate is among them. Through its exquisite final form, however, we can surmise that America's favorite cheery Christian neighbor would've likely paid similar attention to the quality of the hot chocolate itself. This meant rich cream, chopped chocolate, and cocoa powder, and a hint of espresso powder to amp up the flavors. The result is ding-dong-diddly delicious.

VERDICT: This is a top-notch hot cocoa recipe. The toppings are fun but tedious to actually eat and drink.

---

2 cups whole milk

1 cup heavy cream

1 cup evaporated milk

¼ cup unsweetened Dutch-process cocoa powder

4 ounces dark chocolate, chopped, plus 1 ounce for grating

½ cup sugar

½ teaspoon instant espresso powder

¼ teaspoon ground cinnamon

1 teaspoon kosher salt

Canned whipped cream, for serving

4 chocolate sugar wafer cookies

4 marshmallows

IN A large saucepan, combine the whole milk, cream, and evaporated milk and heat over medium heat until steaming (about 190°F). Reduce the heat to medium-low and add the cocoa powder, chopped chocolate, sugar, espresso powder, cinnamon, and salt. Whisk gently until completely combined and creamy.

DIVIDE THE hot chocolate among four mugs. Top each mug with a large swirl of whipped cream and finely grate the remaining chocolate over the whipped cream. Push 1 cookie into each mound of whipped cream, then press 1 marshmallow onto the top of each cookie. Using a culinary torch, toast the marshmallows until browned and serve.

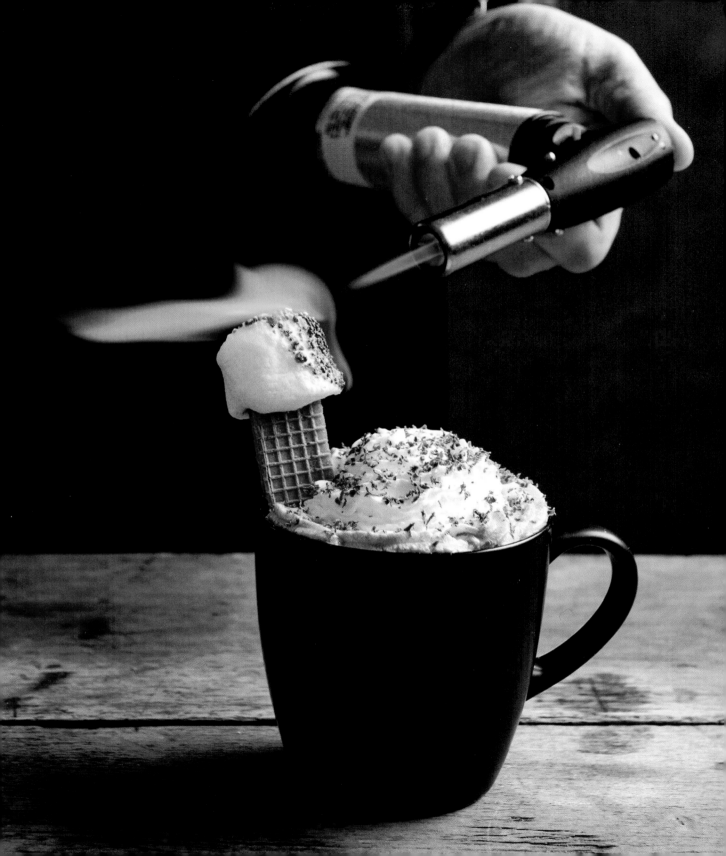

PEKING DUCK

SERVES 4

I had long dreaded the idea of making Peking duck, because I knew that it would involve the inflation of a whole dead animal's carcass. This is a cookbook, Andy, take it down a notch. But it's the unappetizing truth: real Peking duck is blown up like the Michelin Man before being roasted, as the separation of the meat and skin results in a crispier bird. With Christmas approaching, however, I decided it was time to bite the bullet and blow me up a duck. I ordered an air compressor off Amazon, sourced a frozen Peking duck in Chinatown, and was dismayed when I was dressed up and ready to shoot, only to find out that the compressor I had ordered was designed for a car's cigarette lighter. I frantically called every hardware store in the borough, eventually finding one that carried a reasonably sized wall-outlet compressor, just in time to get the episode done before the holiday. It was a Christmas miracle.

VERDICT: This is an effective way of making Peking duck at home, but comes with its fair share of challenges. The bird comes out crisp and flavorful, the pancakes thin and chewy, and the sauce thick and rich, everything you want from the (now) Beijing classic.

HOISIN SAUCE

¼ cup soy sauce

2 tablespoons honey

1 (1-inch) knob fresh ginger, peeled and grated

1 garlic clove, grated

2 teaspoons rice vinegar

2 teaspoons sesame oil

1 tablespoon chile-garlic sauce

2 tablespoons smooth peanut butter

1 teaspoon freshly ground black pepper

2 tablespoons dark brown sugar

2 teaspoons cornstarch, for thickening (optional)

PEKING DUCK

3 cinnamon sticks, crushed

1 tablespoon Szechuan peppercorns

1 tablespoon fennel seeds

7 star anise pods

1½ teaspoons whole cloves

1 head-on young fresh Peking duck (about 5 pounds; available at Asian markets)

¼ cup soy sauce

MANDARIN-STYLE PANCAKES

10 ounces all-purpose flour, plus more for dusting

⅔ cup boiling water

Sesame oil, for brushing

2 scallions, julienned and chilled in ice water for 5 minutes, then drained and patted dry

1 small cucumber, thinly julienned

HOISIN SAUCE

IN A medium bowl, whisk together all the sauce ingredients except the cornstarch. If the hoisin sauce is too runny, whisk in up to 2 teaspoons of cornstarch to thicken it. Set aside until ready to use.

PEKING DUCK

IN A dry sauté pan, toast the cinnamon, peppercorns, fennel seeds, star anise, and cloves over medium heat, stirring, until fragrant, 2 to 3 minutes. Remove from the heat and let cool. Transfer to a spice grinder and grind into a fine powder. Set the Chinese five-spice powder aside.

PLACE THE duck on a wire rack set on a rimmed baking sheet. Fill the cavity with about half the hoisin sauce (reserve the rest for serving) and stitch the cavity closed with a skewer.

CUT A slit in the skin at the base of the duck's neck. Wrap the tip of an air compressor hose with plastic wrap and insert the tip of the hose into the slit, facing the body. Turn on the air compressor to inflate the duck and separate the skin from the meat. It should take 20 to 30 seconds to fully inflate the duck. Remove the compressor hose, let the duck deflate, and set aside. (Note: This is obviously tedious and difficult. Skip this step if you don't have a spare air compressor lying around exclusively for food service use.)

IN A large pot, combine 4 cups water, the soy sauce, and ¼ cup of the Chinese five-spice powder (reserve the rest in an airtight container for another use). Bring to a boil. Grip the duck by its head and hold it over the pot. Carefully ladle the boiling liquid all over the duck skin until the skin is golden and tight, about 3 minutes. Refrigerate, uncovered, for at least 24 hours or up to 72 hours.

WHEN READY to cook the duck, preheat the oven to 350°F. Set a wire rack on a rimmed baking sheet.

REMOVE THE duck from the refrigerator and place it on the rack. Let stand at room temperature for 1 hour. Transfer to the oven and roast for 1 to 1½ hours, until the skin is deeply browned and the internal temperature registers at least 175°F. Remove from the oven and let rest for 10 minutes before carving.

MANDARIN-STYLE PANCAKES

IN A large bowl, combine the flour and boiling water and mix with a wooden spoon until a shaggy dough forms. Turn the dough out onto a floured work surface and knead until smooth, about 5 minutes.

ROLL THE dough into a 2-inch-wide log and divide it into 24 equal pieces. Work with one piece at a time and cover the remaining pieces with plastic wrap to prevent them from drying

(recipe continues)

out. Divide the piece of dough in half and roll out each half into a 3-inch round, flouring the work surface as necessary to keep the dough from sticking. Brush one round with a light layer of sesame oil and top with the other round, sandwiching the sesame oil between the two. Roll out to a 7-inch pancake. Heat a nonstick skillet over medium-high heat for about 2 minutes, and cook the pancake until light brown spots appear, 1 to 2 minutes per side. Remove from the heat and wrap in a clean kitchen towel to keep warm. Repeat with the remaining dough.

CHOP THE duck's head off with a meat cleaver to startle your dinner guests. Carve the duck breast into ½-inch-thick slices, keeping the skin attached to each slice. Remove the skin from the thighs and legs; cut the skin into thin slices and shred the meat.

TRANSFER THE duck meat and skin to a platter and let your guests make wraps with the pancakes, scallions, cucumbers, and remaining hoisin sauce.

FUN FACT

Because of the delay caused by the air compressor, I didn't have time to properly air-dry the duck in the fridge, so it browned horribly unevenly. Some light blowtorching made quick work of that, however. I'm sorry for this moment of culinary dishonesty.

No one was really asking for food from *The Wire*, but I had always been curious about the Charm City specialties occasionally showcased in the gut-wrenching drama. Lake trout, paradoxically not from a lake nor featuring any trout, is a bony deep-fried fillet of whiting. Pit beef appears to be a simple-enough spiced roast beef, heavily laden with horseradish, if Bey has anything to say about it. Both presented great opportunities to explore some basic techniques, and both resulted in delicious (if occasionally a bit difficult to eat), distinctly East Coast dishes.

LAKE TROUT

SERVES 2

VERDICT: Bone-in whiting is inexpensive but very difficult to eat, given all the pin-size bones left in the fish—I might recommend subbing another light, flaky white-fleshed fish, deboned of course.

FRENCH FRIES

Vegetable oil, for frying

4 large russet potatoes, peeled and cut into thick batons

2 teaspoons kosher salt

LAKE TROUT

Vegetable oil, for frying

1 cup all-purpose flour

1 cup fine cornmeal

2 teaspoons garlic powder

2 teaspoons onion powder

1 teaspoon cayenne pepper

1 teaspoon Old Bay seasoning

4 cups whole milk

2 large eggs

2 whole whiting or other white-fleshed fish (about 2 pounds), skinned and deboned

Kosher salt

4 slices white sandwich bread

Hot sauce, for serving

(recipe continues)

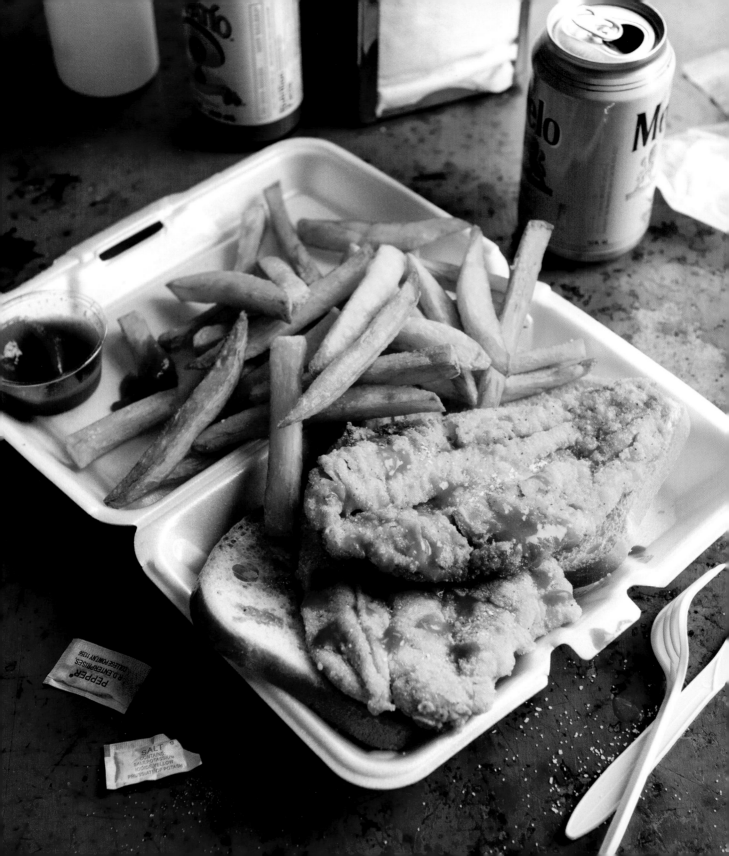

FRENCH FRIES

FILL A large Dutch oven with vegetable oil to a depth of 2 inches. Heat over medium-high heat to 350°F. Line a rimmed baking sheet with paper towels.

WORKING IN batches as necessary to avoid crowding the pan, add the potatoes to the hot oil and fry, flipping occasionally, until just beginning to turn golden, 5 to 7 minutes. Using a mesh spider, drain and remove the fries and transfer to the paper towels, spacing them apart to make sure the fries aren't overlapping. Reserve the oil in the Dutch oven. Let the fries cool for 10 minutes, then freeze for at least 4 hours. (Note: Once frozen, the fries can be stored in a resealable plastic bag for up to 3 months.)

PREHEAT THE oven to 225°F.

REHEAT THE vegetable oil in the Dutch oven over medium-high heat to 350°F, adding fresh oil as needed to bring the oil level back to 2 inches.

WORKING IN batches as needed, add the frozen fries to the hot oil and fry for 5 to 7 minutes, until golden brown and crisp. Transfer the fries to a wire rack set over paper towels and let drain for 2 to 3 minutes. Reserve the oil in the Dutch oven. Transfer the fries to a large bowl and toss with the salt. Transfer to a rimmed baking sheet and keep warm in the oven until ready to serve.

LAKE TROUT

REHEAT THE vegetable oil in the Dutch oven to 350°F, adding fresh oil as needed to bring the oil level back to 2 inches.

IN A large shallow bowl, whisk together the flour, cornmeal, and 1 teaspoon each of the garlic powder, onion powder, and cayenne, and ½ teaspoon of the Old Bay. In another large shallow bowl, whisk together the milk, eggs, remaining 1 teaspoon garlic powder, 1 teaspoon onion powder, and ½ teaspoon Old Bay. Dip the fish in the milk mixture wash and dredge in the seasoned flour, then carefully add to the hot oil and fry until golden brown and cooked through, 2 to 3 minutes. Transfer the fried fish to a wire rack set over paper towels and let drain for 2 minutes before serving. Season with salt while still hot.

DIVIDE THE fries between two Styrofoam containers or two plates. To each serving, add 2 slices of the white bread, top with a fried fish, and drizzle generously with hot sauce.

PIT BEEF

SERVES 4

VERDICT: Pit beef shows an effective way to make inexpensive roast beef and is excellent on its own, but also delicious slathered with horseradish.

---

1 tablespoon kosher salt

1 (3-pound) beef eye of round roast

1 tablespoon vegetable oil

2 teaspoons seasoned salt

1 tablespoon freshly ground black pepper

1 teaspoon smoked paprika

4 sandwich rolls, split

1 small onion, thinly sliced

4 tablespoons prepared horseradish

SPRINKLE THE kosher salt all over the beef. Wrap in plastic wrap and refrigerate for 24 hours. Remove from the refrigerator and let stand at room temperature for 1 hour.

PREHEAT THE oven to 225°F.

IN A large stainless-steel skillet, heat the vegetable oil over medium-high heat until nearly smoking. Sear the roast until evenly browned, about 2 minutes per side. Transfer the roast to a rimmed baking sheet.

IN A small bowl, combine the seasoned salt, pepper, and paprika. Sprinkle the spice mixture all over the roast and insert a temperature probe into the thickest part of the roast. Bake for 1 to 1½ hours, until the internal temperature registers 120°F. Remove from the oven and let rest for 10 minutes.

SLICE SOME of the beef as thinly as possible and divide between the bottom halves of the sandwich rolls. (Reserve the remaining beef for another use.) Top the beef with the onion, and spread 1 tablespoon of the horseradish on the top halves of each roll. Close the sandwiches and serve warm.

SKINNER'S STEW

SERVES 6

There's nothing quite so intimidating as the re-creation of a dish that's deemed by the character himself as impossible to re-create. Principal Skinner laments being driven nearly mad trying to find a jungle delicacy he was "forced to subsist on," a delicious-sounding concoction of fish, prawns, coconut milk, and four kinds of rice. Though the variety of rice seems superfluous, the stew sounds incredible, and reminiscent of *tom kha goong*. Yes, *tom kha* is a Thai dish, but the regions share a number of flavors, and Vietnamese coconut-based soups seem to be few and far between.

So my best guess was that these soldiers were making their favorite Thai dish. Why they would make it with four kinds of rice, however, escapes me.

VERDICT: *Tom kha gai* is an absolutely delicious, deeply flavorful, light-yet-rich seafood stew, and deserves a place in every home cook's repertoire for a quick and comforting meal. Try making your rice in a pressure cooker under low pressure—use the ratio of rice to liquid on the packaging, but divide the cooking time in half.

4 RICES

½ cup brown rice

½ cup red rice

½ cup jasmine rice

½ cup green jade rice

STEW

1½ teaspoons extra-virgin olive oil

2 garlic cloves, minced

1 (1-inch) knob fresh ginger, peeled and grated

1 (2-inch) piece lemongrass, minced

½ pound green beans, cut into 2-inch pieces

¼ pound shiitake mushrooms, sliced

Prawn Stock (recipe follows)

6 makrut lime leaves, or 1 lime, quartered

3 tablespoons green curry paste

1 (8-ounce) can bamboo shoots, drained

1 small red bell pepper, sliced

2 Thai bird's-eye chiles, thinly sliced (optional)

¼ cup fish sauce

1 (14-ounce) can coconut milk

½ cup fresh Thai basil, julienned, plus more for garnish (optional)

½ teaspoon ground cardamom

½ teaspoon cayenne pepper

1 tablespoon light brown sugar

(ingredients continue)

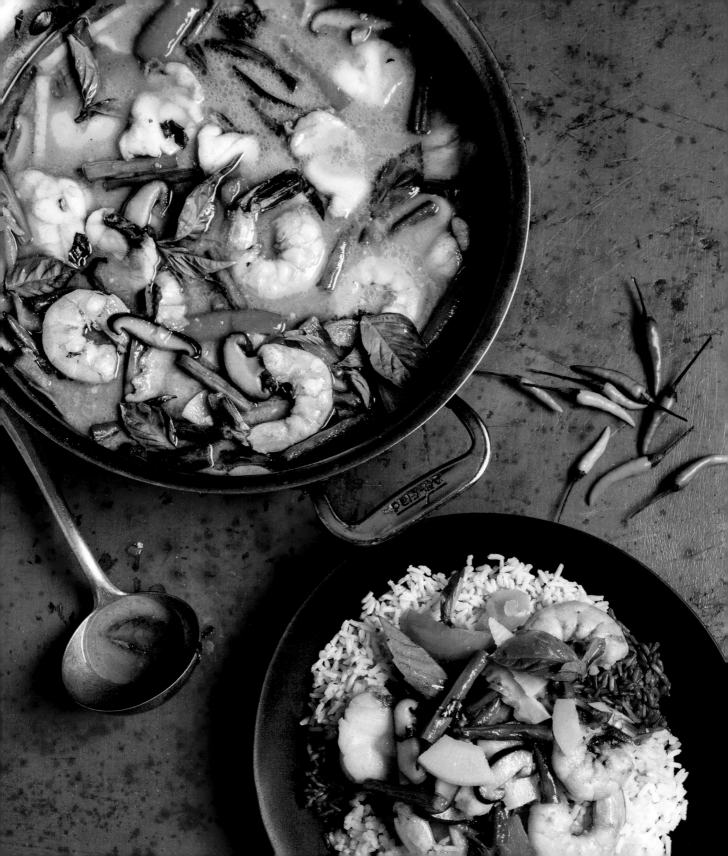

½ pound monkfish fillets, cleaned and cut into 1-inch chunks

1 pound shrimp, peeled and deveined (shells reserved for stock)

Kosher salt and freshly ground black pepper

FOUR RICES

PREHEAT THE oven to 200°F.

COOK EACH rice separately, according to its package directions. Keep warm in the oven until the stew is ready. (Note: The four types of rice are for accuracy. Feel free to cook just one kind of rice.)

STEW

IN A deep sauté pan, heat the olive oil over medium-high heat until shimmering. Add the garlic, ginger, lemongrass, green beans, and mushrooms and cook, stirring, until fragrant, 3 to 5 minutes. Add half the stock and cook, stirring and scraping up all the browned bits from the bottom of the pan. Add the lime leaves, curry paste, bamboo shoots, bell pepper, chiles, fish sauce, coconut milk, remaining stock, and the basil. Bring to a simmer, then add the cardamom, cayenne, and brown sugar. Stir until completely incorporated. Add the monkfish and prawns, reduce the heat, cover, and simmer for 10 minutes, or until the seafood is fully cooked. Season with salt and black pepper.

FOR EACH serving, put a scoop of each type of rice in a shallow bowl and ladle over the fish stew. Garnish with more basil, if desired, and serve.

PRAWN STOCK
MAKES ABOUT 2½ CUPS

1½ teaspoons extra-virgin olive oil
4 scallions, cut into 3-inch lengths
Shells from ½ pound prawns or large shrimp
½ cup dry white wine

IN A large Dutch oven, heat the olive oil over medium-high heat until shimmering. Add the scallions and prawn shells, and sauté for 2 to 3 minutes, until the shells are pink and fragrant. Add the white wine and 2 cups water, and simmer for 45 minutes, until the prawn stock is deeply flavored. Strain and discard the solids.

FUN FACT

This episode was made to accompany my appearance on *Good Mythical Morning*, where Rhett, Link, and I "teamed up" to make a very accurate re-creation of Ralph Wiggum's crayon-and-thumbtack sandwich.

"MOROCCAN" PASTA

SERVES 4

I had been anxiously awaiting the opportunity to make something from one of my favorite sleeper series, *Peep Show*, a devastatingly uncomfortable comedy from across the pond. Food was never a distinct centerpiece in the lives of Mark and Jez, but became the focus of an episode where Mark, predictably, royally screws everything up. What starts as a charming meal for two quickly becomes a harried meal for six, expanding a small serving of pasta Alfredo with beans, eggs, and lovely "filling" lettuce. Gross-out potential aside, this created an interesting challenge: could I make a palatable version of Mark's improvised pasta? By swapping lettuce for spinach, canned beans for crispy chickpeas, Alfredo for a Moroccan-inspired ragout, and upping the presentation factor a bit, I think these darling pasta "nests" accomplish just that.

VERDICT: While an admittedly strange combination of flavors, eggs baked into pasta nests can inspire a wealth of ideas in the home kitchen. This iteration is pleasant enough, transforming some kitchen staples into a surprisingly elegant main course.

CRISPY ROAST CHICKPEAS

1 (14-ounce) can chickpeas, drained, rinsed, and patted dry

1 tablespoon extra-virgin olive oil

2 teaspoons kosher salt

1 teaspoon paprika

MOROCCAN RAGOUT

1 tablespoon extra-virgin olive oil

1 small onion, diced

1 small red bell pepper, diced

1 garlic clove, minced

½ teaspoon ground cumin

½ teaspoon cayenne pepper

½ teaspoon ground turmeric

¼ teaspoon smoked paprika

1 (28-ounce) can whole peeled DOP San Marzano tomatoes, with their juices

1 teaspoon kosher salt

½ cup crumbled feta cheese

(ingredients continue)

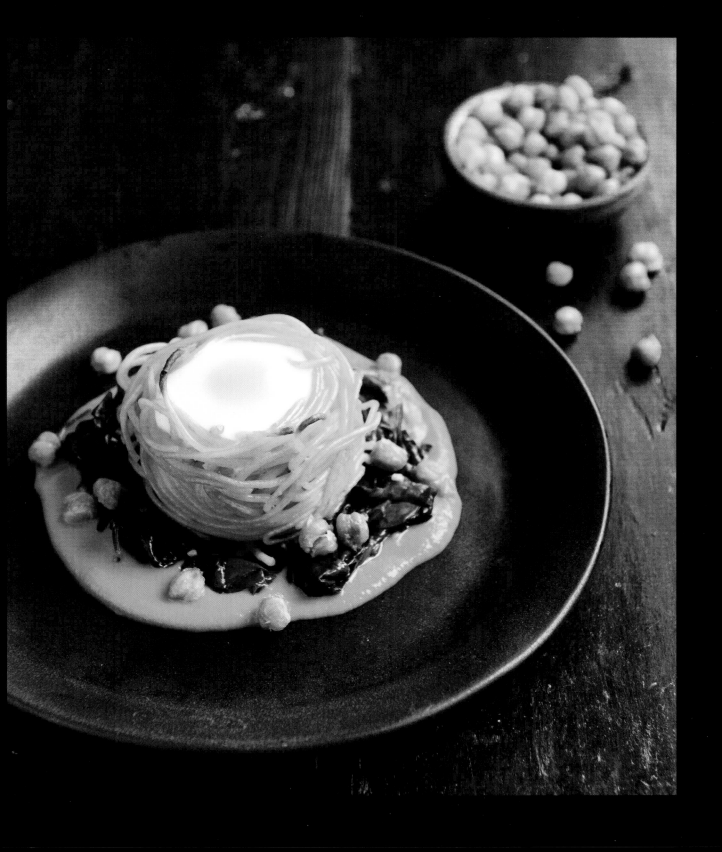

PASTA NESTS

1 tablespoon unsalted butter, plus more for greasing

8 ounces baby spinach

1 garlic clove, minced

1 teaspoon kosher salt

½ teaspoon freshly ground black pepper

1 pound spaghetti, cooked according to the package directions

4 large eggs

CRISPY ROAST CHICKPEAS

PREHEAT THE oven to 400°F.

IN A medium bowl, toss the chickpeas with the olive oil and salt. Spread evenly over a rimmed baking sheet. Roast for 20 to 30 minutes, until browned and crisp. Return the chickpeas to the bowl and toss with the paprika while still warm. Set aside to cool; keep the oven on.

MOROCCAN RAGOUT

IN A large Dutch oven, heat the olive oil over medium-high heat until shimmering. Add the onion and cook, stirring, until translucent, about 2 minutes. Add the bell pepper and garlic and cook, stirring, until fragrant, about 1 minute. Add the cumin, cayenne, turmeric, and smoked paprika and cook, stirring, for 30 seconds to toast the spices. Add the tomatoes and their juices, crushing them with a wooden spoon. Stir and add the salt. Bring to a simmer, reduce the heat to medium-low, and cook gently for 30 minutes.

CAREFULLY TRANSFER the ragout to a high-powered blender and puree for 1 minute, or until very smooth (be careful when blending hot liquids). Pour half the ragout into a saucepan and keep warm for serving. Add the feta to the remaining ragout in the blender. Blend on high speed for 15 seconds, or until the feta is completely incorporated. Set the feta ragout aside.

PASTA NESTS

IN A nonstick pan, melt the butter over medium heat until the foaming subsides. Add the spinach and cook, stirring, until soft and wilted, about 3 minutes. Add the garlic and cook, stirring, for 1 minute. Season with the salt and pepper.

BUTTER FOUR 8-ounce ramekins. Toss the pasta with the feta ragout. Twirl one-quarter of the spaghetti into a nest with a carving fork and place in a prepared ramekin. Repeat with the remaining pasta. Using a spoon, create a well in the center of each pasta nest. Crack 1 egg into each well, transfer the ramekins to a rimmed baking sheet, and bake for 10 to 15 minutes, until the egg whites are set but the yolks are still runny. Remove from the oven.

RUN A butter knife around the ramekins and invert each pasta nest onto a plate. For each serving, spoon a pool of the reserved ragout onto a serving plate and top with one-quarter of the spinach. Place 1 pasta nest, egg-side up, on the spinach and serve.

EVERY-MEAT BURRITO

SERVES 8 TO 10

I had decided that million-subscriber-celebration episodes should be similarly outlandish as the Taco Town episode, and for inspiration, I had to look no further than *Regular Show*. But how to re-create a burrito that supposedly contains every imaginable meat, including but not limited to crow, jackal, and naked mole rat? The answer lay in Brooklyn, at a specialty meat purveyor called Paisanos, the back of which featured several freezers filled to the brim with most every (legal) exotic meat. I cannot conscionably recommend anyone ever doing this again, ever, as the result was nothing short of revolting. I decided, instead, that an "every pork" burrito featuring as many porcine pieces as possible might be a more promising prospect. Who would have guessed that a burrito filled with cheese, rice, and five different kinds of pork would be delicious? Everyone? Oh.

VERDICT: This is an every-meat burrito worth craving—with layers upon layers of flavor that, while difficult to re-create simultaneously, all stand on their own as solid recipes worth trying.

CHICHARRÓNES

3 pounds skin-on pork belly

2 teaspoons kosher salt

1 teaspoon baking powder

CARNITAS

2 pounds boneless pork shoulder, cut into 1-inch cubes

1 large orange, halved and seeded

2 small serrano chiles, halved lengthwise and seeded

1 small onion, chopped

3 tablespoons vegetable oil

2 teaspoons kosher salt

2 teaspoons freshly ground black pepper

4 bay leaves

6 garlic cloves, halved

2 cinnamon sticks

PORK AL PASTOR

5 guajillo chiles, stemmed and seeded

5 pasilla chiles, stemmed and seeded

2 cups water

1 teaspoon onion powder

4 garlic cloves

2 tablespoons ground annatto seeds

2 teaspoons Mexican oregano

1 teaspoon ground cumin

½ teaspoon kosher salt

(ingredients continue)

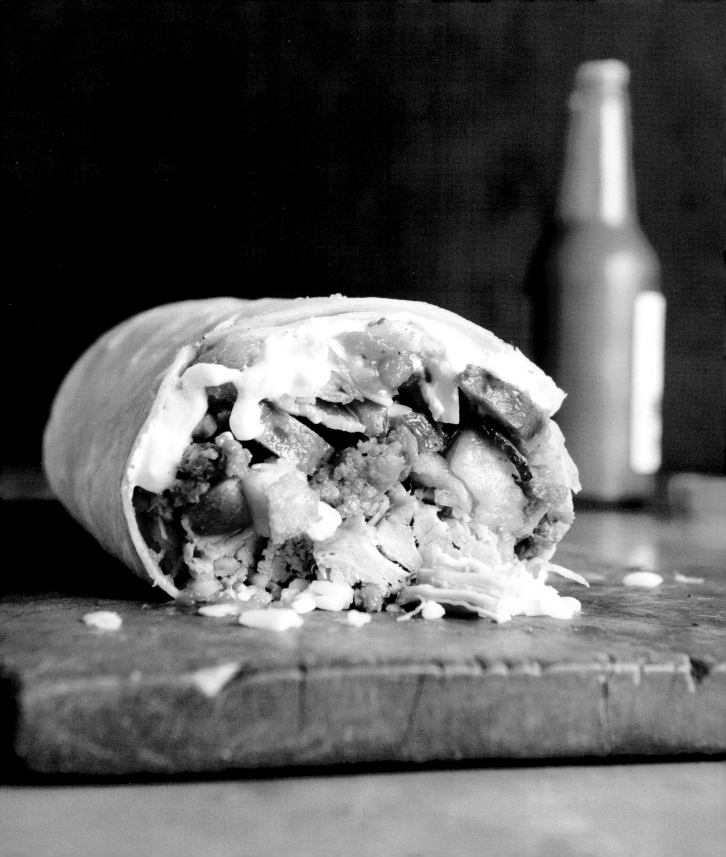

½ teaspoon freshly ground pepper

2 pounds boneless pork shoulder, sliced ½ inch thick

1 large fresh pineapple

TO ASSEMBLE

2 tablespoons vegetable oil

8 large flour tortillas, warmed

4 cups cooked long-grain rice

2 fresh pork chorizo links, cooked and sliced

1 pound bacon, cooked

8 ounces Monterey Jack cheese, shredded

½ cup salsa

½ cup sour cream

CHICHARRÓNES

PLACE THE pork belly on a wire rack set on a rimmed baking sheet. In a small bowl, combine the salt and baking powder and sprinkle the mixture evenly all over the pork belly. Set the pork belly skin-side up on the rack and refrigerate, uncovered, for 2 to 24 hours.

CUT THE pork belly into ½-inch cubes and transfer to a large wok or heavy-bottomed Dutch oven. Add water to barely cover the pork and bring to a simmer over medium-high heat. Reduce the heat and simmer for 2 to 3 hours, until the water has evaporated and the pork is frying in its own fat, about 10 minutes. Cook over medium heat for 15 to 30 minutes more, until the pork is crispy. Using a slotted spoon, transfer the pork to paper towels to drain. The chicharrónes can be served immediately, or let cool to room temperature.

CARNITAS

PREHEAT THE oven to 275°F.

PLACE THE pork in a large bowl. Squeeze in the juice from the orange halves and drop in the rinds. Add the serranos, onion, vegetable oil, salt, pepper, bay leaves, garlic, and cinnamon sticks and toss well to combine. Transfer to a 9 x 13-inch baking dish. Cover tightly with aluminum foil and bake for 3½ hours, or until the pork is fork-tender.

TRANSFER THE pork to a rimmed baking sheet and spread it out. Discard the orange rinds, bay leaves, and cinnamon sticks. Using two forks, shred the pork completely, then cover and refrigerate until ready to use.

PORK AL PASTOR

IN A medium saucepan, combine the chiles and water. Cover and bring to a boil over medium heat. Remove from the heat and let stand for 15 minutes.

TRANSFER THE chiles and their soaking liquid to a blender. Add the onion powder, garlic, annatto, oregano, cumin, salt, and pepper. Blend on high for 1 minute, or until the spice paste is very smooth. Transfer to a large bowl, add the pork, and massage with your hands to completely coat each slice of pork with the spice paste. Cover with plastic wrap and refrigerate for 2 hours, or up to overnight.

(recipe continues)

PREHEAT THE oven to 350°F with a rack in the lowest position.

CUT A 1-inch-thick slice from the bottom of the pineapple. Place it flesh-side up on a rimmed baking sheet. Insert two wooden skewers, 2 inches apart, into the pineapple slice so they stand straight up. Peel and slice the remaining pineapple into ½-inch-thick rounds. Impale the marinated pork on the skewers, adding a pineapple ring every five layers or so, until the skewers are completely covered. You should now have a "column" of pork and pineapple, resembling shawarma on a spit. Bake the pork as close as possible to a rear corner of the oven, rotating the column frequently, until the exterior of the pork is charred and the internal temperature registers at least 165°F on an instant-read thermometer. Remove from the oven and cover with foil to keep warm until ready to serve.

ASSEMBLY

HEAT THE vegetable oil in a large sauté pan over high heat for 1 minute. In batches, add the chicharrónes and cook, stirring, for 1 to 2 minutes, until crisp, lowering the heat to medium if necessary to keep them from burning. Repeat with the carnitas.

UNWRAP THE pork al pastor and, using a long, sharp knife, carve the column of pork and pineapple. (Alternatively, carve off 1 inch from the exterior of the column, then return it to a rear corner of the oven and roast at 400°F for 15 to 20 minutes, rotating the column frequently to crisp the exterior, then carve off another layer. Repeat until all the pork is carved.)

FOR EACH burrito, place a tortilla on a work surface. Add a base layer of rice, then top with some of the carnitas, chicharrónes, pork al pastor, chorizo, bacon, cheese, salsa, and sour cream. Wrap the burrito, cut in half, and serve.

> ## FUN FACT
> The seventeen exotic meats rung in at $576, crowning this the most expensive episode at the time, unseated only by the more recent *Red Dead Redemption* episode, which clocked in at over $1,000.

RUM FRENCH TOAST

SERVES 4 TO 6

Don Draper likes most anything soaked in booze, so when his daughter mistakes rum for maple syrup on his French toast, it doesn't stop him from devouring the most important meal of the day. While this sounds appealing, the reality is less appetizing—French toast is really just a vehicle for syrup, so when the sweet tree sap is removed from the equation and replaced with alcohol, the result is harsh and bitter. Incorporating rum into every part of the dish and (mostly) cooking off the alcohol, however, is a far better utilization of the Caribbean spirit. Since this episode was one of two filmed in a remote cabin in Vermont, a trip whose purpose was to explore bread baking, it only made sense to make the brioche from scratch. The result was underproofed and close-textured, which, while unappealing as brioche, made for halfway decent French toast.

VERDICT: Rum incorporated into every step of the French toast process yields a flavorful, saucy result. It's also a good use for crappy brioche, but I'd recommend going for the good stuff, or at least baking some properly.

1 Brioche (recipe follows), sliced 1 inch thick

3 large eggs

½ cup heavy cream

3 tablespoons granulated sugar

2 tablespoons dark rum

½ teaspoon kosher salt

½ teaspoon pure vanilla extract

¼ teaspoon freshly grated nutmeg

¼ teaspoon ground cinnamon

1 tablespoon unsalted butter

Rum Whipped Cream (recipe follows)

Confectioners' sugar, for serving

Rum Maple Syrup (recipe follows)

PREHEAT THE oven to 200°F. Line a rimmed baking sheet with a wire rack.

PLACE THE brioche slices on the rack and bake for 30 to 40 minutes, until dried. Remove the bread; keep the oven on.

IN A large bowl, whisk together the eggs, cream, granulated sugar, rum, salt, vanilla, nutmeg, and cinnamon until completely combined. Pour into a 9 x 13-inch baking dish for easy dipping.

(recipe continues)

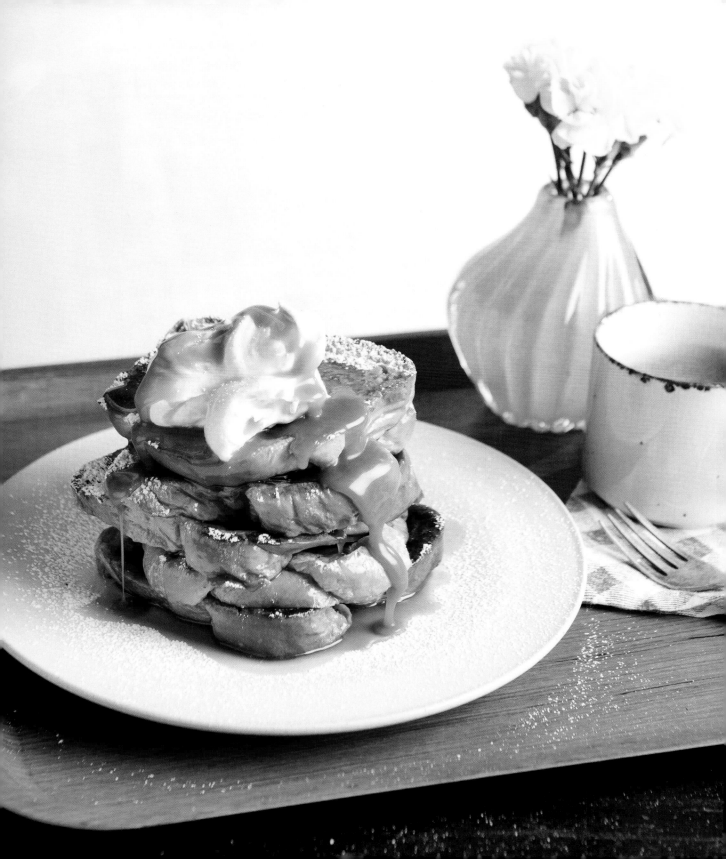

Soak the brioche slices in the mixture for 30 to 60 seconds on each side, until saturated.

IN A large nonstick or cast-iron skillet, melt the butter over medium heat until the foaming subsides. In batches, fry the soaked brioche until browned and crisp, 1 to 2 minutes per side. Transfer the French toast to the wire rack on the baking sheet and keep warm in the oven until ready to serve.

FOR EACH serving, place 3 slices of French toast on a plate, dollop with whipped cream, and dust with confectioners' sugar. Pass the rum maple syrup at the table.

BRIOCHE

MAKES ONE 10-INCH LOAF

4 large eggs, plus 1 egg, lightly beaten, for egg wash

⅓ cup whole milk

1 (¼-ounce) packet active dry yeast

15 ounces all-purpose flour (about 3½ cups), plus more as needed

⅓ cup sugar

2 teaspoons kosher salt

¾ cup (1½ sticks) unsalted butter, at room temperature, plus more for greasing

LIGHTLY BEAT 1 egg. In a small saucepan, heat the milk over medium-low heat to 110°F. Pour into a large bowl and add the yeast, 1 cup (about 4¼ ounces) of the flour, and the beaten egg. Mix with a wooden spoon until a wet mass forms. Top this mass with 1 cup of the flour and let rest for 30 minutes.

ADD THE sugar and salt to the bowl. Lightly beat 3 more eggs, add to the bowl, and mix with a wooden spoon until just incorporated. Add the remaining 10¾ ounces of flour and mix until the wooden spoon is no longer effective, then knead by hand in the bowl for 10 minutes, or until a smooth dough forms, adding 1 to 2 tablespoons more flour if the dough is too sticky.

TURN THE dough out onto a work surface and cut it into 2 equal pieces. Cover one piece with plastic wrap to keep it from drying out. Using your hands, flatten the other piece into about an 8-inch round and place the sticks of butter in the center. Wrap the dough around the butter and knead until a sticky, horrible mess forms, about 10 minutes. Top with the other piece of dough and knead together until a very tacky dough forms that barely pulls away from the work surface when kneaded, about 10 minutes. Place in a large, well-buttered bowl, cover with plastic wrap, and let rise in a warm place for about 2 hours, or until doubled in size.

GENTLY FOLD the dough onto itself to deflate it. Cover with plastic wrap and refrigerate the dough overnight.

BUTTER AND line a 10-inch loaf pan with parchment paper, leaving a 4-inch overhang on each of the long sides. Divide the chilled dough into 16 equal balls. Arrange the dough balls in the prepared pan, cover loosely with plastic

(recipe continues)

wrap, and let rise in a warm place for 1 to 1½ hours, until nearly doubled in size.

PREHEAT THE oven to 375°F.

UNWRAP THE risen loaf, brush with the egg wash, and bake for 30 to 40 minutes, rotating once halfway through the baking time, until the internal temperature registers 200°F at its thickest point. Use the parchment paper to remove the loaf from the pan and let cool completely, about 2 hours, before slicing.

RUM WHIPPED CREAM
MAKES ABOUT 2 CUPS

1 cup heavy cream
⅓ cup sugar
1 teaspoon pure vanilla extract
2 tablespoons dark rum

COMBINE ALL the ingredients in a medium bowl. Using a handheld mixer, beat on medium speed until soft peaks form. Refrigerate until ready to serve.

RUM MAPLE SYRUP
MAKES ABOUT 1 CUP

½ cup pure maple syrup
¼ cup dark rum
1 tablespoon unsalted butter
¼ cup heavy cream

IN A small saucepan, bring the maple syrup and dark rum to a simmer over medium heat. Reduce the heat and simmer for 5 minutes, until the mixture has thickened and the smell of alcohol has dissipated. Remove from the heat and whisk in the butter and cream until completely incorporated. Transfer to a container with a spout and set aside until ready to serve.

FUN FACT
The internet connection in the cabin was (understandably) slow, so it took nearly fourteen hours to upload the 3-gigabyte 4K video file. Needless to say, that was a nervous day.

EGGS IN A NEST

SERVES 6 TO 10

If you thought apple pie was prolifically featured throughout film and television, you haven't kept an eye open for eggs in a nest or, as it's otherwise called: toad in a hole, spit in the ocean, one-eyed jack, eggy in a basket, gashouse eggs, and more. First appearing in *Mary Jane's Pa*, the simple yet sumptuous breakfast can easily be made with little more than a slice of bread, an egg, and a pat of butter. Even though it's decidedly fussier, making homemade bread not only yields a softer and more delicate texture, but allows you to control the thickness of the slices. I was surprised (especially after the five loaves of failure I experienced) to find that not only did scores of viewers re-create this dish for themselves, they elected to make the bread from scratch.

VERDICT: Eggs in a nest, even in its simplest form, is a comforting breakfast that's rightfully endured for generations. Homemade sandwich bread is easy enough to make (once the ingredients are measured by weight, not volume) and adds a homespun flair to the dish.

---

100 milliliters warm water (110°F)

1 (¼-ounce) packet active dry yeast

650 grams all-purpose flour, plus more for dusting

50 grams sugar

45 grams unsalted butter, at room temperature, plus 45 grams (or more, if desired) melted

5 grams kosher salt

300 milliliters room-temperature water

Vegetable oil, for greasing

2 tablespoons bacon fat and/or butter

10 large eggs

Kosher salt and freshly ground black pepper

IN A large bowl, combine the warm water, yeast, 325 grams of the flour, the sugar, the room-temperature butter, and the salt. Mix using a whisk or wooden spoon until combined. Add the room-temperature water and mix until the consistency resembles pancake batter. Add the remaining 325 grams flour and stir until a shaggy dough forms. Turn out onto a lightly floured work surface and knead until a smooth, supple dough forms, 7 to 9 minutes.

(recipe continues)

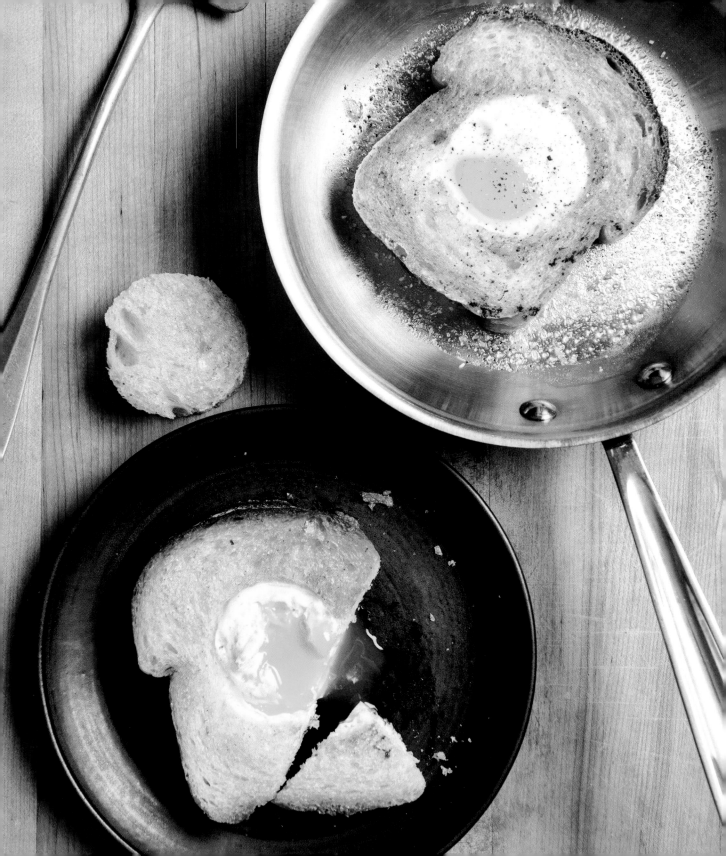

Generously oil a large bowl and roll the dough around in it to coat with oil. Cover with plastic wrap and let rise at room temperature until doubled in size, 45 minutes to 1 hour.

TURN THE dough out onto a lightly floured work surface and punch it down, folding it over on itself to form a loaf shape. Oil a 4-inch loaf pan and line it with parchment paper, leaving a 4-inch overhang on each of the long sides. Tuck the dough under itself to stretch out the top, making it taut and smooth. Place the dough in the prepared pan, seam-side down. Brush the top of the loaf with the melted butter. Cover loosely with plastic wrap and let rise at room temperature for about 1 hour, until doubled in size.

PREHEAT THE oven to 400°F.

REMOVE THE plastic wrap and bake the loaf for 25 to 35 minutes, until deeply browned and the internal temperature registers 190°F at its thickest point. Use the parchment paper to remove the loaf from the pan. If desired, brush the loaf again with more melted butter. Let cool completely, about 2 hours.

SLICE THE loaf into ½-inch-thick slices. Using a drinking glass or small biscuit cutter, stamp out a round from the center of each slice and set the bread rounds aside.

IN A large nonstick skillet, heat ½ tablespoon of the bacon fat over medium high heat until shimmering. In batches, add the slices of bread to the pan, flipping immediately to lightly coat both sides with the fat. Fry on one side until browned, about 90 seconds. Flip, crack 1 egg into the center of each bread slice, and cook for another 90 seconds, or until the egg whites are mostly set. Flip once more and cook for 15 seconds, or until the egg whites are set but the yolks are still runny. Season the egg in the nest with salt and pepper, transfer to a plate, and serve. Repeat with the remaining bread and eggs, adding more bacon fat and/or butter as needed. If desired, toast the bread rounds and serve on the side for dipping.

"We need to cook" takes on a nefarious new meaning when grumbled by television's arguably best-ever antihero, Walter White. While *Breaking Bad* puts less emphasis on food as a character than other media in this book, it's still frequently utilized as an effective plot device. Whether it's a stew lovingly prepared by Gus or a pizza angrily hurled onto a rooftop by Walt, food and drink are used to frighten, coerce, and even kill throughout the chaotic series. The show is even bookended by food, its two-year timeline conveyed with bacon decoratively arranged atop Walter's birthday breakfasts. Okay, I take back what I said; food might be as integral to the world-building of *Breaking Bad* as any other great drama about the human condition. I don't feel like going back and changing that sentence—this is a learning process for both of us, okay?

DIPPING STICKS

SERVES 6

VERDICT: The dipping sticks are easy to make and a spitting image of the soft, cheesy, garlicky breadsticks popularized by Pizza Hut. Candy meth was omitted from this book, as it is a hazard to your mouth integrity.

1 (¼-ounce) packet active dry yeast

¼ cup nonfat dry milk

1 tablespoon sugar

1½ cups warm water (110°F)

17½ ounces all-purpose flour (about 4 cups plus 2 tablespoons), plus more for dusting

3 teaspoons kosher salt

⅓ cup plus 2 tablespoons vegetable oil

Butter-flavored nonstick cooking spray

¼ cup powdered Parmesan cheese (from a can or jar)

2 tablespoons garlic powder

1 tablespoon onion powder

1 tablespoon dried oregano

1 tablespoon dried basil

1 teaspoon freshly ground black pepper

Marinara sauce, warmed, for dipping

(recipe continues)

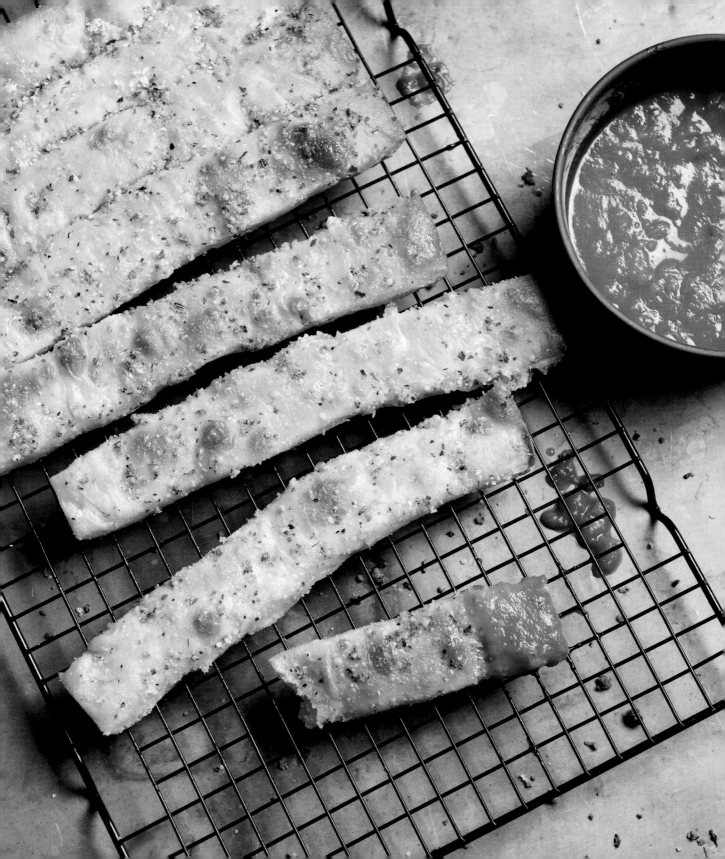

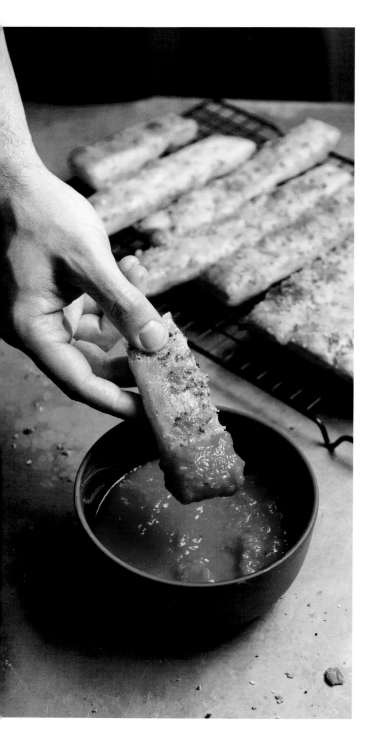

IN THE bowl of a stand mixer fitted with the paddle attachment, combine the yeast, dry milk, sugar, and warm water. Mix on low speed until combined, then let rest for 10 minutes, or until foamy. Replace the paddle with the dough hook. Add the flour, 1 teaspoon of the salt, and 2 tablespoons of the vegetable oil and knead on medium speed for 5 to 8 minutes, until a tacky, smooth ball of dough forms.

TURN THE dough out onto a lightly floured work surface, pressing and stretching it out into a 9 x 13-inch rectangle. Pour the remaining ⅓ cup vegetable oil into a 9 x 13-inch baking dish. Place the dough on top, pressing and stretching it until the dough fills the dish. Cover with plastic wrap and let rise at room temperature for 1 to 1½ hours, until doubled in size.

PREHEAT THE oven to 475°F.

REMOVE THE plastic wrap and, using a bench scraper, cut the dough in the baking dish into 13 or 14 equal sticks, each about 1 inch wide and 9 inches long. Generously spray the tops with cooking spray.

IN A small bowl, combine the Parmesan, garlic powder, onion powder, oregano, basil, pepper, and remaining 2 teaspoons salt. Sprinkle evenly over the dough sticks and bake for 15 to 20 minutes, until puffed up and brown.

USING A large spatula, transfer the dipping sticks to a wire rack and let cool for 10 minutes. Separate the sticks, transfer to a platter, and serve with the warmed marinara sauce.

PAILA MARINA

SERVES 6

VERDICT: *Paila Marina* is an incredibly easy-to-make Chilean comfort food, converting even a cilantro-hater like me with its subtle and complex flavors.

---

2 tablespoons vegetable oil

1 small onion, finely chopped

4 garlic cloves, thinly sliced

½ cup dry white wine

4 cups seafood stock or double batch of Prawn Stock (see page 221)

1 pound boneless, skinless cod fillets

1 pound shrimp, peeled and deveined (shells reserved for stock)

½ pound sea scallops

½ pound cleaned squid, sliced into bite-size pieces

1 pound mussels, scrubbed

1 pound Manila clams

2 cups boiling water

Kosher salt and freshly ground black pepper

Torn fresh cilantro, for garnish (optional)

IN A large pot, heat the vegetable oil over medium-high heat until shimmering. Add the onion and cook, stirring occasionally, until translucent around the edges, 1 to 2 minutes. Add the garlic and cook, stirring, until fragrant, about 30 seconds. Add the wine and stock, stirring and scraping up all the browned bits from the bottom of the pot. Bring to a simmer and add all the seafood. Add water if necessary to nearly submerge the seafood. Reduce the heat to medium-low, cover, and cook until the mussels and clams have opened, 5 to 8 minutes. Discard any mussels and clams that do not open.

SEASON LIBERALLY with salt and pepper. Ladle into bowls, garnish with cilantro (if that's your thing), and serve.

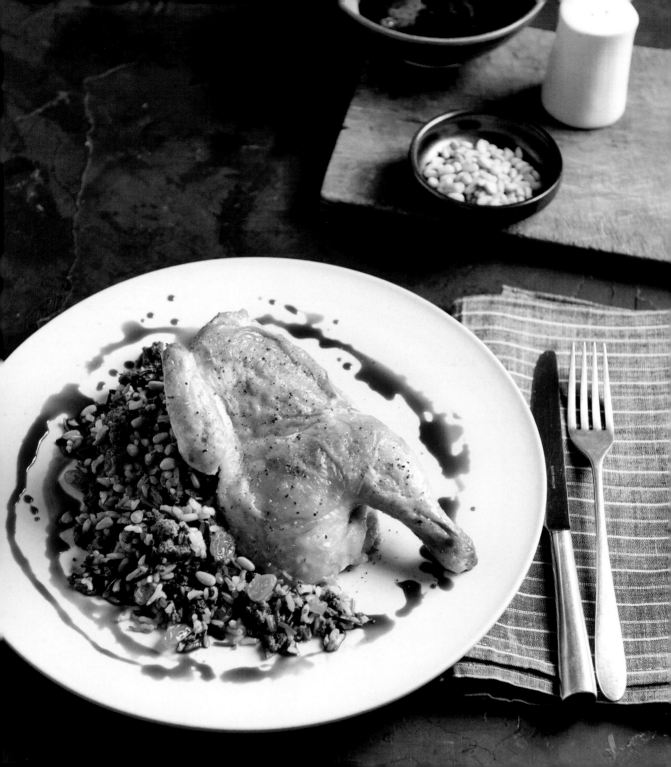

Finally, the show is allowed to come full circle as we explore one of the many fussy dishes featured on my favorite show of all time, *Frasier*. Unbeknownst to my younger viewers, the original theme song of *Binging with Babish* was an excerpt from the sitcom's end credits, sung by Kelsey Grammer himself. It made sense to incorporate, as it was both a reference to pop culture and used food as a metaphor for its mixed-up plotlines. Though I was spoiled for choice, I decided to try to tackle the dishes featured at a dinner party in season 10, as it came together to form a cohesive meal. While yellowtail carpaccio was merely mentioned, Frasier's (literally) bloodred pomegranate honey sauce was more vividly seen and described. It was also perfect Frasier: pretentious, fussy, and referred to as his "signature" sauce.

CORNISH GAME HENS WITH POMEGRANATE SAUCE

SERVES 4

VERDICT: Frasier's signature pomegranate sauce, properly sweetened and balanced with homemade stock, is an excellent accompaniment to a Mediterranean style meal.

CORNISH GAME HENS

4 Cornish game hens

3 tablespoons kosher salt

1 teaspoon baking powder

HEN STOCK

1 tablespoon vegetable oil

1 carrot, cut into 3-inch lengths

1 onion, quartered

1 celery stalk, cut into 3-inch lengths

4 fresh thyme sprigs

2 fresh rosemary sprigs

2 fresh parsley sprigs

1 garlic clove

Nonstick cooking spray

POMEGRANATE HONEY SAUCE

½ cup pomegranate juice, unsweetened

2 tablespoons honey

(ingredients continue)

WILD RICE STUFFING

2 cups wild rice

1 teaspoon extra-virgin olive oil

1 pound ground lamb

1 small onion, finely chopped

2 garlic cloves, minced

½ teaspoon ground cardamom

¼ teaspoon ground cinnamon

¼ teaspoon ground allspice

¼ cup currants

¼ cup golden raisins

Kosher salt and freshly ground black pepper

CORNISH GAME HENS

BUTTERFLY THE Cornish game hens: For each bird, using a pair of sturdy poultry shears, cut along each side of the backbone. Remove the backbones and reserve them for the hen stock. Flip the birds over and press down between the breasts to flatten.

IN A small bowl, combine the salt and baking powder and sprinkle the mixture evenly all over the birds. Place the hens on a wire rack set on a rimmed baking sheet and refrigerate, uncovered, for 4 to 24 hours.

HEN STOCK

IN A large saucepan, heat the vegetable oil over medium-high heat until shimmering. Add the reserved hen backbones and cook until browned on all sides, about 8 minutes total. Add the carrot, onion, celery, thyme, rosemary, parsley, and garlic and cook, stirring, until the vegetables have browned slightly, about 5 minutes. Cover with about 4 cups cold water and bring to a bare simmer over high heat. Reduce the heat to keep the stock at a bare simmer. Simmer until the stock is flavorful, 4 to 6 hours. Strain, discard the solids, and set aside (or let

cool, transfer to an airtight container, and refrigerate for up to 2 days, if making ahead of time). You should have 2 cups of stock for the pomegranate honey sauce, plus more for the wild rice stuffing.

PREHEAT THE oven to 500°F with a rimmed aluminum baking sheet inside it.

REMOVE THE hens from the refrigerator, brush off any excess salt, and let stand at room temperature for 30 minutes. Lightly spray the hens with cooking spray. Place the hens skin-side down on the preheated baking sheet. Roast for 10 minutes, remove from the oven, and flip the hens over. Preheat the broiler to high for 5 minutes. Broil the hens on the second-highest rack for 5 to 8 minutes, until the skin is browned and crisp and the breasts register 165°F.

POMEGRANATE HONEY SAUCE

IN A wide saucepan, combine 2 cups of the hen stock, the pomegranate juice, and the honey. Whisk until incorporated. Bring to a gentle boil over medium-high heat. Reduce the heat and simmer for 30 minutes to 1 hour, until the sauce has reduced and is thick and syrupy.

WILD RICE STUFFING

COOK THE wild rice according to the package directions, replacing the water called for with hen stock.

IN A large sauté pan, heat the olive oil over medium-high heat until shimmering. Add the lamb and cook, breaking it up with a wooden spoon as it cooks, until browned, 5 to 7 minutes. Transfer the lamb to a bowl. Add the onion to the pan and cook over medium heat, stirring, until softened, 2 to 3 minutes. Add the garlic and cook, stirring, until fragrant, about 1 minute. Add the cardamom, cinnamon, allspice, currants, and raisins and season with salt and pepper. Reduce the heat to medium-low and cook, stirring, until the lamb is cooked through and the rice is fragrant.

ASSEMBLY

TRANSFER EACH hen to a plate, spoon some of the pomegranate honey sauce alongside, or decoratively around the plate, add a scoop of wild rice stuffing and serve.

YELLOWTAIL CARPACCIO

SERVES 4

VERDICT: Yellowtail carpaccio is an elegant starter and an excellent introduction to the (occasionally) magic results of fusion.

Juice of ½ blood orange

Juice of ½ lemon

½ cup high-quality extra-virgin olive oil

Small bunch fresh chives, minced

2 scallions, thinly sliced into 2-inch strips

½ pound boneless, skinless sushi-grade yellowtail fillet

2 radishes, thinly sliced

1 jalapeño, thinly sliced

1 blood orange, peeled, quartered, and sliced crosswise ¼ inch thick

Flaky sea salt

Freshly ground black pepper

IN A small bowl, combine the blood orange juice, lemon juice, olive oil, and chives. Whisk with a fork or tiny whisk until the mixture forms a creamy emulsion. Set the vinaigrette aside.

FILL A small bowl with ice water. Add the scallions and let soak until they curl, about 2 minutes. Drain the scallions and pat dry.

USING A very sharp knife, slice the yellowtail as thinly as possible.

FOR EACH serving, arrange the fish in a flower pattern on a plate and decoratively arrange some of the radishes, jalapeño, and blood orange slices on top. Drizzle the vinaigrette sparingly over the carpaccio. (Reserve the rest of the vinaigrette for other use and refrigerate for up to 5 days.) Garnish with sea salt and the scallions, season with pepper, and serve immediately.

CHOCOLATE LAVA CAKES

SERVES 8

Well, folks, it's all downhill from here—meeting my hero, receiving a prop from one of my favorite movies, having all my wildest dreams validated, all coming together to form the greatest day of my life. When I wrote an email to Jon Favreau's team, I never expected a response, much less that he'd offer to come on the show as a guest, along with Roy Choi, *Chef*'s culinary consultant and architect of the food truck renaissance. In a moment I will continue to replay in my mind whenever I'm in a rut, Jon brought out the carving fork from the *pasta aglio e olio* scene in *Chef*—the fork I have tattooed on my arm—and presented it to me as a gift. When I stayed up late after work making pasta for a single camera, alone in my apartment, I never could have imagined what it would eventually lead to. Just shy of two years later, Jon Favreau himself was showing me how a winter Olympian wearing an *Iron Man* helmet had tagged him on Instagram, remarking that this is the magic of making something: seeing the ways it can touch, inspire, and enliven others. The excitement and possibility that comes from connecting with an audience. I couldn't agree more.

VERDICT: Oh, snap, I didn't talk about the cake at all—it's really good. Like, really good. A bit of whipped cream, fruit, and a dusting of cocoa powder are necessary to liven up the plate a bit, but the star of the show is the liquid ganache flowing out onto the plate after the first forkful.

---

14 ounces high-quality dark chocolate, chopped

½ cup heavy cream

¾ cup (1½ sticks) unsalted butter, cut into pieces, plus more for greasing

6 large eggs

½ cup packed light brown sugar

1 teaspoon pure vanilla extract

1 tablespoon Grand Marnier

6 tablespoons all-purpose flour

Raw sugar, for coating the ramekins

8 large strawberries, sliced decoratively

1 pint blueberries

Confectioners' sugar, for dusting

Cocoa powder, for dusting

Whipped Cream (see page 186), for serving

(recipe continues)

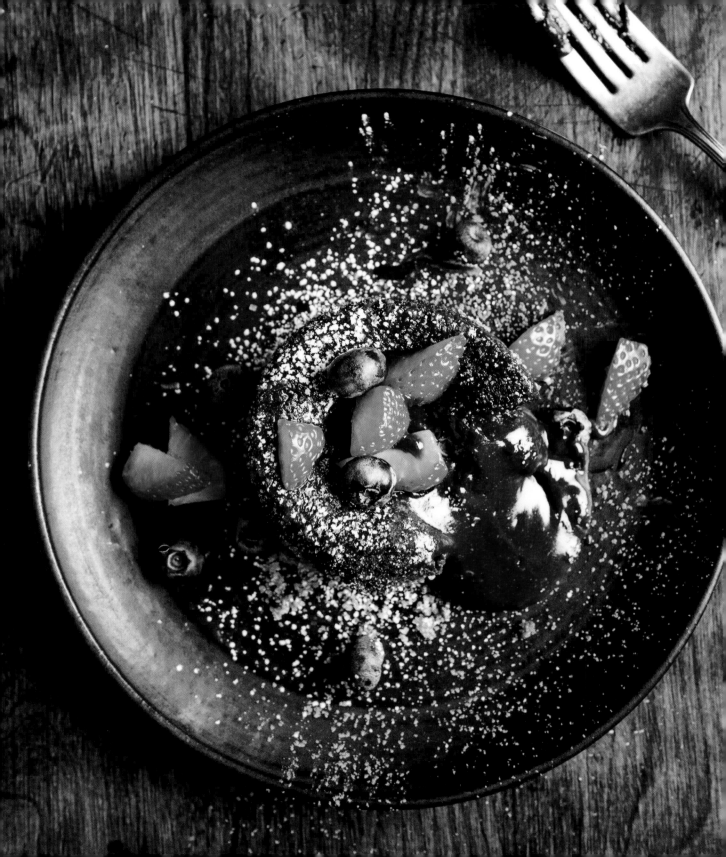

MAKE THE ganache: Place 4 ounces of the dark chocolate in a double boiler or a heatproof bowl set over a small saucepan of simmering water, making sure the bottom of the bowl does not touch the water. Melt the chocolate, stirring with a rubber spatula. Slowly stream in the cream, whisking continuously, until completely combined. Remove from the double boiler, cover with plastic wrap, and freeze until hardened, about 2 hours.

MAKE THE batter: Combine the remaining 10 ounces chocolate and the butter in another heatproof bowl and set it over the saucepan of simmering water. Stir until the chocolate and butter are melted and combined. Remove the mixture from the heat.

IN A large bowl, whisk together the eggs, brown sugar, vanilla, and Grand Marnier until light and fluffy. While whisking continuously, very slowly drizzle the chocolate mixture into the egg mixture. Add the flour 1 tablespoon at a time and whisk to combine.

PREHEAT THE oven to 425°F. Generously butter eight 8-ounce ramekins. Add raw sugar to each and rotate over a bowl (to catch the excess) until the insides are completely coated with the sugar. Transfer the ramekins to a rimmed baking sheet.

FILL EACH ramekin one-third full with the batter. Using a 2-tablespoon ice cream scoop, scoop a small ball of the frozen ganache into the center of each ramekin. Add more batter to fill each ramekin to the inner lip, leaving about ¼ inch of headroom. Bake on the baking sheet for 11 minutes, or until the cakes are set but the centers are molten. Remove from the oven and transfer to a wire rack.

RUN A knife around the outside of the cakes and immediately turn each cake out onto a plate, tapping and gently shaking as necessary to loosen it from the ramekin. Garnish with strawberries and blueberries and, using a sieve, dust with confectioners' sugar and then cocoa powder. Top with whipped cream and serve immediately.

FUN FACT
Jon Favreau can crack an egg with one hand better than Roy Choi.

TAMALES

SERVES 12 +

At the time of this episode's production, I hadn't yet seen *Coco*, so I had no idea the emotional whirlwind of weeping and smiling I was in for. I had, however, seen a TV spot for the film, in which a doting *abuela* excitedly stacks tamales in front of little Miguel, and I knew one thing: I wanted some tamales. Having sampled a wide variety in my day, from very good to very bad, I was determined to make that perfectly toothsome dough, laced with spices and stretching with cheese. After my usual process of trawling through blog posts and popular recipes, I realized that tamales were a daunting task—not for their

difficulty, but for their time commitment. To that, I said pish-posh—I could crank out a batch of these suckers before my red-eye flight to Zurich. To that, I now say pish-posh—I nearly keeled over halfway through, and left the country with a sinkful of dishes needing doing. Set aside a Saturday for this one, folks.

VERDICT: Great tamales come down to the correct consistency of the dough, flavorful fillings, and proper cooking. They're delicious any time of day, freeze beautifully, and are a great opportunity to learn more about Mexican comfort food.

---

20 dried corn husks (available at Mexican markets)

6 guajillo chiles, stemmed and seeded

6 pasilla chiles, stemmed and seeded

4 garlic cloves

2 tomatillos, quartered

Juice of ½ orange

Juice of 1 lime

1 teaspoon dried Mexican oregano

1 teaspoon ground cumin

2 teaspoons kosher salt

1 teaspoon freshly ground black pepper

3 pounds boneless pork shoulder, cut into 1-inch cubes

2 poblano peppers, halved lengthwise, deveined and seeded

4 ounces Oaxaca cheese, pulled apart into 3-inch-long strips

20 ounces masa harina (about 4¼ cups)

3 cups hot (not boiling) water

14 ounces lard or shortening (about 1¾ cups)

1½ teaspoons baking powder

1 cup chicken stock, warmed

Tomatillo Salsa (see page 62), for serving

(recipe continues)

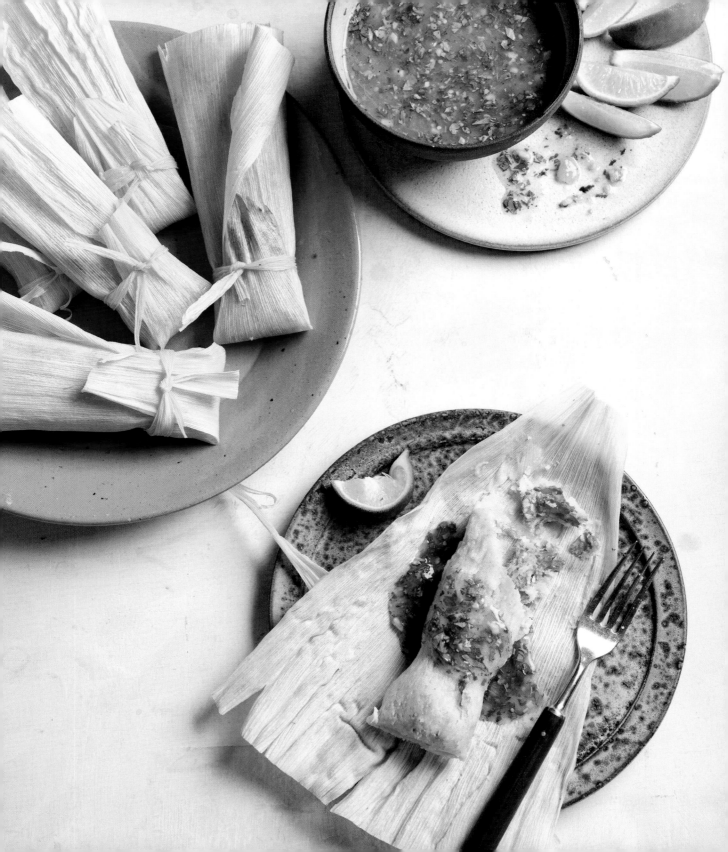

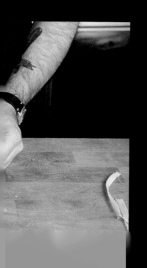
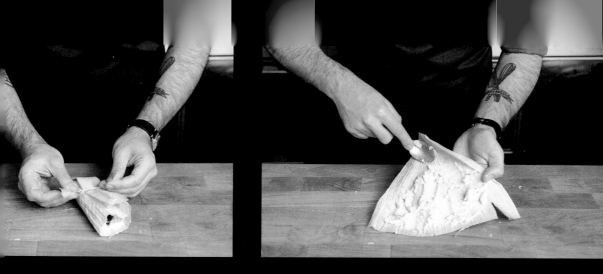
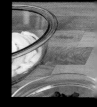
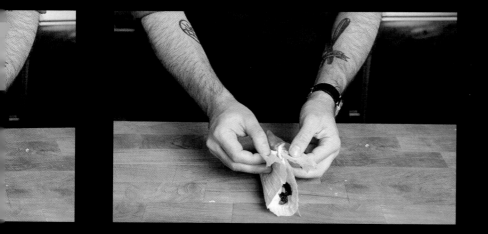
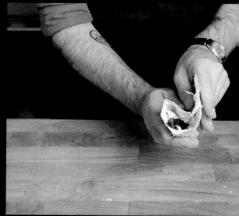
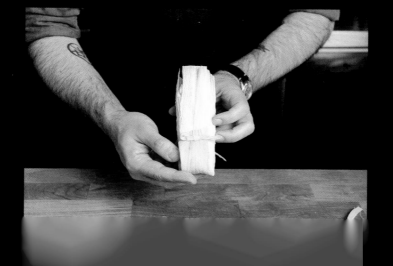
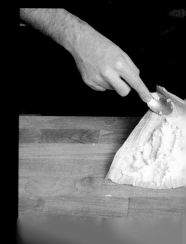

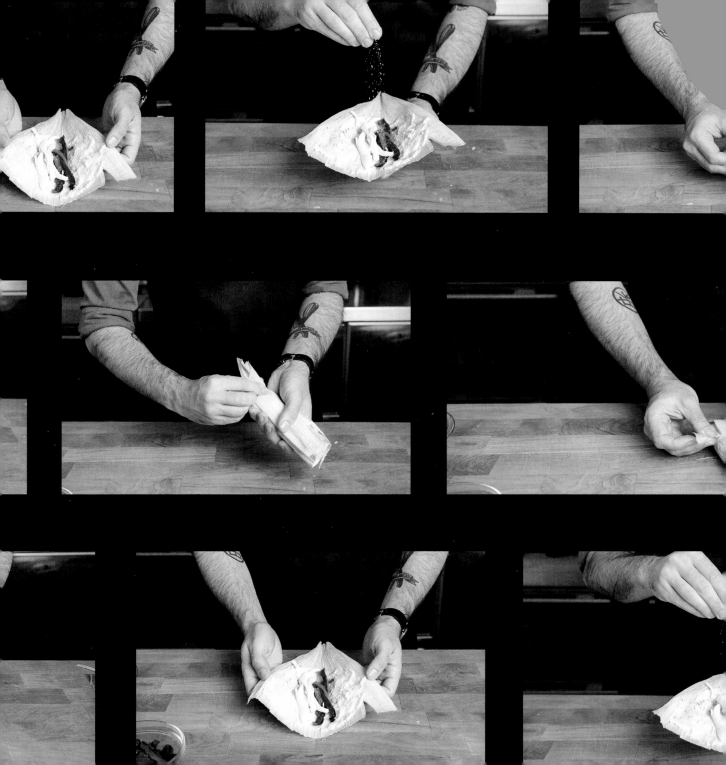

PLACE THE corn husks in a clean bucket or large bowl. Cover with water and top with a heavy plate to keep them submerged. Soak for at least 3 hours or up to overnight.

MEANWHILE, MAKE the pork filling: Place the dried chiles in a large saucepan with 2 cups water, cover, and bring to a boil over high heat. Remove from the heat and soak for 10 minutes, until softened. Transfer the chiles and their soaking liquid to a blender. Add the garlic, tomatillos, orange juice, lime juice, oregano, cumin, 1 teaspoon of the salt, and the black pepper. Puree until very smooth and let the spice paste cool completely, about 30 minutes.

COMBINE THE spice paste and pork in a large resealable plastic bag, seal, and massage to completely coat the pork with the spice paste. Refrigerate for 3 hours or up to overnight.

WHEN READY to cook the pork, preheat the oven to 275°F.

TRANSFER THE pork and spice paste to a 9 x 13-inch baking dish, cover tightly with aluminum foil, and bake for 3 hours, until the pork is very tender. Transfer the pork to a platter; switch the oven to broil. Shred the pork using two forks and moisten it with some of the braising liquid. Let cool.

MEANWHILE, MAKE the poblano filling: Place an oven rack in the highest position. Line a rimmed baking sheet with aluminum foil.

PLACE THE poblanos skin-side up on the lined baking sheet. Broil for 4 to 5 minutes, until the poblanos are blackened all over, rotating halfway through the cooking time. Remove from the oven. Wrap the poblanos in foil and set aside for 10 minutes to let them steam and soften. Unwrap and, wearing nitrile gloves, rub the blackened skins off the poblanos. Discard the skins and slice the poblanos into 1-inch-wide strips. Transfer to a plate, add the Oaxaca cheese, and season both with ½ teaspoon of the salt.

MAKE THE tamales: In a large bowl, combine the masa harina and hot water. Mix with a wooden spoon until combined, cover with plastic wrap, and let rest for 15 minutes.

IN THE bowl of a stand mixer fitted with the paddle attachment, beat the lard on medium-high speed for 2 minutes, or until light and fluffy. Add the baking powder and ½ teaspoon of the salt. Mix on low speed until combined. With the machine running on the lowest speed, add the soaked masa harina one handful at a time, scraping down the sides of the bowl frequently. With the machine running on medium speed, slowly stream in the stock until well combined. Cover and refrigerate the tamale dough for 1 to 12 hours.

DRAIN THE corn husks and pat dry with kitchen towels. Sort out any broken or damaged husks and pull them apart into ¼-inch-wide strips. On the inside of each whole husk, evenly spread about ¼ cup of the tamale dough, leaving a 2-inch border on each side except the top. Fill half the husks with 2 tablespoons of the pork each; fill the remaining husks with 2 or 3 strips each of the poblanos and Oaxaca cheese each. Fold in the long sides of each husk, overlapping them to enclose the filling. Fold the tapered end of the husk up, leaving the wide end open. Using a torn strip of husk, tie up each tamale to secure the tapered end. Arrange the tamales in a large steamer basket, open-end up, and set the basket in a large pot with 2 inches of simmering water in it. Cover and steam over medium-low heat for 45 minutes.

REMOVE FROM the heat and transfer the tamales to a serving platter. Let rest for 15 to 30 minutes, then unwrap and serve with salsa.

CLEMENTINE CAKE

SERVES 8

The Secret Life of Walter Mitty, a charming film that unfortunately comes off like a two-hour commercial for the litany of products placed front and center in its wanderlust story line, gracefully features one food item not emblazoned with a corporate logo: Walter's mother's clementine cake. Featuring the slightly sharper flavor of the titular fruit in both its cake and its icing, delightfully chewy candied clementines, and not much else, it's a simple and elegant homespun dessert. It also just rolls off the tongue so nicely! *Clementine cake*. Almost as nicely as Cinnabon's new slogan: "That's frosted heroin!"

VERDICT: This is a simple, sweet, tart little cake, the kind that puts a graceful period on the end of a meal's sentence. Did that make any sense? No? Whatever, it's pretty good. Just make it.

---

3 clementines, thinly sliced

38 ounces sugar (about 5¼ cups)

Juice of 1 clementine plus ¾ cup plus 3 tablespoons fresh clementine juice

15¾ ounces cake flour (about 3¾ cups)

1 teaspoon fine salt

¾ teaspoon baking powder

¾ teaspoon baking soda

1½ cups (3 sticks) unsalted butter, at room temperature

6 large eggs

2 teaspoons pure vanilla extract

Zest of 5 clementines

1¼ cups buttermilk

Nonstick cooking spray

5½ ounces confectioners' sugar, sifted

BRING A large saucepan of water to a rolling boil and fill a large bowl with ice and water. Add the clementine slices to the saucepan and poach for 1 minute. Using tongs, transfer the clementines to the ice bath to stop the cooking. Drain the clementines and set aside.

IN A wide Dutch oven, combine 14 ounces (about 2 cups) of the sugar, the juice of 1 clementine, and 1 cup water. Whisk to combine and bring to a simmer over medium heat. Add the poached clementine slices in a single layer, making sure none overlap. Simmer for 1½ hours,

(recipe continues)

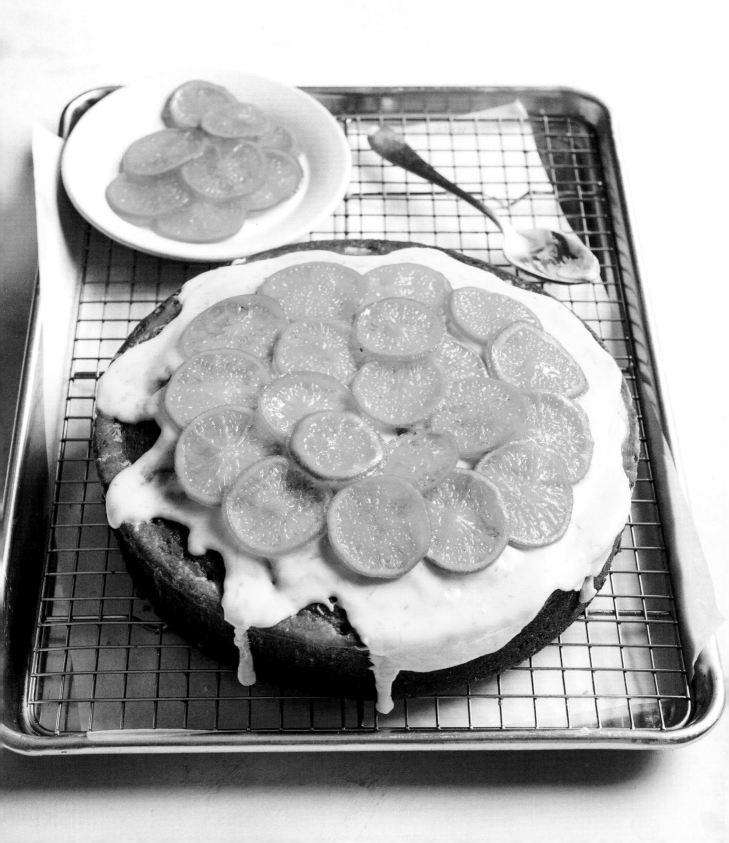

flipping every 30 minutes, until soft and translucent. Using a spider or tongs, transfer the clementines to a wire rack set on a rimmed baking sheet and let drain. Reserve the clementine syrup in the pot and let cool.

IN A large bowl, whisk together the cake flour, salt, baking powder, and baking soda.

IN THE bowl of a stand mixer fitted with the paddle attachment, beat together the remaining 24 ounces sugar and the butter on medium-high speed until fluffy, about 2 minutes. Scrape down the sides of the bowl. Add the eggs and vanilla and mix on medium-low speed until well combined. Add the ¾ cup clementine juice and the zest of 4 clementines and mix again on medium-low speed until combined. Add the dry ingredients and buttermilk and mix on low speed until just combined, about 1 minute.

PREHEAT THE oven to 350°F. Spray a 9-inch round cake pan with cooking spray and line the bottom with a round of parchment paper cut to fit.

FILL THE prepared pan with the batter and bake for 45 minutes, until a cake tester or paring knife inserted into the center comes out with a few crumbs clinging to it.

INVERT THE cake to remove it from the pan, then flip it right-side up and place it on a wire rack. While the cake is still warm, pierce the top all over with a skewer and generously brush with the reserved clementine syrup. Let cool completely.

IN THE bowl of a stand mixer fitted with the whisk attachment, combine the confectioners' sugar, 2 tablespoons of the remaining clementine juice, and all of the remaining clementine zest. Start mixing at low speed, then slowly increase the speed to medium and mix until the glaze is smooth and well combined. If the glaze is too thick for your liking, mix in the remaining tablespoon of clementine juice.

GENTLY POUR the glaze over the top of the cake so it drips down the sides. Garnish with the candied clementines and let the glaze set. Transfer to a platter, slice, and serve.

PINEAPPLE-CURRY FRIED RICE

SERVES 6

Food Wars! gave me pause for a considerable amount of time—its unusually high upskirt-to-dialogue ratio led me to believe that it was kind of terrible. After watching it, however, I concluded that . . . I wasn't entirely wrong. But I also realized that the show is very tongue-in-cheek, features some beautiful animation, and some genuinely funny content. Additionally, the series has a distinct affection for food, creating fantastical exaggerations of the magic of flavor, portraying wildly imaginative, fistfight-level-intensity cook-offs with bravado and humor. That being said, there are an awful lot of close-ups of female body parts undulating in uncontrollable arousal upon tasting food. So it's still weird.

VERDICT: Pineapple fried rice is delicious, but in its form on the show has some unnecessary steps. As the notes describe below, there is no need to bake the rice in a salted pineapple, as a taste test determined that it has little to no effect on the flavor.

---

3 or 4 dried Chinese red chiles

2 teaspoons cumin seeds

1 teaspoon coriander seeds

1 teaspoon cardamom seeds

1 teaspoon mustard seeds

1 teaspoon whole black peppercorns

1 cinnamon stick, crushed

1 pineapple

3 tablespoons vegetable oil

2 large eggs, lightly beaten

1 red bell pepper, diced

1 carrot, diced

1 Thai bird's-eye chile (optional)

1 (1-inch) knob fresh ginger, peeled and grated

1 (1-inch) knob fresh turmeric, peeled and grated, or 1 teaspoon ground turmeric

1 garlic clove, minced

2 cups short-grain rice, such as sushi rice, cooked and chilled overnight

1 tablespoon rice vinegar

1 tablespoon fish sauce

1 tablespoon sesame oil

1 tablespoon soy sauce

Kosher salt and freshly ground black pepper

2 scallions, thinly sliced

2 ounces cashews, toasted and chopped

Unsalted butter, for greasing

(recipe continues)

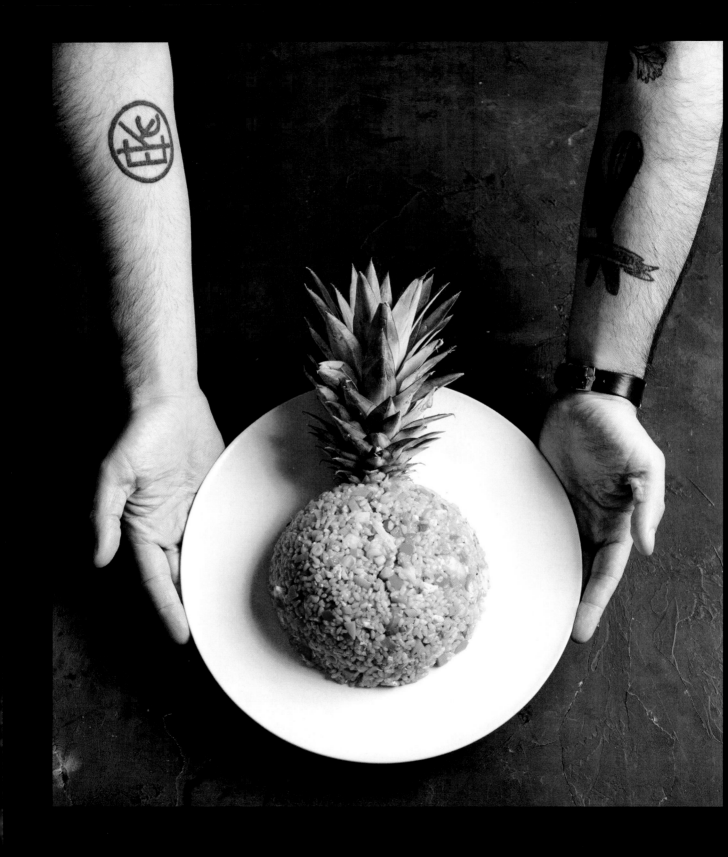

HEAT A large sauté pan over medium heat for 1 minute. Add the dried chiles, cumin, coriander, cardamom, mustard seeds, peppercorns, and cinnamon and toast, shaking frequently, until very fragrant, about 2 minutes. Remove from the heat and let cool for 10 minutes. Transfer to a spice grinder and grind into a fine powder. Set aside 2 tablespoons of the spice powder and reserve the rest for another use—it can be kept in an airtight container for several months.

CUT THE pineapple in half lengthwise. Carve out the center of each half, leaving about 1 inch of flesh all around the inside of the rind to create 2 pineapple bowls. Discard the core, chop the pineapple flesh, and set aside. Reserve the leafy top of one pineapple bowl. If you choose the optional step of baking the fried rice (steps follow), reserve both pineapple bowls and preheat the oven to 375°F.

IN A large wok, heat the vegetable oil over high heat until nearly smoking. Add the eggs and, using chopsticks, stir continuously until barely cooked. Add the bell pepper, carrot, bird's-eye chile, ginger, turmeric, and garlic and cook, stirring, until fragrant and the vegetables have softened, about 2 minutes. Add the rice, the 2 tablespoons spice powder, vinegar, fish sauce, sesame oil, soy sauce, and reserved chopped pineapple. Cook, stirring, until the flavors are well incorporated. Lightly season with salt and pepper. Add the scallions and cashews and stir to combine.

IF DESIRED, to be show-accurate, bake the fried rice inside the pineapple. Lightly salt the inside of each pineapple half. Fill each with the fried rice and join the two halves to enclose the rice. Transfer to a rimmed baking sheet and bake for 30 minutes. (Note: This makes virtually no difference in the flavor of the fried rice. You can skip this step and proceed to the next step.)

BUTTER A medium bowl and pack the fried rice inside. Invert the bowl onto a large plate and remove it to reveal a dome of rice. Garnish with the reserved leafy top of the pineapple, so the presentation mimics the shape of a pineapple. Serve immediately.

CHICKEN PARM HEROS

SERVES 4

Here we continue the series of episodes dreamed up as an excuse to make my favorite foods, chief among which may be [fill in the blank] Parmesan. In either its entrée or sandwich form, a deep-fried cutlet of something smothered in cheese and sauce has got to be one of the greatest pleasures ever imagined by our species. Finding Parm heros in fiction proved to be difficult, with none distinctly highlighting or showing the sandwich to the extent that it deserved re-creation, so an anthology episode was the only answer. As I'm writing this, I just had the idea to bread and deep-fry meatballs for use in a meatball Parm. Excuse me, I gotta go.

VERDICT: Chicken, veal, and meatball Parmesan are the apex of the human experience, and these iterations are no exception. Layering the sauce on top of the cheese makes for a less-classic look, but also makes for less-soggy breading, which I think is a small price to pay for perfection.

Vegetable oil, for frying

1 cup all-purpose flour

1 teaspoon dried basil

1 teaspoon dried oregano

½ teaspoon onion powder

½ teaspoon garlic powder

1 cup panko bread crumbs

2 large eggs, beaten

8 chicken tenders, lightly pounded

½ cup (1 stick) unsalted butter, at room temperature

2 garlic cloves, grated or minced

¼ cup finely chopped fresh parsley

4 large hero rolls, split lengthwise

Kosher salt and freshly ground black pepper

1 (8-ounce) ball fresh mozzarella cheese, sliced

4 ounces Parmesan cheese, grated

½ cup homemade or jarred tomato sauce, warmed

(recipe continues)

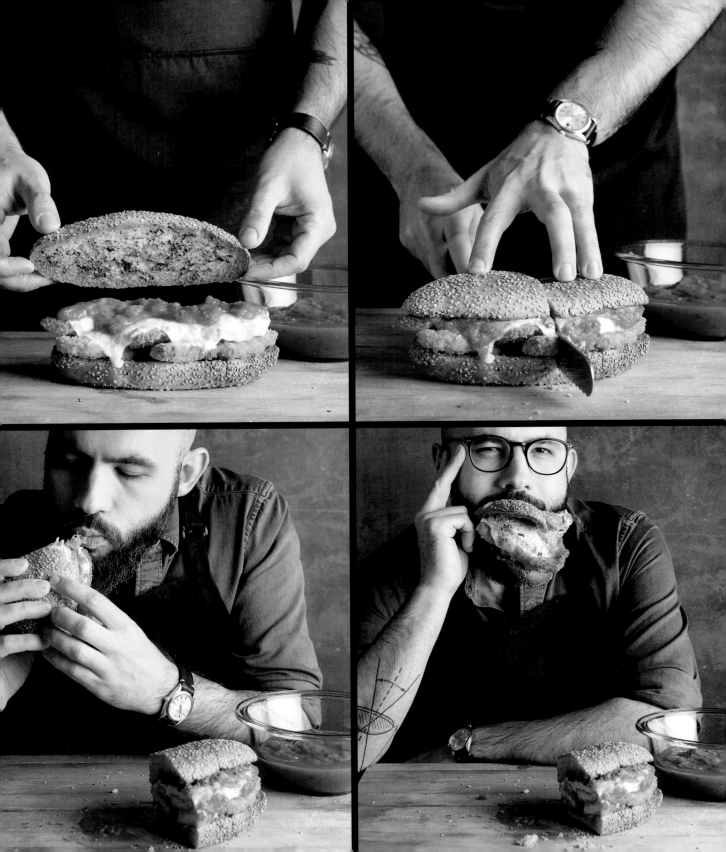

FILL A large saucepan with vegetable oil to a depth of 2 inches. Heat over medium-high heat to 350°F. Set a wire rack over paper towels or a brown paper bag.

MEANWHILE, IN a wide shallow bowl or cake pan, whisk together the flour, basil, oregano, onion powder, and garlic powder until combined. Place the bread crumbs and eggs in their own separate shallow bowls. Dredge the chicken in the seasoned flour, dip in the eggs, then dredge in the bread crumbs. Transfer the chicken to a wire rack as you go. Carefully lower the chicken tenders into the hot oil and fry until golden brown and cooked through, 5 to 8 minutes. Transfer the chicken to the wire rack and let drain.

IN A small bowl, mix together the butter, garlic, and parsley with a rubber spatula. Set the compound butter aside.

PREHEAT THE oven to 400°F. Line a baking sheet with aluminum foil.

EVENLY SPREAD a thin layer of the compound butter on the split sides of each roll. Lightly season with salt and pepper, place on the lined baking sheet, and toast in the oven for 3 to 5 minutes, until lightly browned.

REMOVE THE rolls from the oven. Move an oven rack to the highest position and preheat the broiler to high. Arrange the chicken cutlets on the bottom halves of the rolls. Top with mozzarella slices and Parmesan and broil for 2 to 3 minutes, until the cheese is lightly browned and bubbling. For each roll, spread 3 to 4 tablespoons of the tomato sauce onto the cheese, close the sandwich, cut in half, and serve.

NOTE: *You can adapt this recipe to your desired filling: Substitute thinly pounded veal for the chicken. Or salt eggplant slices and let drain for 30 minutes, then pat dry with paper towels before breading and frying. Or instead of deep-frying, fill the heros with meatballs in red sauce (see page 26).*

FUN FACT

I ate all three Parm heros, having made a deal with myself to not have any more for three months after. I made it two weeks.

LASAGNA BOLOGNESE

SERVES 12

With little more than a drippy sack of ricotta cheese, so began the internet bromance betwixt Brad and Babby. I was ecstatic to hear that the *Bon Appétit* team was a fan of the show and beyond excited to meet one of my YouTube heroes, Brad Leone. Brad and Vinny's show was unlike anything I'd ever seen, deftly mixing Brad's larger-than-life personality with humor built entirely in the edit room. Upon visiting the *BA* test kitchens in 1 World Trade Center, I was a bit nervous, having only previously been there to visit a friend who worked a few floors up. That nervousness definitely came across in the video, especially when my relatively low-key vibe was pitted against Brad's steamroller of physicality and humor. But, much like a first date, any anxiety was quashed by love at first sight, and Brad, Vinny, Sawyer, and I have been boys ever since.

VERDICT: This is about as good as classic lasagna gets: lovingly simmered Bolognese, homemade pasta and ricotta, melty mozzarella, and a bit of bromance.

LASAGNA

2 recipes Fresh Pasta (see page 26)

Bolognese Sauce (recipe follows)

12 ounces low-moisture mozzarella cheese, shredded (not preshredded)

4 ounces Parmesan cheese, grated

8 ounces Fresh Ricotta Cheese (recipe follows)

4 fresh basil leaves, torn

PREHEAT THE oven to 375°F.

ROLL OUT the pasta and cut into eight 4 x 12-inch lasagna noodles.

IN A deep 9 x 13-inch baking dish, ladle 1 cup of the Bolognese sauce, spreading it to evenly cover the bottom. Line the dish with a layer of lasagna noodles, making sure to cover the sauce completely. Add a layer of mozzarella and sprinkle with Parmesan. Layer with one-quarter of the ricotta and 1 cup of the sauce, followed by another layer of noodles. Repeat until the baking dish is nearly filled to the brim. Top with a light layer of sauce and mozzarella and sprinkle with Parmesan. Transfer to a rimmed baking

(recipe continues)

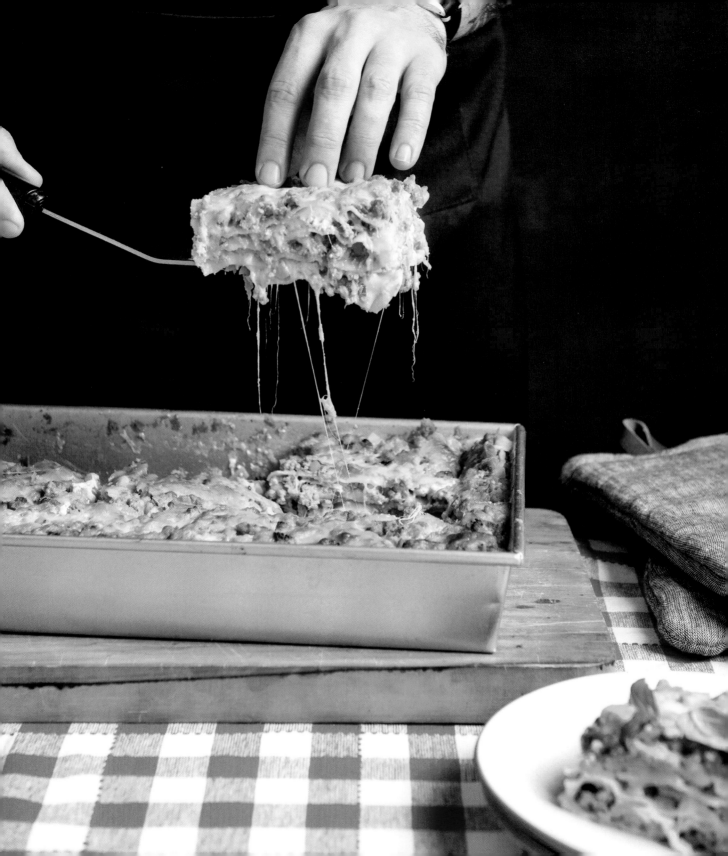

sheet and bake, uncovered, for 45 minutes, or until browned and bubbling.

REMOVE FROM the oven and let rest for at least 30 minutes. Garnish with the torn basil, cut into 12 pieces, and serve.

BOLOGNESE SAUCE

2 cups chicken stock

3 (1¼-ounce) packets unflavored powdered gelatin

1 tablespoon extra-virgin olive oil

1 pound ground pork

1 pound ground veal

1 pound ground beef

1 medium onion, finely chopped

2 celery stalks, finely chopped

1 carrot, finely chopped

4 garlic cloves, finely chopped

1 teaspoon dried oregano

Pinch of red pepper flakes (optional)

2 cups dry white wine

1 (28-ounce) can whole peeled DOP San Marzano tomatoes, with their juices

1 (14-ounce) can diced tomatoes, with their juices

1½ cups whole milk

2 fresh basil sprigs, plus 10 large basil leaves, finely chopped

2 or 3 fresh sage leaves, finely chopped

2 bay leaves

½ cup heavy cream

3 ounces Parmesan cheese, grated

Kosher salt and freshly ground black pepper

IN A medium bowl, stir together the stock and gelatin powder. Let sit at room temperature for 15 minutes.

MEANWHILE, IN a large, nonreactive pot with a heavy bottom (such as a Dutch oven), heat the olive oil over medium heat until shimmering, about 2 minutes. Add the pork, veal, and beef and cook, breaking up the meat with a wooden spoon and stirring as it cooks, until the meat is browned and a large amount of fat has rendered off, about 5 minutes. Using a slotted spoon, transfer the meat to a colander set over a bowl and let drain, reserving about 1 tablespoon of the fat in the pot.

RETURN THE pot to medium heat. Add the onion and cook, stirring, until softened, about 2 minutes. Add the celery, carrot, garlic, oregano, and red pepper flakes and cook, stirring well, until fragrant, about 2 minutes. Add the wine and cook, stirring and scraping up all the browned bits from the bottom of the pot. Add the stock-gelatin mixture, both canned tomatoes and their juices, the milk, basil sprigs, sage, and bay leaves. Stir well to combine and bring to a simmer over medium-high heat. Reduce the heat to maintain a bare simmer and cover the pot with the lid ajar. Simmer for 4 hours, occasionally skimming fat from the surface, until the sauce is dark, thick, and rich. (Alternatively, bake the sauce instead of cooking it on the stovetop: After bringing the sauce to a simmer, cover the pot with the lid ajar, and transfer to a preheated 325°F oven. Cook for 4 hours. Remove from the oven and skim the fat from the surface before continuing.)

(recipe continues)

REMOVE AND discard the basil sprigs and bay leaves. Add the chopped basil, cream, and Parmesan. Season with salt and black pepper. Stir until completely incorporated, then taste and adjust the seasonings, if necessary.

FRESH RICOTTA CHEESE

MAKES ABOUT 2 CUPS

4 cups whole milk (not ultra-pasteurized)

1 cup heavy cream (not ultra-pasteurized)

1 tablespoon kosher salt

5 tablespoons distilled white vinegar or fresh lemon juice

IN A large, heavy-bottomed Dutch oven, combine the milk and cream. Heat the mixture over medium heat to 200°F. Remove from the heat and stir in the salt and vinegar. Let the mixture stand, undisturbed, for 15 to 20 minutes, until large curds have formed and separated from the translucent whey.

LINE A fine-mesh sieve with three or four layers of cheesecloth and set the sieve over a bowl. Pour the ricotta into the sieve and let drain for 15 minutes. Gently squeeze the cheese to remove any excess whey. Transfer to an airtight container and refrigerate until ready to use or up to 2 days.

CRÈME BRÛLÉE

SERVES 6

I was excited when folks began suggesting this classic custard dessert from *Amélie*, not only because it gave me an excuse to break out the blowtorch, but because I had cut my teeth as a teenager making brûlée for a little crêperie in my hometown of Rochester, NY. It had been years since I had last retrieved a jiggling ramekin from its water bath, but I hoped that it would be like riding a bike. It wasn't—I spilled water into the custards, dropped one trying to get it out of the bain-marie, and had a pretty unevenly torched topping on my first go-round. A little practice made perfect however, opting instead for wider ramekins and a more aggressive torching technique. If you can set aside your fears of boiling water, curdled custard, and burnt sugar, these little frozen ponds of sugar and vanilla are a timeless and elegant dessert for almost any occasion.

VERDICT: It's an established scientific fact that crème brûlée is awesome, no matter how many times it must be copy/pasted due to all the diacritical marks festooning its name. This is a relatively easy and reliable recipe—maybe make a few extra so you can practice with a torch.

---

2 cups heavy cream

⅔ cup plus 1 tablespoon granulated sugar

1 large vanilla bean, split lengthwise and seeds scraped out

6 large egg yolks

½ to ¾ cup raw sugar

PREHEAT THE oven to 300°F.

IN A medium saucepan, combine the cream, granulated sugar, and vanilla bean pod and seeds and bring to a bare simmer over medium heat, stirring continuously. As soon as the cream begins to simmer, remove from the heat. Remove and discard the vanilla bean pod, pour the cream into a spouted medium bowl, and let cool for 15 minutes.

IN A large bowl, whisk the egg yolks until lightened in color. While whisking continuously, pour half the hot cream into the eggs in a very

(recipe continues)

267

slow, steady stream to temper the eggs. Add the remaining cream all at once. Whisk until the custard is well combined.

LINE A 9 x 13-inch baking dish with a clean kitchen towel. Place 6 shallow 5-ounce ramekins on the towel. Fill each ramekin nearly to the brim with the custard. Add enough boiling water to the baking dish to reach two-thirds of the way up the sides of the ramekins. Carefully transfer the baking dish to the oven and bake for 24 to 40 minutes (depending on the size and depth of your ramekins), until the custard registers 175°F.

CAREFULLY REMOVE the ramekins from the water bath and let cool completely on a wire rack, about 1 hour. Wrap with plastic wrap and refrigerate until completely chilled, about 4 hours.

DEPENDING ON the size of your ramekins, sprinkle 1 to 2 tablespoons of the raw sugar over each custard, until lightly and evenly coated, tapping out any excess. Carefully caramelize the sugar with a kitchen torch. Serve immediately or refrigerate for up to 45 minutes until ready to serve.

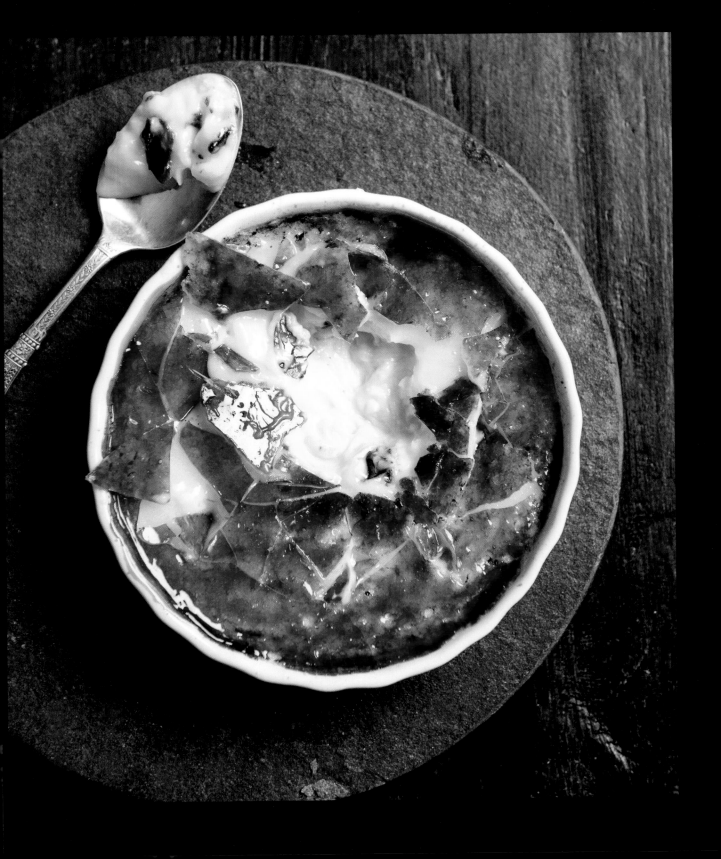

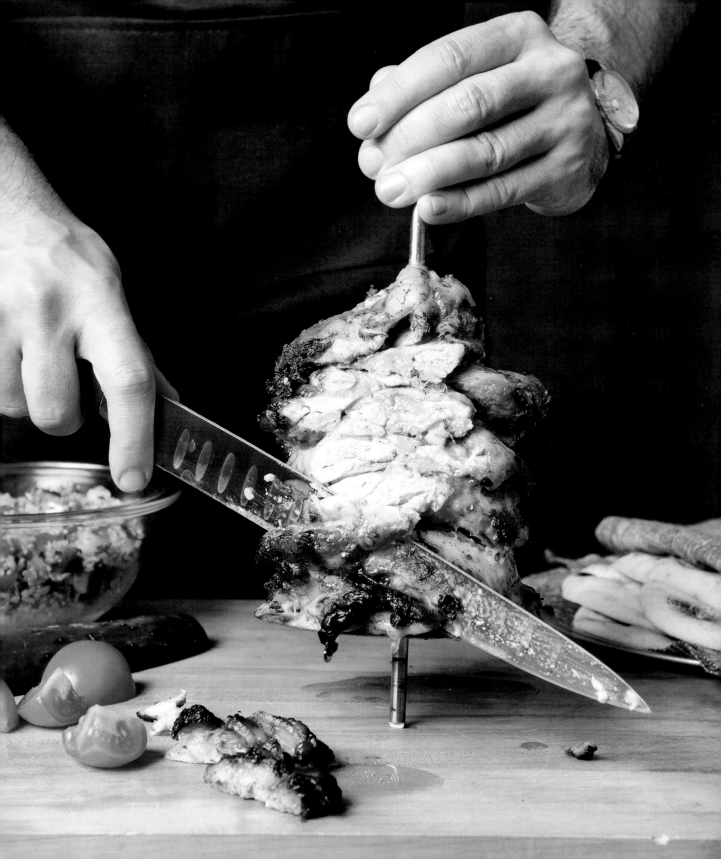

CHICKEN SHAWARMA

SERVES 8

Tony Stark is just the type of guy who would never have heard of shawarma, but would somehow crave it. I can't deny I felt the same way the first time I saw the glowing neon sign emanating from a street cart hocking the towering pillars of meat. At first, I balked at the challenge of re-creating this Middle Eastern fête in the comfort of my own home, but after the success wrought by Tasty's *al pastor* technique, I figured it was accomplishable. Following a brief perusal of Amazon, however, I realized that there are home shawarma solutions available to the consumer. Vertical rotisserie ovens will run you about $100, aren't very useful outside of grilling spinning meats, and take up way too much space on your countertop—but I'm here to bite that bullet in the interest of science. The results were stupendous, but a very similar outcome can be achieved with a little oven ingenuity. Some ovengenuity. Sorry.

VERDICT: Shawarma at home is certainly more difficult than popping down to the halal cart, but without the providence of living in New York City, this is a close approximation. If you don't want to spring for a vertical rotisserie, see the method of roasting meat for the pork al pastor in the Every-Meat Burrito (page 225).

SHAWARMA

Marinade (see page 73)

2 pounds skinless, boneless chicken thighs

Pita Bread (recipe follows)

Tzatziki Sauce (recipe follows)

Tahini Sauce (recipe follows)

Tabbouleh Salad (recipe follows)

Sliced cucumbers, for serving

Chopped tomatoes, for serving

COMBINE THE marinade and chicken in a large resealable plastic bag, seal, and massage to evenly coat the chicken in the marinade. Refrigerate overnight.

SHAKE OFF the excess marinade from each chicken thigh and impale them on the skewers of a shawarma machine. You should now have a "column" of chicken. Cook the shawarma

(recipe continues)

according to the manufacturer's instructions. When the outside of the chicken is browned and crisp, use a long, sharp knife to shave slices off the exterior. Continue to cook the shawarma and shave off the outer layer when it becomes browned and crisp.

FOR EACH serving, pile some sliced chicken into a pita. Top with some of the tzatziki, tahini sauce, and tabbouleh salad. Transfer to a plate, garnish with sliced cucumbers and chopped tomatoes, and serve.

PITA BREAD

MAKES 8 TO 10 PITAS

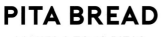

1 (¼-ounce) packet active dry yeast
1 cup warm water (110°F)
11¾ ounces (about 2¾ cups) all-purpose flour, plus more for dusting
1½ tablespoons extra-virgin olive oil
1¾ teaspoons kosher salt
Vegetable oil, for greasing

IN THE bowl of a stand mixer, whisk together the yeast, warm water, and 1 cup of the flour to combine. Cover and let stand for 15 to 20 minutes, until the mixture begins to bubble and foam.

ADD THE remaining flour, the olive oil, and the salt. Fit the mixer with the paddle attachment and mix on low speed until a shaggy dough forms. Replace the paddle with the dough hook

and knead for 7 to 10 minutes, until a soft, tacky dough forms. If the dough doesn't pull away from the sides of the bowl, add 1 tablespoon more flour every minute of the kneading process until it does.

GENEROUSLY GREASE a large bowl with oil. Using floured hands, remove the dough from the stand mixer and form it into a taut ball. Toss the dough around in the bowl to evenly coat the dough with oil, cover the bowl with plastic wrap, and let the dough rest for 1½ to 2 hours in a warm place, until doubled in size.

DUST A baking sheet lightly with flour. Turn the dough out onto a lightly floured work surface and punch it down. Roll it into a 12-inch-long cylinder. Cut it crosswise into 8 equal pieces and form each piece into a smooth, taut ball. Place the dough balls on the prepared baking sheet. Cover with oiled plastic wrap and let rise at room temperature for 30 minutes, or until puffed up but not doubled in size.

HEAT A nonstick skillet over medium-high heat for about 2 minutes. Working with one ball at a time (keep the remaining balls covered), roll out the dough to a 6-inch round on a lightly floured work surface. Place the dough in the pan and cook, letting it bubble up and rise, until large brown spots appear on the bottom of the dough, about 2 minutes. Flip and cook for 1 to 2 minutes, until the pita has puffed and browned in spots. Transfer to a plate and keep warm under a kitchen towel. Repeat with the remaining dough balls. Keep warm until ready to serve.

TZATZIKI SAUCE

MAKES ABOUT 1¾ CUPS

1 cup Greek yogurt
1 English cucumber, seeded and finely chopped
2 garlic cloves, grated
Juice of 1 lemon
½ cup packed fresh dill, finely minced
Kosher salt and freshly ground black pepper

IN A bowl, stir together the yogurt, cucumber, garlic, lemon juice, and dill. Taste and season with salt and pepper. Cover and refrigerate until ready to use.

TAHINI SAUCE

MAKES ABOUT 1 CUP

1 cup sesame seeds
2 to 4 tablespoons vegetable or sesame oil

HEAT A heavy skillet over medium-high heat for 1 minute. Add the sesame seeds and toast, stirring continuously, until they begin to turn golden brown and are fragrant, 2 minutes. Transfer to a plate immediately (sesame seeds tend to burn quickly) and let cool completely.

TRANSFER THE sesame seeds to a food processor. With the machine running, slowly stream in 2 tablespoons of the oil through the feed tube until the sauce is smooth and creamy, but still pourable. Add up to 2 more tablespoons to reach your desired consistency.

TABBOULEH SALAD

MAKES 1½ CUPS

¾ pound cherry tomatoes
2 teaspoons kosher salt, plus more as needed
¼ cup bulgur wheat
1 cup fresh parsley, finely chopped
¼ cup fresh mint, finely chopped
1 English cucumber, seeded and finely diced
2 scallions, finely chopped
2 tablespoons extra-virgin olive oil
¼ teaspoon ground coriander
¼ teaspoon ground allspice
¼ teaspoon ground cumin
⅛ teaspoon ground cinnamon
Juice of 1 lemon
Freshly ground black pepper

FINELY CHOP the tomatoes, toss with the salt, and let drain in a sieve set over a bowl for about 1 hour. Set the tomatoes aside. You should have about ½ cup of liquid in the bowl—add water to make ½ cup if necessary. Transfer the liquid to a small saucepan and bring to a boil over medium-high heat. Remove from the heat, add the bulgur wheat, and cover. Let the bulgur soften for 1 hour. Drain any unabsorbed liquid.

IN A medium bowl, combine the bulgur, tomatoes, parsley, mint, cucumber, scallions, olive oil, coriander, allspice, cumin, cinnamon, and lemon juice. Toss well, taste, and season with salt and pepper.

COVER AND refrigerate until ready to serve.

CHATEAUBRIAND

SERVES 6 TO 10

Joe Pantoliano plays the exact character you'd expect him to play in *The Matrix*, swapping Tastee Wheat for digital steak in maybe the film's sole appetizing scene. Cypher chows down on a gorgeously cooked, gigantic piece of what could only be filet mignon, based on its uniformity and fat content. Even though I was still eating my meat medium-well when the movie came out (I was twelve, give me a break), the "ignorance is bliss" muttered between mouthfuls made me hungry for a steak. I endeavored to find the best way to re-create that rosy gradation at home, and the answer lay in the most traditional method: sear, roast, slice, serve. Reverse-searing, while creating a more uniform result, has an inferior texture. I know that doesn't quite make sense, but beef tenderloin is so lean, the end result becomes slippery if undercooked by even a few degrees.

VERDICT: Traditional searing-then-roasting seems to work best for whole tenderloin roasts, where a bit of gray around the outside edge is actually a welcome variance in the texture and presentation of the beef.

---

1 whole beef tenderloin, trimmed and tied

Kosher salt and freshly ground black pepper

3 tablespoons vegetable oil

1 pound whole cipollini or pearl onions, peeled

2 shallots, finely chopped

1 cup chicken stock

1 cup dry red wine

3 tablespoons unsalted butter

LIBERALLY SEASON the tenderloin with salt and pepper—2 to 4 tablespoons of each, depending on the size of the roast. Place on a wire rack set on a rimmed baking sheet and refrigerate, uncovered, for 24 hours.

PREHEAT THE oven to 450°F, with a rimmed baking sheet on the lowest rack.

IN A large stainless-steel roasting pan, heat 2 tablespoons of the vegetable oil over medium-high heat until nearly smoking. Add the tenderloin and sear until evenly browned on all sides, including the ends, about 2 minutes per side. Remove from the heat, insert a temperature probe into the thickest part of the tenderloin,

(recipe continues)

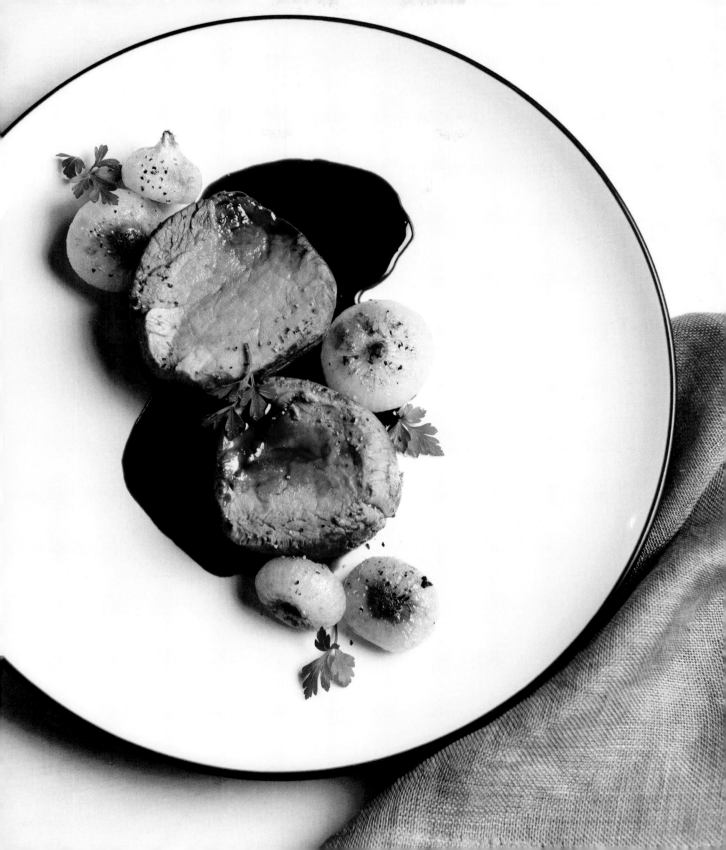

and roast on the highest rack for 20 to 25 minutes, until the internal temperature registers 125°F.

MEANWHILE, IN a large, microwave-safe bowl, toss the cipollini onions with 1 tablespoon water, the remaining 1 tablespoon oil, and 1 teaspoon each of salt and pepper. Microwave on high for 30 to 60 seconds, until just softened. Pour out onto the preheated baking sheet and roast for 9 to 12 minutes, flipping halfway through, until browned and caramelized.

REMOVE THE roast from the oven and transfer to a carving board. Tent with aluminum foil to keep warm and let rest for 10 minutes.

PLACE THE roasting pan over medium-high heat. Add the shallots and cook, stirring, until soft and translucent, about 3 minutes. Add the stock and wine and cook, stirring and scraping up all the browned bits from the bottom of the pan. Bring to a simmer and cook, whisking occasionally, until reduced by half, about 5 minutes. Remove from the heat, whisk in the butter, and season with salt and pepper.

CARVE THE steak into large medallions, transfer to plates, and serve with the pan sauce and onions.

CHICKEN PAPRIKASH

SERVES 4

While this episode might have not been the final one featuring my kitchen, it was the final episode filmed there. That didn't make sense. I shot the last three episodes out of order, is what I mean, and this was the last one I filmed. It was bittersweet, cooking in the last few pots and pans not yet wrapped and packed into a myriad of boxes. I knew there were better things ahead but that kitchen had given me the best two years of my life thus far, and I knew I'd miss the times we shared together.

It seemed only fitting to end with my favorite kind of meal—something simple, comforting, and wholesome. Like Wanda Maximoff said, "Spirits lifted." So long, Harlem—see you again soon.

VERDICT: Chicken paprikash, while a new concept to me, can be immediately recognized for the homestyle comfort it is. Rich, delicately spiced, with perfectly al dente dumplings, it's a cold-weather classic.

¼ cup vegetable oil

1 whole (3- to 5-pound) chicken, broken down into 10 pieces

1 small Spanish onion, finely minced

2 plum tomatoes, cored, seeded, and finely chopped

1 Italian frying pepper, stemmed, seeded, and finely chopped

3 tablespoons paprika, plus more for garnish

2 cups chicken stock

Kosher salt and freshly ground black pepper

Dumplings (recipe follows)

¼ cup sour cream, for serving

¼ cup chopped fresh parsley, for garnish

PREHEAT THE oven to 350°F. In a large, high-walled, ovenproof skillet, heat the vegetable oil over medium-high heat until nearly smoking. Working in batches, add the chicken pieces skin-side down in a single layer and cook, undisturbed, until the skin is deeply browned, about 5 minutes. Flip and cook until lightly browned underneath, about 2 minutes more. Transfer the chicken to a large plate.

ADD THE onion to the pan and cook, stirring, until soft and translucent, about 2 minutes. Add the tomatoes and frying pepper and cook,

(recipe continues)

277

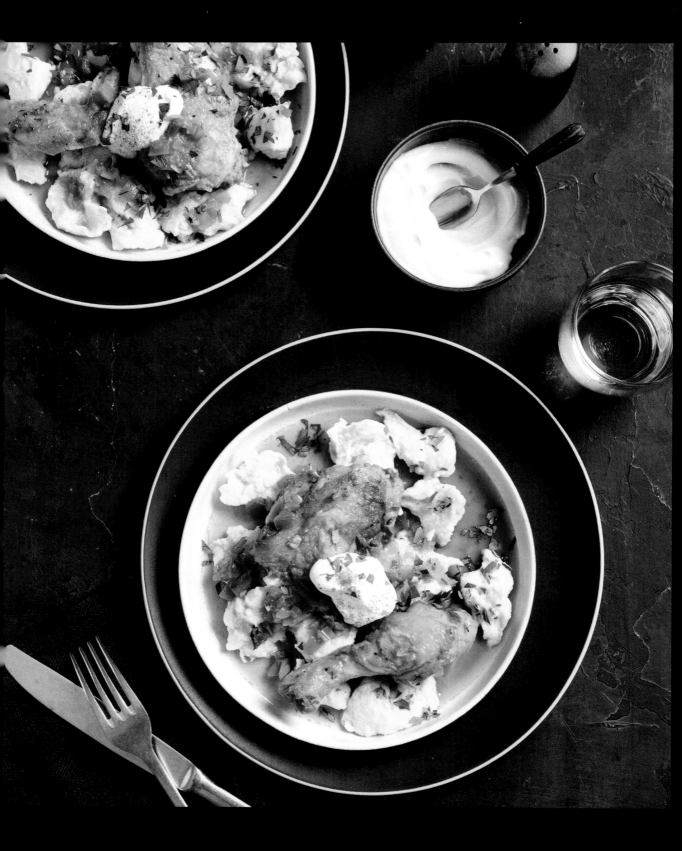

stirring, for 1 minute. Add the paprika and toast, stirring, for no more than 15 seconds. Add the stock, stirring and scraping up all the browned bits from the bottom of the pot. Season with salt and pepper and return all the chicken pieces to the pot, skin-side up, and any accumulated juices from the plate—make sure the chicken skin sits above the liquid and remove excess liquid if the skin is submerged. Braise in the oven, uncovered, for 30 to 40 minutes, until the internal temperature registers 155°F for the white meat and 175°F for the dark meat, at their thickest points.

DIVIDE THE dumplings evenly among four plates, add the chicken pieces, and spoon the sauce over the top. Dollop each plate with the sour cream, garnish with a pinch of paprika and chopped parsley, and serve.

FUN FACT
My friend Ari's mom apparently makes the best paprikash. She approved of my recipe.

DUMPLINGS
SERVES 4

4 large eggs

2 tablespoons sour cream

2 teaspoons kosher salt

1½ cups all-purpose flour, plus more as needed

2 tablespoons unsalted butter

Kosher salt and freshly ground black pepper

IN A large bowl, beat together the eggs, sour cream, and salt with a fork until well incorporated. Slowly beat in the flour until the mixture resembles a thick pancake batter.

BRING A large pot of salted water to a boil over high heat. Using two spoons, drop in about ½ tablespoon of batter for each dumpling. Reduce the heat to maintain a boil and cook until the dumplings are tender but firm, 6 to 10 minutes. Drain, toss with the butter, and season with salt and pepper, keeping warm until ready to serve

SLOPPY JESSICA

MAKES 1 SANDWICH

The Sloppy Jessica is appropriately named—it takes a look at the sloppy joe, and says, "No. Not sloppy enough. We gotta add mac and cheese. No, I'm not done, you think that's sloppy enough? Not after you've had it between two French bread pizzas. Yeah, that's it. Pass me the joint." The sandwich itself is a torpedo headed at high-velocity toward the sinking dinghy of an abandoned diet, as depicted with reckless abandon by Chelsea Peretti. In fact, the sandwich can only be properly consumed when yelling "I gave up so easy!" to jealous friends and coworkers.

VERDICT: This is an inappropriate sandwich for any occasion. Don't make it. Unless you want to—I'm not your mom.

---

3 cups Chili (recipe follows)

3 cups Mac and Cheese (recipe follows)

French Bread Pizza (recipe follows)

PLACE THE chili and mac and cheese in a large bowl and toss to combine. Pile the mixture onto the French bread pizza, close the sandwich, and cut into 8 even pieces. Consume at your own risk.

CHILI

MAKES 4 CUPS

4 ancho chiles, stemmed and seeded

1 cup boiling water

2 teaspoons ground cumin

2 teaspoons ground coriander

2 teaspoons smoked paprika

1 canned chipotle chile in adobo sauce

1 tablespoon vegetable oil

1 pound ground beef

1 small onion, finely chopped

2 garlic cloves, minced

1 (14-ounce) can diced tomatoes, with their juices

Kosher salt and freshly ground black pepper

(recipe continues)

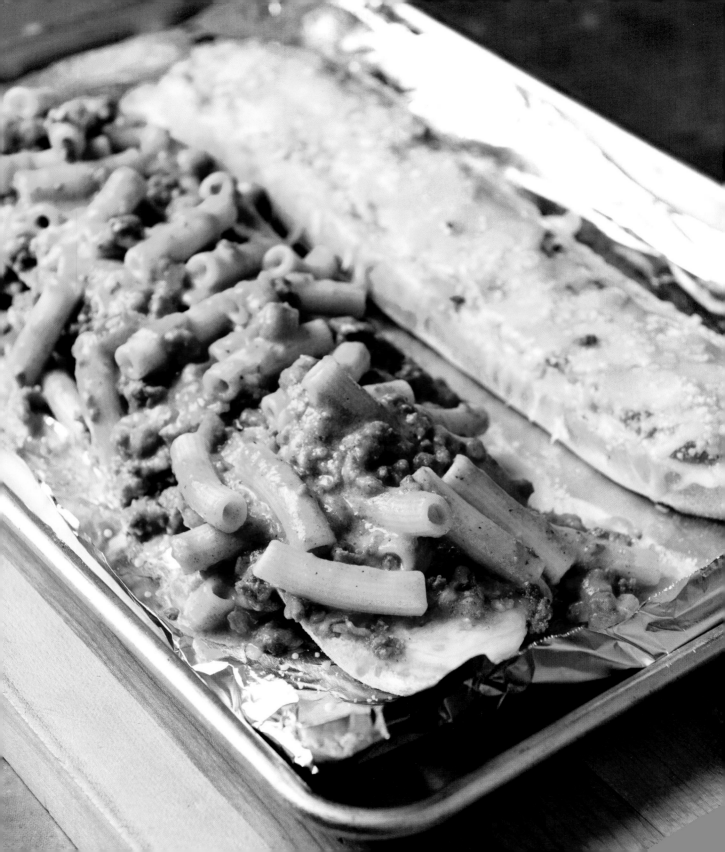

HEAT A small sauté pan over medium heat for 2 minutes. Add the ancho chiles and toast until fragrant, about 2 minutes. Remove the pan from the heat and let cool for 1 minute, then add the boiling water. Cover and let steep for 10 minutes.

TRANSFER THE anchos and their soaking liquid to a blender. Add the cumin, coriander, paprika, and chipotle. Blend on high speed or until the spice paste is smooth, about 1 minute.

IN A large high-walled skillet, heat the vegetable oil over medium-high heat until shimmering, about 2 minutes. Add the beef and cook, stirring, until browned, about 5 minutes. Transfer the beef to a bowl and pour off all but 1 tablespoon of the fat from the skillet. Add the onion to the skillet and cook, stirring, until soft and translucent, about 3 minutes. Add the garlic and cook, stirring, for 1 minute more. Add the spice paste, beef, and tomatoes and their juices to the pan. Stir well to combine. Reduce the heat to low and simmer until the vegetables have softened and the flavors have developed, about 30 minutes. Season with salt and pepper, remove from the heat, and keep warm until ready to use.

MAC AND CHEESE
MAKES ABOUT 5 CUPS

3 tablespoons unsalted butter
3 tablespoons all-purpose flour
3 cups whole milk
1 teaspoon mustard powder
2 teaspoons hot sauce
1 pound sharp cheddar cheese, shredded
6 ounces Parmesan cheese, grated
Kosher salt and freshly ground black pepper
1 pound ziti, cooked

IN A large saucepan, heat the butter over medium-high heat until it melts and the foaming subsides, about 1 minute. Add the flour and cook, whisking continuously, until the smell of raw flour dissipates, about 30 seconds. While whisking continuously, slowly stream in the milk, making sure to whisk apart any clumps that form. Reduce the heat to medium and bring to a bare simmer. Add the mustard powder, hot sauce, and cheeses and cook, whisking continuously, until the cheese has melted and been incorporated. Reduce the heat to low and cook until thickened, about 3 minutes. Season with salt and pepper. Add the pasta and toss until evenly coated. Remove from the heat and keep warm until ready to use.

FRENCH BREAD PIZZA

MAKES 2 PIZZAS, ENOUGH TO SERVE 4

2 tablespoons extra-virgin olive oil

1 small onion, finely chopped

2 garlic cloves, minced

1 (14-ounce) can tomato puree

1 (14-ounce) can diced tomatoes, with their juices

1 teaspoon dried oregano

1 fresh basil sprig

Kosher salt and freshly ground black pepper

1 large loaf supermarket French bread

1 pound low-moisture mozzarella cheese, shredded

4 ounces Parmesan cheese, grated

IN A large high-walled skillet, heat the olive oil over medium heat until shimmering, about 2 minutes. Add the onion and cook, stirring, until soft and translucent, about 3 minutes. Add the garlic and cook, stirring, until fragrant, about 1 minute. Add both canned tomatoes and their juices, oregano, and basil and bring to a simmer. Reduce the heat and cook at a bare simmer until the flavors have mellowed and the pizza sauce has thickened, about 45 minutes. Season with salt and pepper and remove from the heat.

PREHEAT THE oven to 425°F. Line a rimmed baking sheet with aluminum foil.

WITHOUT CUTTING all the way through the loaf, split the French bread lengthwise and open it up like a book. Lay the bread split-sides up on the lined baking sheet. Sprinkle half the mozzarella over the top and spread 1½ cups of the pizza sauce evenly over the cheese. (Reserve the remaining sauce for another use or refrigerate in an airtight container for up to 1 week.) Top with the remaining mozzarella and the Parmesan. Bake for 10 to 15 minutes, until the bread is toasted and the cheese is melted and browned in spots. Remove from the oven and set aside until ready to assemble the sandwich.

As I write these recipes, I'm realizing that maybe a third of them are my personal confrontation with recipes that intimidate me. *Waitress* was no exception—in fact, it was a shining example, as pie will continue to intimidate me for the rest of time. Gracefully, two of these pies aren't pies at all, but a chocolate tart and a cheesecake. Jenna was even good enough to specify the cheesecake as "New York–style," which borders on my favorite dessert. It was an opportunity to make one of those towering, creamy, chestnut-hued confections normally dancing their carousel around the rotating display in a diner. Ultimately, I knew I had to pull off this episode just right, as my cousin is a *Waitress* fanatic and I didn't want to piss her off.

BAD BABY QUICHE

SERVES 8

VERDICT: Bad Baby Quiche is flawed by its construction, but by chopping up the brie a bit, it makes for a solid (if unrefined) quiche.

Pie Dough (see page 40)

4 large eggs

½ cup heavy cream

2 teaspoons kosher salt

1 teaspoon freshly ground black pepper

8 ounces Brie, sliced

1 (4-ounce) slab cooked ham, chopped

ROLL OUT the pie dough to a 13-inch round. Roll the round onto your rolling pin and unroll it over a 9-inch pie plate. Without stretching the dough, ease it into the pie plate, leaving a 1-inch overhang all around. Crimp the edges decoratively if desired. Refrigerate for 30 minutes.

PREHEAT THE oven to 425°F.

LINE THE pie crust with aluminum foil and fill with pie weights, dried beans, or uncooked rice. Bake for 15 minutes, or until the crust is just beginning to brown. Remove from the oven and let cool on a wire rack for 30 minutes. Reduce the oven temperature to 350°F and place a rimmed baking sheet in the oven to preheat for 10 minutes.

MEANWHILE, IN a medium bowl, whisk together the eggs, cream, salt, and pepper. Line the bottom of the piecrust with the Brie. Scatter the ham over the top and pour in the egg mixture. Bake for 30 to 40 minutes on the preheated baking sheet, until the eggs are set and lightly browned on top. Remove from the oven, transfer the pie plate to a wire rack, and let cool for 30 minutes. Slice the quiche into wedges and serve.

FUN FACT

My niece is obsessed with *Waitress*, and I thought it'd be funny to freak her out if she happens across this note. Hi, Claire!

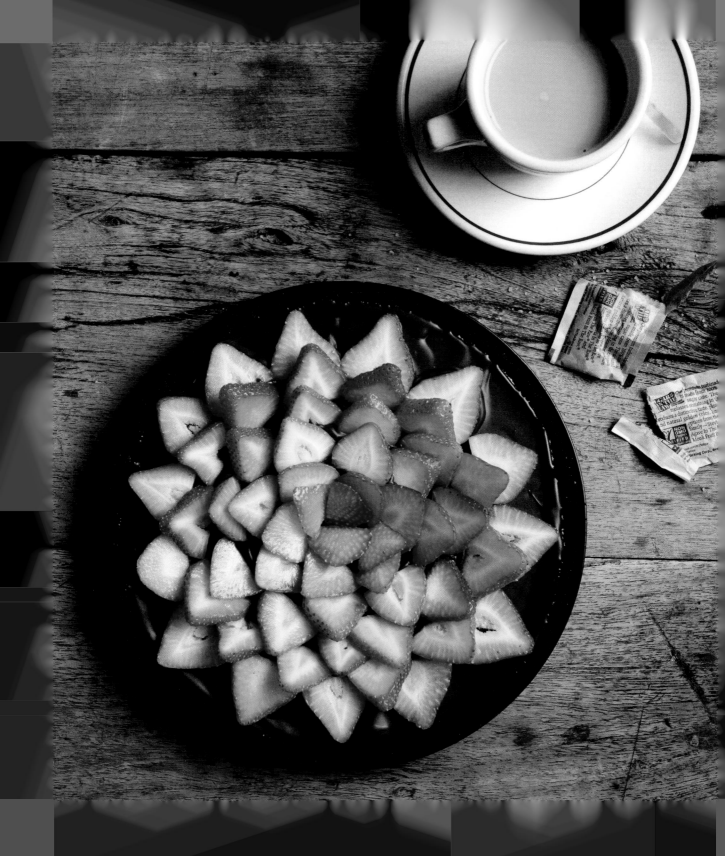

CHOCOLATE STRAWBERRY OASIS PIE

SERVES 8

VERDICT: Chocolate Strawberry Oasis pie is as lovely to look at as it is to eat.

- 25 chocolate sandwich cookies, such as Oreos (including the filling)
- ½ cup (1 stick) unsalted butter, melted, plus 4 tablespoons (½ stick) cubed and chilled
- 1¼ cups heavy cream
- 1 teaspoon instant espresso powder
- ½ teaspoon ground allspice
- ¼ teaspoon ground cinnamon
- 11 ounces dark chocolate, chopped
- 2 large eggs, lightly beaten
- 1 tablespoon hot water
- 1 pint strawberries, hulled and thinly sliced

PREHEAT THE oven to 350°F.

PLACE THE cookies in a food processor and process into fine crumbs. With the machine running, stream in 5 tablespoons of the melted butter, until the mixture resembles wet sand. Transfer the crumbs to a 9-inch tart pan with a removable bottom. Using the bottom of a ramekin or a drinking glass, press the crumbs evenly over the bottom and up the sides of the pan until smooth and flat. Bake for 8 minutes, or until the crust begins to set. Remove from the oven and let cool completely on a wire rack. Reduce the oven temperature to 250°F.

IN A large saucepan, combine the cream, espresso powder, allspice, and cinnamon and bring to a bare simmer. Place 9 ounces of the chocolate in a large heatproof bowl and pour in the hot cream. Whisk gently until melted and incorporated. Add the cold butter and whisk until incorporated and cooled. Whisk in the eggs until completely incorporated. Pour into the tart shell, filling it to the top, and place on a rimmed baking sheet to catch any drips. Bake for 30 to 35 minutes, until the filling is jiggly but set. Remove from the oven and let cool completely on a wire rack.

(recipe continues)

PLACE THE remaining 2 ounces chocolate in a medium bowl. Heat the remaining 3 tablespoons melted butter in a small saucepan until bubbling, then pour it over the chocolate. Cover and let stand for 30 seconds. Whisk to combine. Add 1 tablespoon hot water and whisk slowly until incorporated. Pour the glaze over the chocolate tart, using an offset spatula to smooth the top.

WHILE THE glaze is still soft, decorate the top of the tart with the strawberries. Let cool completely. Remove the side of the tart pan, slice the tart into wedges, and serve.

BABY SCREAMING ITS HEAD OFF IN THE MIDDLE OF THE NIGHT AND RUINING MY LIFE PIE

SERVES 8

VERDICT: BSIHOITMOTNARML Pie, AKA cheesecake, is light, creamy, and impossible to resist.

GRAHAM CRACKER CRUST

6 graham crackers (about 3 ounces), broken up

2⅓ ounces light brown sugar (about ⅓ cup packed)

2½ ounces all-purpose flour (about ½ cup)

1 teaspoon fine salt

7 tablespoons unsalted butter, melted

CREAM CHEESE FILLING

2½ pounds cream cheese, cut into 1-inch pieces, at room temperature

11 ounces sugar (about 1½ cups)

1 teaspoon fine salt

⅓ cup sour cream

Juice of ½ lemon

1 teaspoon pure vanilla extract

2 large egg yolks

6 large eggs

Melted butter, for greasing

2 tablespoons brandy

4 ounces chopped pecans, toasted

GRAHAM CRACKER CRUST

PREHEAT THE oven to 325°F.

IN A food processor, combine the graham crackers and brown sugar and process into fine crumbs, about 20 seconds. Add the flour and salt and pulse five or six times until incorporated. With the machine running, drizzle the melted butter through the feed tube and process until the mixture resembles wet sand.

TRANSFER THE crumbs to a tall 9-inch spring-form pan. Using the bottom of a ramekin or a drinking glass, press the crumbs evenly over the bottom of the pan until smooth and flat. Bake for 12 to 15 minutes, until the crust just begins to brown. Remove from the oven and let cool on a wire rack. Reduce the oven temperature to 200°F.

(recipe continues)

CREAM CHEESE FILLING

IN THE bowl of a stand mixer fitted with the paddle attachment, combine the cream cheese, half the sugar, and the salt. Mix on medium speed until just combined, about 1 minute. Scrape down the sides of the bowl, add the remaining sugar, the sour cream, lemon juice, and vanilla and mix on medium speed for 1 minute. Scrape down the sides of the bowl again, add the egg yolks, and mix on medium speed for 1 minute. Add the whole eggs, two at a time, and mix until fully incorporated. Press the filling through a fine-mesh sieve set over a spouted large bowl.

GENEROUSLY BUTTER the sides of the spring-form pan, place the pan on a rimmed baking sheet, and pour in the filling. Bake for 45 minutes, then remove from the oven and pop any bubbles on the surface with a skewer. Bake for 2 hours 45 minutes more, or until the center of the cheesecake registers 165°F, rotating the pan twice during the cooking time.

INCREASE THE oven temperature to its maximum (or to 500°F) and bake for 6 to 10 minutes more, until the top of the cheesecake is well browned. Remove from the oven and run a paring knife around the outside of the cheesecake to help it release later on, but do not remove it from the pan. Transfer the pan to a wire rack and let the cheesecake cool for at least 3 hours. Wrap in plastic wrap, then refrigerate for 4 hours.

BRUSH THE top of the cake with the brandy and sprinkle with the pecans, pressing lightly to help them adhere. Remove the sides of the springform pan, slice the cheesecake into wedges, and serve.

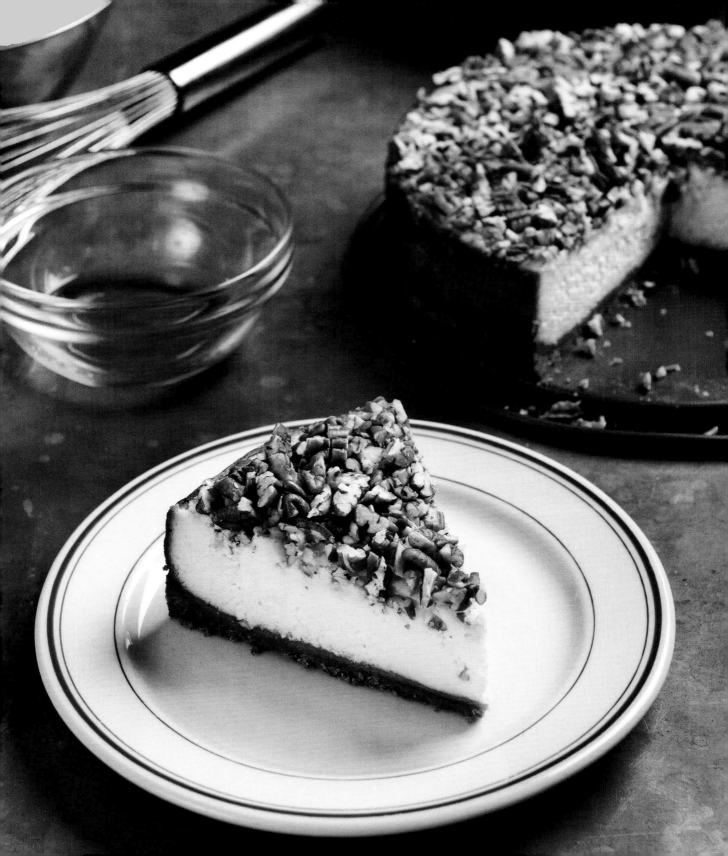

Here we have some Liz Lemon–inspired grossness in the form of Cheesy Blasters, the frozen kids' snack with the forethought to combine hot dogs, pizza, and Jack cheese. Thanks, Meat Cat! I traveled upstate to my high school alma mater, the Harley School, at the behest of the Tang Gang, a group of student food enthusiasts. I got to experience the most magical moment when I walked into a room behind them, where they were watching my show on a laptop. I snuck up and asked, "What are y'all watching?"—it was my little moment to feel like a celebrity. Afterward, they did me the favor of eating all the outcomes of the episode, which my arteries continue to thank them for.

CHEESY BLASTERS

SERVES 4

VERDICT: I don't know, ask the Tang Gang. They said it was good.

---

2 hot dogs, split lengthwise and griddled
4 ounces Monterey Jack cheese, shredded

1 frozen pizza, baked according to the package directions

" *You take a hot dog, stuff it with some Jack cheese, fold it in a pizza . . . You've got cheesy blasters!* "
—LIZ LEMON

FUN FACT
Back in high school, I was also part of a food enthusiast group, the GUC (Gluttonous Union of Competitors). We would go to Chinese buffets and see who could eat the most plates. Gross, I know.

"CHEESY BLASTERS" CALZONE

SERVES 4

1 recipe New York–Style Pizza Dough (see page 33)

½ cup Pizza Sauce (see page 34), plus warmed sauce for serving

8 ounces low-moisture mozzarella cheese, shredded

4 ounces whole-milk ricotta cheese, drained

2 ounces hot Italian sausage, crumbled and cooked

2 ounces sliced pepperoni

2 ounces thinly sliced Genoa salami

2 ounces thinly sliced spicy coppa ham

1 large egg, lightly beaten

PREHEAT THE oven to 450°F.

DIVIDE THE pizza dough into 4 equal pieces. Work with one piece at a time and keep the rest covered in plastic wrap to prevent them from drying out. Roll the dough out into an 8-inch round. Spread 2 tablespoons of sauce on the round, leaving a 2-inch border. Layer one-quarter of each filling (both cheeses, sausage, pepperoni, salami, and ham) in the center of the round. Brush the exposed border around half the round with the beaten egg. Fold over into a half-moon and crimp the edges to enclose the filling. Brush the top of the calzone with the beaten egg and, using a serrated knife, make three small slits in the top to allow steam to escape. Repeat with the remaining dough and fillings. Transfer the calzones to a rimmed baking sheet and bake for 10 to 15 minutes, until the crust is golden brown and the cheese has melted. Serve with warm pizza sauce on the side.

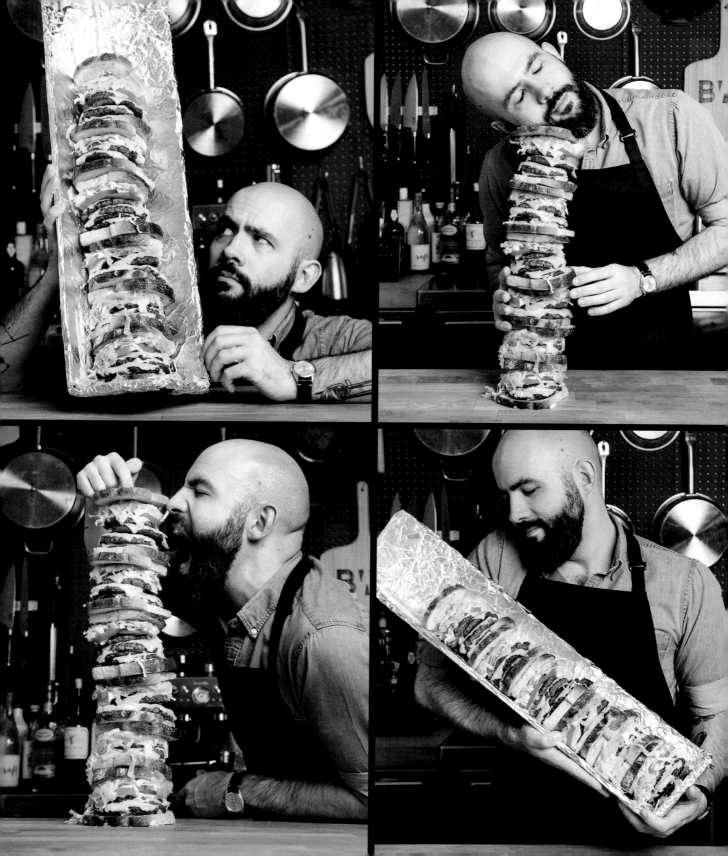

After two happy years in Harlem, I decided to invest in myself and the business I wanted to grow. I hired my best friend Sawyer as my business partner, moved to the only apartment with a commercial kitchen I could find, and set up shop. I knew I had to start things off with a bang, so a (theoretical) 24-patty burger from *SpongeBob SquarePants* seemed like the obvious choice. Someone on 4chan had decoded the secret menu jargon rattled off by Bubble Bass, the pickle-hiding antagonist with the ugliest laugh in recorded human history: "I'll take a double triple [6 burgers] bossy [all-beef] deluxe [everything on it], on a raft [on Texas toast], four by four [4 patties, 4 slices of cheese], animal style [fried in mustard], extra shingles [extra toast] with a shimmy and a squeeze [unknown], light axle grease [lightly buttered toast], make it cry [extra onions], burn it [well done], and let it swim [extra sauce]." Yikes.

THE BUBBLE BASS KRABBY PATTY— ORIGINAL ORDER

SERVES 6

VERDICT: The literal interpretation of Bubble Bass's original order is an exercise in absurdity, but if made for a crowd (and not stacked into one giant burger), it's a solid burgers-for-the-masses recipe. Bass's second, fussier order is definitely more refined, but still caloric enough for him to maintain his figure.

½ cup vegetable oil

8 large Spanish onions, halved and thinly sliced

4 tablespoons (½ stick) unsalted butter

12 slices thick-cut sandwich bread

4½ pounds ground beef

Kosher salt and freshly ground black pepper

½ cup yellow mustard

24 slices American cheese

3 large tomatoes, thinly sliced

1 head iceberg lettuce, cored and shredded

3 dill pickles, thinly sliced

12 tablespoons Special Sauce (recipe follows)

(recipe continues)

ON A large flat-top griddle or pancake griddle, heat ¼ cup of the vegetable oil over medium heat. Add the onions, reduce the heat to medium-low, and cook, moving the onions and reducing the heat as necessary to prevent them from browning, until jammy, soft, and caramelized, 30 minutes to 1 hour. Add ¼ cup water as necessary if the onions become dry during cooking. Transfer to a bowl and set aside.

WIPE THE griddle clean and increase the heat to medium-high. Evenly coat the griddle with the butter and heat until the foaming subsides. Working in batches if necessary, add the bread in a single layer and flip immediately to coat both sides with butter. Toast for 1 to 3 minutes per side, until golden brown. Transfer to a plate.

WIPE THE griddle clean. Increase the heat to medium-high and add the remaining ¼ cup oil and heat until nearly smoking.

FORM THE beef into 24 equal balls and season with salt and pepper. Working in batches, place the beef balls several inches apart in the skillet and smash them down using a large spatula. Press down firmly on the spatula with a rolling pin or the handle of another spatula until the patties are thin and craggy. Spread 1 teaspoon of the mustard on each patty and cook for about 1 minute, until browned and lacy around the edges. Flip, immediately top each patty with a slice of cheese, and heat for 1 minute more, or until the patty is cooked and the cheese has melted.

TO ASSEMBLE the "burger," stand up a large metal trough vertically. Stack the burger ingredients in the trough in the following order: 1 slice of the bread, 4 beef patties, tomato, lettuce, caramelized onions, 3 or 4 pickle slices, 2 tablespoons of the Special Sauce, 1 slice of the bread. Repeat until it stands 6 quad-burgers tall, and serve.

NOTE: *Obviously, this recipe is ridiculous. It's best made as double-patty burgers for a crowd, one to four burgers at a time.*

SPECIAL SAUCE

MAKES ABOUT 1¼ CUPS

½ cup ketchup
½ cup mayonnaise
1 teaspoon garlic powder
1 teaspoon onion powder
½ teaspoon paprika
1 teaspoon kosher salt
¼ cup sweet pickle relish

IN A medium bowl, stir together all the ingredients until completely combined. Cover and refrigerate until ready to serve.

THE BUBBLE BASS KRABBY PATTY— FANCY ORDER

SERVES 2

2 tablespoons unsalted butter

4 slices thick-cut sandwich bread

2 tablespoons vegetable oil

24 ounces ground beef

2 teaspoons smoked paprika

1 teaspoon Himalayan pink salt

6 ounces aged Gouda cheese, shredded

1 tomato, thinly sliced

½ head iceberg lettuce, shredded

1 small onion, halved and thinly sliced

1 dill pickle, thinly sliced

¼ cup Special Sauce (see page 296)

ON A flat-top griddle or pancake griddle, heat the butter over medium-high heat until the foaming subsides. Add the bread in a single layer and flip immediately to coat both sides with butter. Toast for 1 to 3 minutes per side, until golden brown. Transfer to a plate.

WIPE THE griddle clean and increase the heat to medium-high. Add 1 tablespoon of the oil and heat until nearly smoking.

FORM THE beef into 8 equal balls. Place 4 balls several inches apart in the skillet, and smash down using a large spatula. Press down firmly on the spatula with a rolling pin or the handle of another spatula until the patties are thin and craggy. Cook for about 1 minute, until browned and lacy around the edges. Flip, sprinkle with 1 teaspoon of the paprika, ½ teaspoon of the Himalayan salt, and half the Gouda, and heat for 1 minute more, or until the patty is cooked and the cheese has melted. Repeat with the ingredients to make 4 more patties.

FOR EACH quad burger, stack 4 patties on 1 slice of the bread and top with half the tomatoes, lettuce, onion, pickle, and special sauce. Close the burgers and serve.

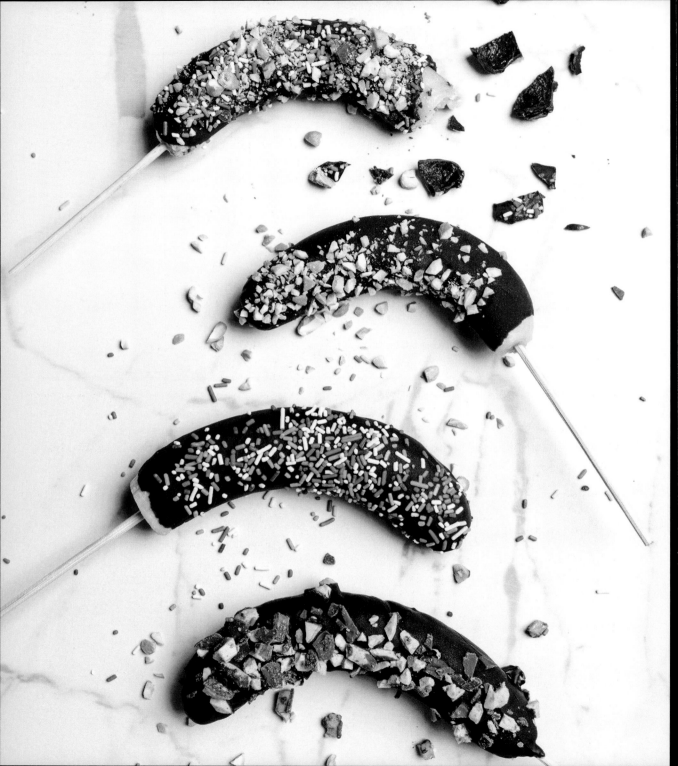

An *Arrested Development* special was hotly requested, and my original intention was to make the Skip's Scramble (a giant platter containing every item on the menu). With a large portion of the menu visible in a freeze-frame, this was accomplishable, but would be wildly difficult to pull off—so, chocolate-dipped bananas anyone? While I might've taken the easier road, I still endeavored to make the Babish version of everything from the show, including hot ham water, which took the form of *tonkotsu* ramen broth. Sean Evans was kind enough test drive my recipe for homemade Magic Shell—after previously subjecting him to a Krispy Kreme doughnut burger, I was happy to help get some fruit into his diet.

FROZEN BANANAS

SERVES 12

VERDICT: Frozen bananas are a fun and easy summertime snack,
and Magic Shell is a breeze to make.

12 bananas, peeled

42 ounces dark chocolate, chopped

½ cup refined coconut oil

Sprinkles, chopped nuts, and/or toffee bits,
   for topping

LINE A baking sheet with parchment paper.

SKEWER EACH banana on a large wooden dowel and transfer to the lined baking sheet. Freeze completely, at least 4 hours.

BRING A few inches of water to a boil in a large saucepan. Place the chocolate in a heatproof glass bowl—large enough so the bottom of the bowl does not touch the water when set over the pan. Melt the chocolate, stirring continuously with a rubber spatula. When it's half melted, add the coconut oil and stir until completely melted and combined, about 1 minute. Remove from the heat and keep the chocolate warm. Remove the bananas from the freezer and line the baking sheet with a fresh sheet of parchment paper. Dip each banana in the melted chocolate, spooning the chocolate over the banana if necessary to coat it entirely. Immediately sprinkle with your desired toppings before the chocolate hardens. Place on the prepared baking sheet and let the chocolate harden 15 seconds, then serve.

CORNBALLS

SERVES 6

VERDICT: My cornballs might more closely resemble hush puppies than the dough balls being tossed about by Michael Bluth, but they're a tastier way to pay fan service.

4¼ ounces cornmeal (about 1¼ cups)

3 ounces all-purpose flour (about ¾ cup)

1½ teaspoons baking powder

½ teaspoon baking soda

1 teaspoon kosher salt

½ teaspoon paprika

¾ cup buttermilk

2 large eggs

Vegetable oil, for frying

1 jalapeño, seeded if desired, chopped

1 scallion, thinly sliced

1 cup drained canned corn

Tartar sauce, for serving

IN A large bowl, whisk together the cornmeal, flour, baking powder, baking soda, salt, and paprika until combined. In a medium bowl, whisk together the buttermilk and eggs until well combined. Gently whisk the wet ingredients into the dry ingredients until a lumpy batter forms. Let rest for 10 minutes.

FILL A Dutch oven or deep fryer with vegetable oil to a depth of 2 inches. Heat over medium-high heat to 350°F.

ADD THE jalapeño, scallion, and corn to the batter and gently fold in until combined. Using a small ice cream scoop or two large spoons, scoop out 2-tablespoon rounds of the batter and carefully drop them into the hot oil. Fry, flipping halfway through, until golden brown and crisp, 5 to 7 minutes. Using a spider or slotted spoon, transfer the cornballs to paper towels to drain. Serve hot, with tartar sauce.

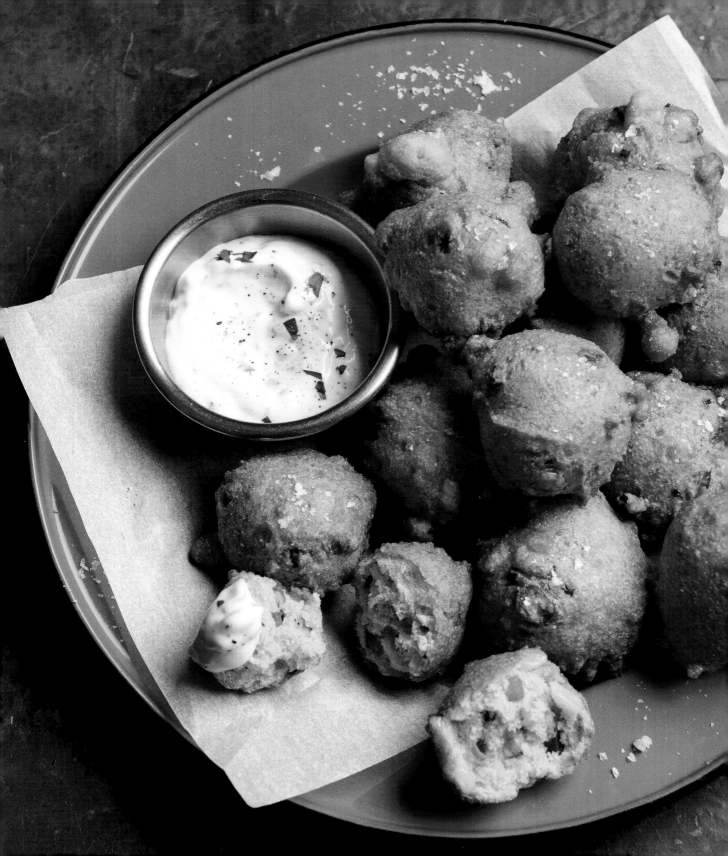

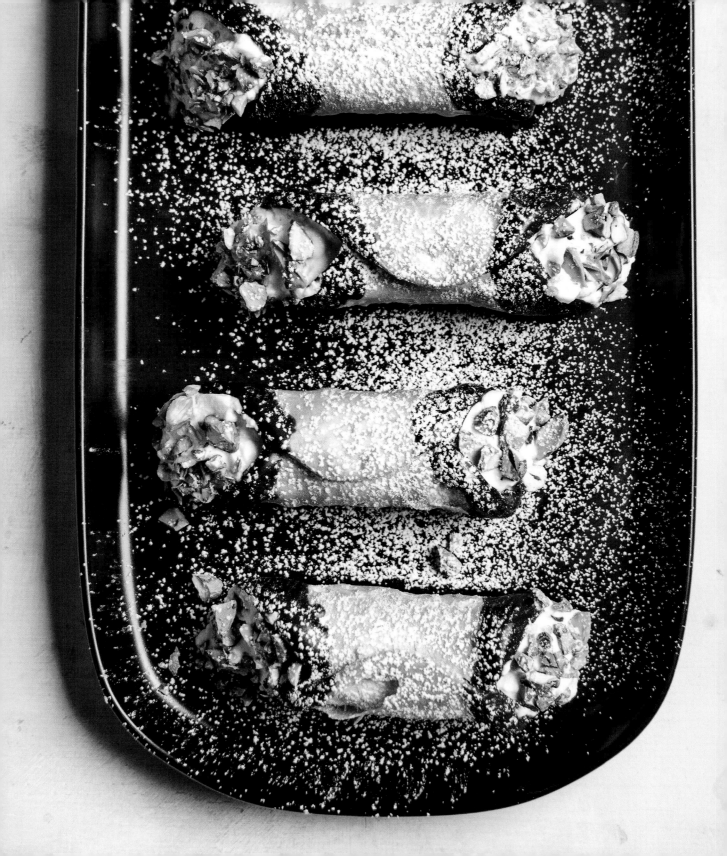

CANNOLI

SERVES 10

"Leave the gun, take the cannoli"—an instantly recognizable quote from a movie composed of the world's most instantly recognizable quotes. We might never see the cannoli in question, but its mere mention was enough to make it one of the more requested episodes in recent memory. I normally cower at the mention of any recipe that's been perfected by a grandmother from the old country, but I trusted that my (quarter) Italian heritage would reward me with instinctual expertise. Like Alton Brown, I detest "unitaskers," or tools that only serve one possible purpose. Unlike Alton Brown, however, I didn't mastermind some clever repurposed gadget to stand in for cannoli molds; I caved almost immediately and ordered them off Amazon. I suppose you could use them to make cannoli-shaped taco shells. That's not a bad idea, actually.

VERDICT: This is a solidly traditional cannoli recipe, made extra-traditional by its use of lard as the deep-frying fat. An addition of Marsala wine darkens the dough slightly, so knowing when they're done frying can be tricky—but lucky for you, this isn't a *Great British Bake Off* technical challenge, and you can test one or two to get the feel for it before frying up the rest.

24 ounces whole-milk ricotta cheese

9 ounces all-purpose flour (about 2 cups plus 2 tablespoons), plus more for dusting

5½ ounces confectioners' sugar (about 1⅓ cups), sifted, plus more for dusting

2 teaspoons unsweetened cocoa powder

1½ teaspoons ground cinnamon

½ teaspoon instant espresso powder

2 tablespoons Marsala wine

2 tablespoons white wine vinegar

2 tablespoons unsalted butter, melted

1 large egg

Lard or vegetable oil, for frying

Nonstick cooking spray or vegetable oil

1 large egg white, beaten

4 ounces dark chocolate, melted

3 ounces chopped pistachios, toasted (optional)

4 ounces mini chocolate chips (optional)

(recipe continues)

PLACE THE ricotta in a fine-mesh sieve set over a large bowl. Cover with plastic wrap and refrigerate for 1 hour to drain.

MEANWHILE, IN a food processor, combine the flour, 1 ounce of the confectioners' sugar, the cocoa powder, 1 teaspoon of the cinnamon, and the espresso powder. Pulse to incorporate. Add the Marsala and vinegar and process until the mixture resembles wet sand. Add the butter and egg and process until a rough ball of dough forms, 30 to 45 seconds. Turn out the dough onto a lightly floured work surface and knead until silky and elastic, 4 to 5 minutes. Wrap tightly in plastic wrap and refrigerate for 1 hour.

FILL A large saucepan with lard (or vegetable oil) to a depth of 3 inches. Heat over medium-high heat to 325°F.

GENEROUSLY COAT the outside of ten cannoli molds with cooking spray or rub with vegetable oil.

ROLL THE chilled dough out on a lightly floured work surface to about 1/16 inch thick. Using a 4-inch biscuit cutter, stamp out 10 rounds of dough. Working with one round (keep the rest covered with plastic wrap), wrap the dough around a cannoli mold, slightly overlapping the ends at the shorter side of the cylinder. Brush one end of the dough round with egg white and press the opposite end on top to seal. Repeat until all the rounds are wrapped. Working in batches to avoid overlapping, carefully lower the molds into the oil and fry, flipping once during cooking if possible, until browned and puffy, 2 to 4 minutes. Using tongs, transfer to a wire rack set over a rimmed baking sheet to drain and let cool completely, about 30 minutes.

GENTLY SQUEEZE the molds to slide off the cannoli shells. Dip the ends of the shells in melted chocolate and return to the rack. Refrigerate for 15 minutes to harden the chocolate.

REMOVE THE ricotta from the refrigerator and, using a wooden spoon, lightly press it against the sieve to squeeze out any remaining liquid; discard the liquid in the bowl. Using a rubber spatula, press the ricotta directly through the sieve into the bowl of a stand mixer. Fit the stand mixer with the whisk attachment. Add the remaining 4½ ounces confectioners' sugar and ½ teaspoon cinnamon and mix on medium speed until completely incorporated, about 1 minute. Spoon the mixture into a pastry bag fitted with a decorative tip. Pipe the ricotta into each cannoli shell, starting at the middle and working toward the ends from each side. If desired, garnish each end of the cannoli with chopped pistachios or mini chocolate chips. Dust the cannoli with confectioners' sugar and serve immediately, or cover and refrigerate for up to 1 day.

PASTA PUTTANESCA

SERVES 4

I make no secret of my distaste for a few things in life: cilantro, screaming children, olives, bad tippers, anchovies, and spiders. Two of those things appear in pasta puttanesca, so I was understandably dreading its eventual re-creation. I mean, they practically spell out the recipe in the narration—I kind of had to, right? Surprisingly, when made correctly, puttanesca becomes a deeply flavorful and not-revolting sauce. In the same way Marmite disappears into the background when incorporated into sauces and meats, the olives and anchovies mellow when

sautéed and serve to only complement the bright tomatoes at the forefront. With that, puttanesca went from compulsory to congenial, surprising me (as food often does) with its ability to change my preconceptions.

VERDICT: Puttanesca takes some of God's repugnant mistakes and makes something downright palatable with them. Finish the pasta in the sauce with a pat of butter if you want to live your life with meaning and purpose.

All-purpose flour, for dusting

16 ounces unshaped pasta dough for Homemade Garganelli (see page 27)

2 tablespoons extra-virgin olive oil

7 garlic cloves, chopped

4 ounces black olives, pitted and sliced

2 tablespoons capers, drained and chopped

1 (2-ounce) can anchovies, drained and chopped

1 (28-ounce) can whole DOP San Marzano tomatoes, with their juices

1 cup fresh parsley, minced

Kosher salt and freshly ground black pepper

2 tablespoons unsalted butter, cut into small pieces

4 ounces Parmesan cheese, grated

DUST A rimmed baking sheet with flour. Roll out the pasta dough, then run it through successively narrower settings on a pasta machine

until it can fit into the pasta cutter. Run the dough through the spaghetti cutter. Toss the pasta with flour, then arrange it into nests on

(recipe continues)

the prepared baking sheet. Cover with plastic wrap and refrigerate until ready to use.

IN A large nonstick sauté pan, heat the olive oil over medium heat for 2 minutes, until shimmering. Add the garlic, olives, capers, and anchovies and cook, stirring, until fragrant, about 1 minute. Add the tomatoes and their juices and crush the tomatoes with a wooden spoon. Bring to a simmer, then reduce the heat and simmer until the raw tomato flavor has subsided and the flavors are incorporated, 30 to 45 minutes. Remove from the heat and stir in the parsley. Season with salt and pepper.

BRING A large pot of salted water to a rolling boil over high heat. Add the pasta and cook until tender, 1 to 3 minutes. Drain, reserving ½ cup of the pasta cooking water, and return the pasta to the empty pot. Add the sauce and

reserved pasta water, toss to combine, and place over low heat. Simmer, tossing, until the sauce thickens and the pasta is evenly coated, 1 to 2 minutes. Remove from the heat and toss with the butter until melted and incorporated.

FOR EACH serving, transfer to a bowl and, if desired, twirl the pasta into a nest with a carving fork. Sprinkle with Parmesan and serve.

FUN FACT

Pasta alla Puttanesca translates literally to "pasta in the style of a whore." Not quite sure what to do with that information? Me neither.

PINEAPPLE AND OLIVE PIZZA

SERVES 4

Olives take a turn for the worse in the form of pizza, ordered up by superhero-level troll Wade Wilson. Olive and pineapple pizza with a burnt crust, to be exact. The toppings were easy enough, but I wanted to address "burning" the crust without actually burning it, which to me meant cold-fermenting the dough. Fermenting pizza dough in the refrigerator not only deepens its flavor, it creates charred bubbles on the resultant crust, reminiscent of a pie from your favorite artisan pizza place. Of course, your oven needs to be in full cooperation, which mine was not—so while the crust had a nicely charred bottom, it was missing the carbonized bubbles characteristic of Neapolitan-style pizzas. After waiting three days and with only twelve hours left to make the episode, I was out of options, but if you can get your oven hot enough, you should see more ideal results.

VERDICT: Cold-fermented pizza dough is how some of the best pizza in the world is made, including the pies at Lucali in Brooklyn. Get your oven wicked hot, keep it hot with a pizza stone/steel inside for at least an hour, and you'll get some fantastic results.

Cold-Fermented Pizza Dough (recipe follows), store-bought dough, or New York–Style Pizza Dough (see page 33) divided into 4 balls

All-purpose flour, for dusting

4 tablespoons semolina flour or cornmeal

½ cup pizza sauce, store-bought or homemade (see page 34)

8 ounces low-moisture mozzarella cheese, shredded

4 ounces black olives, pitted and sliced

4 ounces pineapple, chopped

2 ounces Parmesan cheese, grated

PREHEAT THE oven to its maximum temperature (or 500°F) with a pizza stone or steel on the bottom rack (or the top rack, if your oven is top-heating).

WORKING WITH one ball of dough at a time, press the dough out on a well-floured work surface to form a 6-inch disc. Using a rolling pin or wine bottle, roll out the disc into a roughly

(recipe continues)

10-inch round. Pick up the dough and pass it over your knuckles, stretching out the center and leaving the edges slightly thicker. Continue until you have about a 12-inch round. Place the round of dough on a pizza peel dusted with 1 tablespoon of the semolina flour.

SPREAD 1 ounce of the pizza sauce on the round, leaving a ½-inch border uncovered. Sprinkle 2 ounces of the mozzarella on top, dot with one-quarter each of the olives and pineapple, and sprinkle with one-quarter of the Parmesan. Slide the pizza onto the preheated pizza stone and bake for 5 to 8 minutes, until the cheese has melted and the crust is browned and puffed. Using the pizza peel, remove the pizza from the oven, slice into wedges, and serve. Repeat with the remaining dough balls and toppings, dusting the peel with 1 tablespoon of the semolina before placing the dough on top each time.

FUN FACT
I should have made *chimichangas* instead.

COLD-FERMENTED PIZZA DOUGH
MAKES ENOUGH DOUGH FOR FOUR 12-INCH PIZZAS

9 ounces bread flour (about 2 cups plus 2 tablespoons)
8½ ounces tipo 00 flour or all-purpose flour (about 2 cups), plus more for dusting
2 teaspoons active dry yeast (from one ¼-ounce packet)
1 teaspoon kosher salt
Extra-virgin olive oil, for greasing

IN A large bowl, whisk together the bread flour, 00 flour, and yeast. Add 1¼ cups plus 2 tablespoons water and mix with a wooden spoon until a shaggy dough forms. Cover and let rest for 5 minutes.

MIX THE salt into the dough. Turn the dough out onto a well-floured work surface and knead until no dry clumps remain, 2 minutes.

TRANSFER THE dough to a large, well-oiled bowl, cover with plastic wrap, and let ferment at room temperature for 12 to 24 hours.

TURN THE dough out onto a generously oiled work surface. Oil your hands and knead the dough for 1 minute, until the air is punched out and the dough is smooth. Divide the dough into 4 equal pieces and form each into a smooth, round ball. Generously oil 4 small bowls, about twice the size of the dough balls, and place 1 ball in each bowl. Cover with oiled plastic wrap and refrigerate for 3 days before using.

BREAKFAST CONGEE

SERVES 4

Exploring comfort foods from other cultures has always been a favorite pastime, and congee was one I had been curious about for some time. How could this plain white rice, cooked until broken and soupy, have a place near and dear to so many hearts? As it happens, it's not unlike any other porridge—thoroughly bland, but made personal with a bevy of possible toppings. As it turns out, a single slice of bacon and two eggs is far from enough to make a bowlful of starch exciting.

VERDICT: Much like oatmeal, congee becomes something worth eating with a wealth of toppings offering contrasting flavors and textures, especially when too young or too old to have teeth.

6 cups chicken stock

1 cup long-grain jasmine rice

1 (1-inch) knob fresh ginger, peeled and chopped

1 shallot, finely chopped

1 garlic clove, finely minced

Kosher salt and freshly ground black pepper

8 slices bacon

8 large eggs

1 garlic clove, thinly sliced and fried in vegetable oil until lightly browned, for garnish (optional)

4 ounces shiitake mushrooms, sautéed in butter, for garnish (optional)

Black sesame seeds, toasted, for garnish (optional)

Peanuts, toasted, for garnish (optional)

1 scallion, thinly sliced, for garnish (optional)

Sriracha, for serving (optional)

IN A large saucepan, combine the stock, rice, ginger, shallot, and garlic. Bring to a simmer over medium-high heat, then reduce the heat to barely maintain a simmer. Cook, stirring occasionally, until the rice has broken and formed a creamy porridge, about 1 hour. Season with salt and pepper.

PREHEAT THE oven to 375°F. Line a rimmed baking sheet with a wire rack.

ARRANGE THE bacon on the rack so each strip is curved. Bake for 15 to 20 minutes, until the bacon is crisp and the curved shape has

(recipe continues)

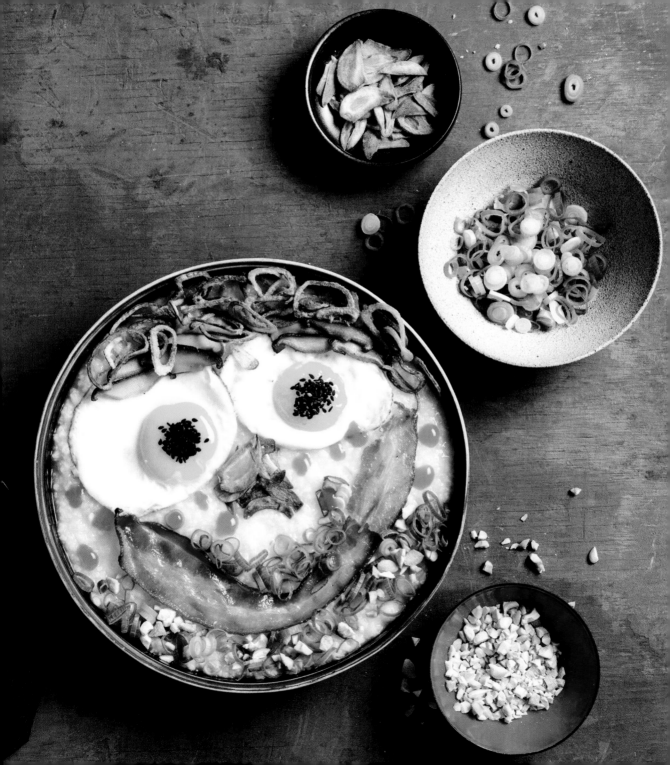

set. Remove from the oven, drain the bacon on paper towels, and reserve the bacon fat.

IN A large nonstick pan, heat 1 tablespoon of the reserved bacon fat over medium-high heat until shimmering. Working in batches and adding more bacon fat as necessary, fry the eggs sunny-side up, then reduce the heat to medium. Fry 3 to 5 minutes, until the whites have set but the yolks are still runny. Transfer to a plate.

FOR EACH serving, ladle the porridge into a large bowl. Arrange two eggs and two strips of bacon on top to create a smiley face. Top with your desired garnishes to create other facial features, and serve with sriracha.

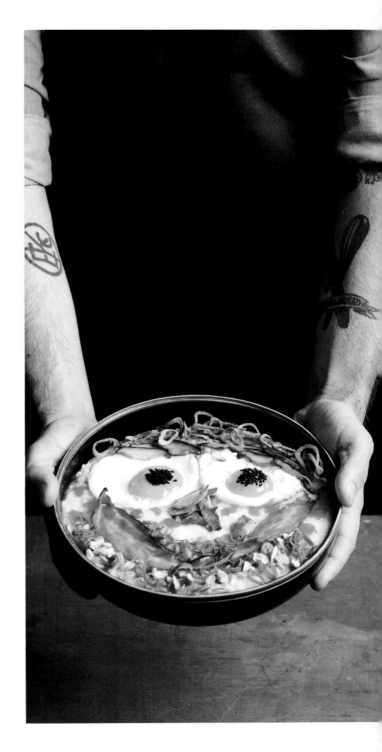

Twenty-one distinct styles of America's favorite seafaring bug, rattled off by America's favorite shrimp enthusiast. How could I resist? Especially when it was the top request from one of my longest and most generous Patreon benefactors, whom I had the pleasure of meeting and sharing some shrimp with. I have to admit that I wasn't the biggest shrimp fan before filming this episode, but by the end, I was converted. The highlight had to be gumbo—I have an affinity for near anything with roots in the Big Easy, and seeing those Low Country flavors meld together in my Yankee kitchen was too exciting not to make again. And again. Three times in two weeks, actually. That's all I have to say about that.

SHRIMP SALAD SANDWICH

SERVES 2

VERDICT: The sandwich is a simple but delicious use for poached or broiled shrimp.

Kosher salt

1 pound small or medium shrimp, peeled and deveined

1 lemon, sliced, plus the juice of 1 lemon

2 bay leaves

¼ cup mayonnaise

¼ cup packed fresh dill, finely chopped

¼ cup packed fresh parsley, finely chopped

1 celery stalk, thinly sliced

2 scallions, thinly sliced

Freshly ground black pepper

2 hoagie rolls, split lengthwise and toasted

4 butter lettuce leaves

1 plum tomato, thinly sliced

BRING A medium pot of salted water to a boil. Fill a large bowl with ice and water. Add the shrimp, lemon slices, and bay leaves to the boiling water, cover, and remove from the heat. Let stand until the shrimp are fully cooked, 8 to 10 minutes. Transfer the shrimp to the ice bath and let cool completely, about 5 minutes. Drain and pat dry with paper towels.

IN A large bowl, combine the mayonnaise, lemon juice, dill, parsley, celery, and scallion. Season with salt and pepper. Add the shrimp and toss to coat. Taste and adjust the seasoning if necessary. Divide the shrimp salad evenly among the bottom halves of the hoagie rolls and top with lettuce and tomato. Close the rolls, cut in half, and serve.

SHRIMP GUMBO

SERVES 8

VERDICT: This gumbo is decidedly labor-intensive, but it pays off in a deeply complex, comforting dish that transports you straight to the bayou.

½ cup plus 1 teaspoon vegetable oil

1 pound medium shrimp, peeled (shells reserved) and deveined

½ cup all-purpose flour

4 celery stalks, finely diced

1 green bell pepper, finely diced

1 small white onion, finely diced

1 cup sliced fresh or frozen okra (thawed, if frozen)

6 garlic cloves, minced

1 teaspoon smoked paprika

½ teaspoon cayenne pepper (optional)

8 ounces andouille sausage or smoked kielbasa, sliced

3 bay leaves

Kosher salt and freshly ground black pepper

8 ounces long-grain white rice, cooked, for serving

½ cup packed fresh parsley, finely chopped

Sliced scallions, for garnish

IN A medium saucepan, heat the 1 teaspoon of vegetable oil over medium-high heat until shimmering, about 2 minutes. Add the shrimp shells and cook, stirring, until pink, about 2 minutes. Add 4 cups water and bring to a simmer. Reduce the heat to medium-low and simmer for 30 minutes. Strain the stock through a fine-mesh sieve and set aside. Discard the shells.

IN A large Dutch oven, heat the remaining ½ cup vegetable oil over medium heat until shimmering, about 1 minute. Add the flour and cook, whisking continuously, until a deep-brown roux resembling dark chocolate forms, 30 to 45 minutes (depending on the temperature). Reduce the heat if the roux darkens too quickly.

ADD THE celery, bell pepper, onion, and okra to the roux and cook over medium heat, stirring continuously, until the vegetables have softened, about 5 minutes. Add the garlic and cook, stirring, until fragrant, about 1 minute. While whisking continuously, slowly stream in the shrimp stock. Don't be discouraged if the gumbo separates—with some brisk whisking,

(recipe continues)

it will smooth out over the following hour of cooking.

WHISK IN the paprika and cayenne. Add the sausage and bay leaves, reduce the heat to maintain a simmer, and cook for 45 minutes to 1 hour, until the flavors are deep and well incorporated. Add the shrimp and simmer for 10 minutes, until the shrimp are cooked through. Remove and discard the bay leaves, and season with salt and black pepper.

FOR EACH serving, mound rice in a bowl and ladle the gumbo around the rice. Garnish with parsley and scallions, and serve.

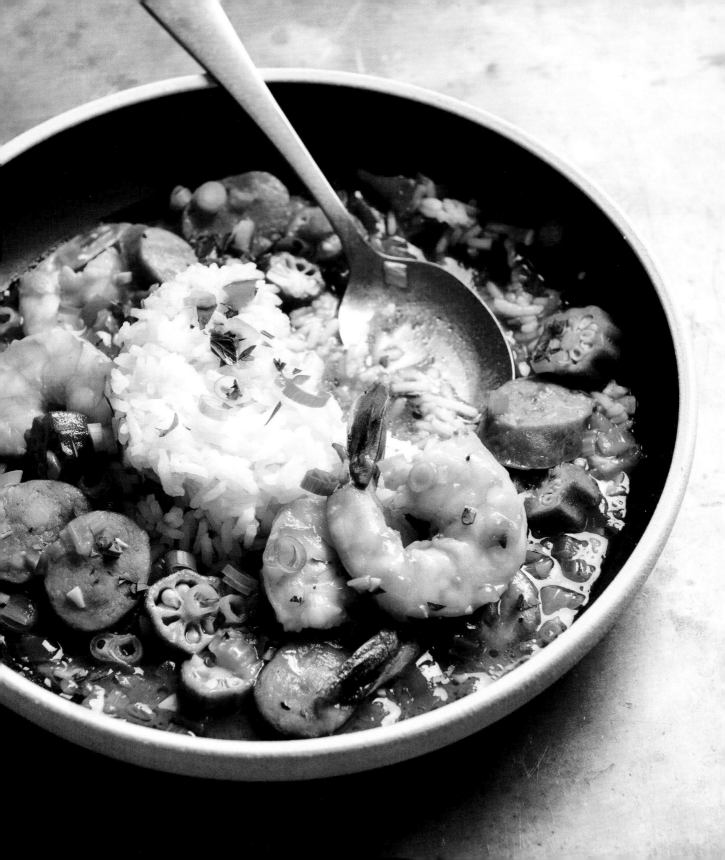

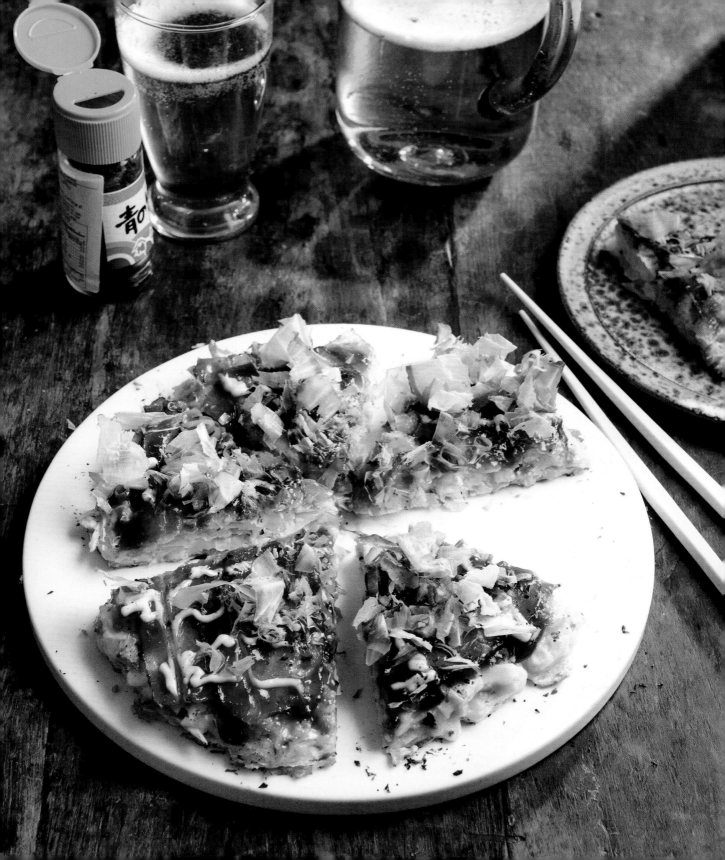

OKONOMIYAKI

SERVES 8

Researching the world of anime exposed me to some delicacies and street foods I might not have ever known existed otherwise. *Sweetness and Lightning* also proved to be a downright wholesome story as well, using the power of food to tell the story of a single father connecting with his young daughter. She's particularly enamored of a popular snack called *okonomiyaki*, which roughly translates to "as you like," illustrating its wide customizability. At its most basic, it's a cabbage pancake made with dashi broth, bonito, and pork belly. Like *takoyaki* (featured later in *Binging with Babish*), the Japanese street treat can be filled with damn near any savory fillings, ranging from shrimp to edamame to cheese. Whatever it's filled with, it can be topped with thinly sliced pork belly or bacon, fried crisp, topped with a savory brown sauce, and drizzled with a lightly sweet Japanese mayo. I may have wanted to visit Japan in the past, but now I think I need to.

VERDICT: *Okonomiyaki* is a very unique combination of flavors and textures, relatively easy to make, and impressive to look at. You don't need to be a single father with a daughter to connect with to enjoy this street food, but I'm sure it wouldn't hurt.

1 cup cake flour

1½ teaspoons baking powder

1 teaspoon dashi powder (available at Asian markets or online)

1 small Japanese mountain yam, grated, or ½ cup milk whisked with 3 tablespoons potato starch

½ head cabbage, cored and shredded

4 scallions, thinly sliced, green and white parts kept separate

¼ cup pickled red ginger, drained and chopped

4 large eggs, lightly beaten

½ cup tenkasu (crunchy tempura bits; available at Asian markets or online) or panko bread crumbs

4 tablespoons vegetable oil

½ pound thinly sliced pork belly or bacon

½ cup Okonomiyaki Sauce (recipe follows)

½ cup Japanese Mayo (recipe follows)

1 ounce bonito flakes (smoked dried tuna; available at Japanese markets), for serving

Aonori (dried green seaweed flakes; available at Asian markets or online) or crumbled dried seaweed, for serving

(recipe continues)

IN A large bowl, whisk together the cake flour and baking powder. In a liquid measuring cup, dissolve the dashi powder in 1 cup water and pour into the bowl. Add the mountain yam and whisk until just combined. Cover and refrigerate for 30 minutes.

REMOVE THE batter from the refrigerator and add three-quarters of the cabbage, the white parts of the scallions, the pickled ginger, eggs, and tenkasu. Gently fold to combine. Add the remaining cabbage as necessary until the mixture resembles coleslaw.

IN A large nonstick pan, heat 2 tablespoons of the vegetable oil over medium-high heat until shimmering, about 2 minutes. Add half the okonomiyaki batter and shape it into a 10-inch pancake with a rubber spatula. Shingle 4 to 6 slices of the pork belly on top and reduce the heat to medium. Cover and cook for 5 minutes, or until well browned.

UNCOVER AND flip the okonomiyaki. Cover and cook for 5 minutes more, or until the batter is cooked through.

INVERT THE okonomiyaki onto a plate so the pork belly faces up. Top with half of the okonomiyaki sauce, spreading it with a spoon to evenly coat the top. Using the squeeze bottle, stripe the entire surface of the pancake with the Japanese mayo. Drag a toothpick or wooden skewer across the top, perpendicular to the stripes, going back and forth to create a feathered pattern. Top with half the bonito, the green parts of the scallions, and the aonori, slice into wedges, and serve hot. Repeat with the remaining batter.

OKONOMIYAKI SAUCE
MAKES ABOUT ½ CUP

¼ cup ketchup
3½ tablespoons Worcestershire sauce
2 tablespoons oyster sauce
1 tablespoon sugar

IN A small bowl, whisk together all the ingredients until well incorporated. Set aside until ready to use.

JAPANESE MAYO
MAKES ABOUT 1 CUP

1 cup mayonnaise
1 tablespoon sugar
2 teaspoons rice vinegar

IN A small bowl, whisk together all the ingredients until well incorporated. Spoon into a squeeze bottle. Refrigerate until ready to serve.

FRIED GREEN TOMATOES

SERVES 4

I have to be honest: I've still never seen *Fried Green Tomatoes*. It seems like one of those movies that's going to make me cry a lot, and I'm saving that for the next time I'm in a relationship and need to show that I'm a sensitive soul. While the connections between some recipes and their source media in this book are tenuous at best, this one might be considered almost too on-the-nose. My dad was in town and craving something fried and salty, so I obliged him with this Southern classic.

VERDICT: These are crisp, juicy, savory fried green tomatoes with a tangy, spicy rémoulade. They're easy, pretty, and a great way to feel like a Southerner anywhere in the world—if you can manage to find green tomatoes.

---

4 large green tomatoes, sliced ¼ inch thick

1 tablespoon plus 1 teaspoon kosher salt

Vegetable oil, for frying

1½ cups all-purpose flour

1 teaspoon onion powder

1 teaspoon garlic powder

½ teaspoon ground white pepper

2 large eggs, beaten

1 cup buttermilk

1 cup medium-grind cornmeal

½ cup bread crumbs

Rémoulade (recipe follows), for serving

PLACE THE green tomatoes on a wire rack set over a rimmed baking sheet. Sprinkle each side evenly with 1 tablespoon of the salt and let them weep moisture for 30 minutes at room temperature.

FILL A deep cast-iron skillet with vegetable oil to a depth of 2 inches. Heat over medium-high heat to 325°F.

MEANWHILE, WHISK together the flour, remaining 1 teaspoon salt, the onion powder, garlic powder, and white pepper in a shallow bowl. In another shallow bowl, whisk together the eggs and buttermilk. In a third shallow bowl, combine the cornmeal and bread crumbs and stir together with a fork.

(recipe continues)

PAT THE tomatoes dry with paper towels and bread each one as follows: dredge in the seasoned flour, dip in the buttermilk mixture, then dredge in the cornmeal crumbs. Transfer to the wire rack until ready to fry.

WORKING IN batches to avoid overlapping, add the tomatoes to the hot oil and fry for about 2 minutes per side, until they are golden brown and float. Using tongs, transfer to the wire rack or to a paper towel–lined plate to drain.

TRANSFER TO a plate and serve hot with the rémoulade.

RÉMOULADE
MAKES ABOUT 1 CUP

¾ cup mayonnaise
1 tablespoon Dijon mustard
1 teaspoon whole-grain mustard
Juice of ½ lemon
2 garlic cloves, grated
1 scallion, finely minced
1 tablespoon capers, drained and minced
2 teaspoons Louisiana-style hot sauce
1 teaspoon Worcestershire sauce
1 teaspoon cayenne pepper
1 teaspoon smoked paprika

IN A small bowl, combine all the ingredients and whisk until completely incorporated. Refrigerate until ready to serve.

TEAMSTER SANDWICH

SERVES 4, PLUS ENOUGH EXTRA BEEF TO SERVE 4

30 Rock returns once more as the sleeper star of the BCU (Babish Comic Universe), second only to *Chef* as the source of the most recipe inspiration. I tend to balk at foods of mysterious origin or disputed provenance, and the Teamster Sandwich had me worried, given that on the show it's brought to NBC's offices from an unknown deli in Brooklyn. After a bit of research, however, I discovered someone intimately involved in the show's production had confirmed that the sandwiches were inspired by one served at Fiore's House of Quality in Hoboken, New Jersey. The sandwich in question features thinly sliced roast beef, peppers marinated with garlic, house-made mozzarella, and, of course, the obligatory dipping jus. While I purchased all the elements necessary from the actual Fiore's for comparison, the following recipe does create an excellent approximation of the real thing. The only shortcoming has got to be the jus—high-volume restaurants have the ability to roast whole joints of beef, collecting a veritable rainstorm of drippings, making flavorful sauces from them. At home, we have to be a bit more industrious—but the results are excellent.

VERDICT: This is not only a solid recipe for restaurant-style prime rib, but for a sandwich that'll knock your bi-curious shoes off.

1 standing rib roast with 3 ribs attached (about 10 pounds)

1 tablespoon dried rosemary

1 tablespoon dried thyme

2 tablespoons kosher salt, plus more for seasoning

1 tablespoon freshly ground black pepper, plus more for seasoning

1 teaspoon onion powder

1 teaspoon garlic powder

1 tablespoon extra-virgin olive oil

1 tablespoon all-purpose flour

4 cups beef stock (preferably homemade), warmed

1 (15-ounce) jar roasted red peppers, drained

4 garlic cloves, minced

1 whole baguette

8 ounces fresh mozzarella cheese, sliced

(recipe continues)

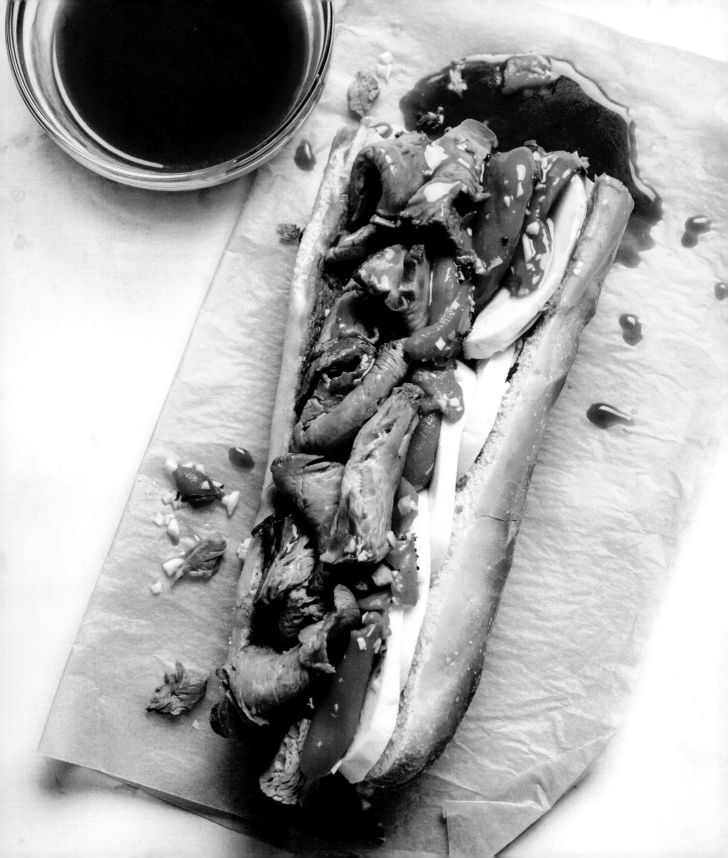

PREHEAT THE oven to 500°F.

USING A long, thin knife, slice the ribs off the roast in one slab. Reserve the slab of ribs. Score the fat cap of the roast at 1-inch intervals in a crosshatch pattern.

IN A small food processor, combine the rosemary and thyme and process for 15 seconds, or until finely ground. (Alternatively, pound the rosemary and thyme in a mortar and pestle until finely ground.) Transfer to a small bowl and whisk in the salt, pepper, onion powder, and garlic powder. Liberally coat the roast all over with the spice mixture. Drizzle with olive oil and rub it into the roast.

PLACE THE roast on its slab of ribs, which will act as a natural roasting rack. Tie the ribs back onto the roast, looping a piece of butcher's twine between each bone and securing it with a knot. Insert a temperature probe into the thickest part of the beef, transfer to a large stainless-steel roasting pan, and roast for 25 minutes. Reduce the oven temperature to 300°F and roast for 30 minutes to 1 hour more (depending on the size of the roast), until the internal temperature registers 115°F. Remove from the oven, transfer the roast to a carving board, tent with aluminum foil, and let rest for 30 minutes.

RESERVE THE drippings and ⅓ cup of the fat in the roasting pan. Set the pan over medium-high heat and whisk in the flour until a slurry forms. Cook for 1 minute, or until the raw flour smell dissipates. While whisking continuously, stream in the stock and whisk until completely incorporated. Cook until slightly reduced, 2 to 3 minutes. Season with salt and pepper. Wrap the roast in plastic wrap, transfer the jus to an airtight container, and refrigerate both for at least 4 hours, or ideally overnight.

MEANWHILE, IN a small bowl, toss the roasted peppers with the garlic. Cover and refrigerate for 4 hours, or ideally overnight.

REHEAT 2 cups of the jus in a medium saucepan until simmering (reserve the rest for another use). Divide the hot jus among four small bowls. Without cutting all the way through, split the baguette lengthwise and open it up like a book. Using a long, thin knife, slice 24 ounces of the beef as thinly as possible and layer onto the baguette. Top with the mozzarella and marinated peppers. Cut the sandwich into 4 equal pieces, transfer to plates, and serve each piece with a bowl of hot jus alongside for dipping.

BEIGNETS

SERVES 8

It seems only fitting that this book concludes with one of my favorite recipes, featured in one of my favorite movies, hailing from one of my favorite cities. Chef Carl Casper continues his father-son bonding offensive with the hot, airy, confectioners'-sugar-laden sweets that Cafe du Monde is rightfully famous for, during their stint in the Crescent City. With his face covered in confectioners' sugar, his son looks at up at him, smiles, and proclaims, "I like New Orleans!" Though on the surface, he's talking about the food, we can tell he's responding to his father finally trying to connect with him on a deeper level than just

seeing *Iron Man 3* again. For comparison, I tried using a box of the selfsame cafe's beignet mix, which turned out disappointingly limp and crunchy. The following recipe, while a bit more labor-intensive than just adding water, yields the light-as-air New Orleanian doughnuts you'll find yourself craving the moment you return from the Big Easy.

VERDICT: Beignets are a simple, indulgent treat, best when liberally mounded with confectioners' sugar and served alongside coffee brewed with chicory.

½ cup whole milk

1½ cups buttermilk, chilled

4 teaspoons active dry yeast

2½ tablespoons granulated sugar

22 ounces bread flour (about 5 cups plus 2 tablespoons), plus more for dusting

½ teaspoon baking soda

½ teaspoon kosher salt

Vegetable oil, for greasing and frying

Confectioners' sugar, for dusting

Honey, for drizzling (optional)

IN A small saucepan, bring the milk just to a boil over medium heat. Pour into a heatproof liquid measuring cup and stir in the buttermilk until tepid. Whisk in the yeast and sugar until dissolved and set aside for 10 minutes.

IN THE bowl of a stand mixer fitted with the whisk attachment, whisk together the flour, baking soda, and salt. Replace the whisk attachment with the dough hook. Add the buttermilk mixture and knead on medium speed

(recipe continues)

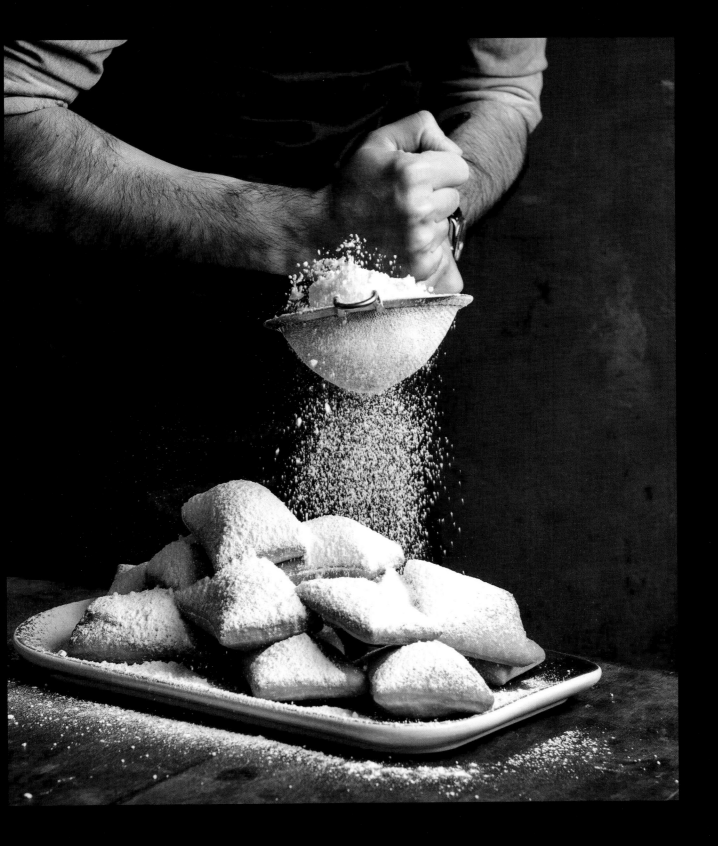

for 4 to 5 minutes, until a sticky dough forms. Transfer to a large oiled bowl, cover, and let rise for 1 hour, or until doubled in size.

FILL A large Dutch oven with vegetable oil to a depth of 3 inches. Heat over medium-high heat to 370°F.

SCRAPE THE dough out onto a well-floured work surface. Roll it out to ¼ to ½ inch thick and, using a pizza cutter, cut it into 3 x 5-inch rectangles. Working in batches to avoid crowding the pot, carefully lower the dough rectangles into the hot oil and fry for 1 to 2 minutes, then flip and fry for 30 seconds more, or until golden brown and puffed. Using a spider, transfer the beignets to a wire rack over paper towels to drain.

TRANSFER THE beignets to a plate, dust with confectioners' sugar, and serve hot. If desired, drizzle with honey for *Princess and the Frog*–style beignets.

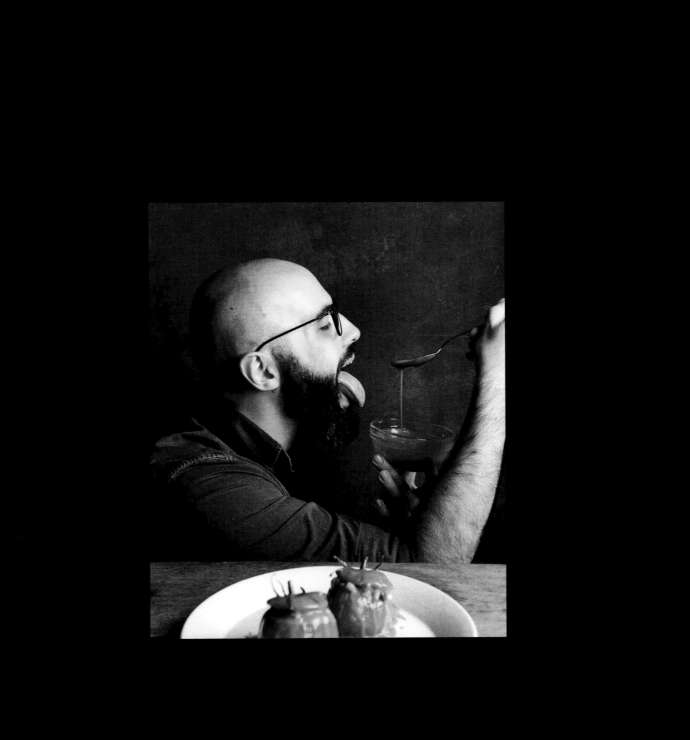

INDEX

Note: Page references in *italics* indicate photographs.

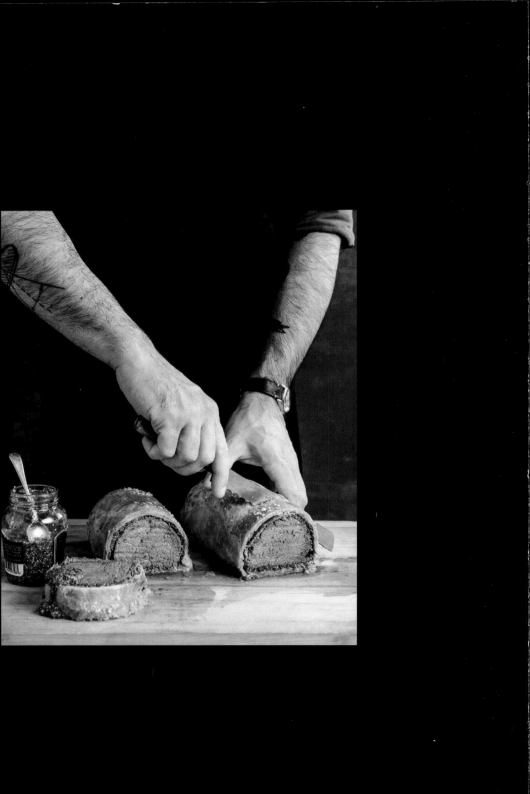